Gender and Respiratory Disease

Editor

MARGARET A. PISANI

CLINICS IN
CHEST MEDICINE

www.chestmed.theclinics.com

September 2021 • Volume 42 • Number 3

ELSEVIER

1600 John F. Kennedy Boulevard • Suite 1800 • Philadelphia, Pennsylvania, 19103-2899

http://www.theclinics.com

CLINICS IN CHEST MEDICINE Volume 42, Number 3
September 2021 ISSN 0272-5231, ISBN-13: 978-0-323-78955-4

Editor: Joanna Collett
Developmental Editor: Karen Justine Solomon

Clinics in Chest Medicine (ISSN 0272-5231) is published quarterly by Elsevier Inc., 360 Park Avenue South, New York, NY 10010-1710. Months of issue are March, June, September, and December. Periodicals postage paid at New York, NY and additional mailing offices. Subscription prices are $396.00 per year (domestic individuals), $1009.00 per year (domestic institutions), $100.00 per year (domestic students/residents), $423.00 per year (Canadian individuals), $1075.00 per year (Canadian institutions), $484.00 per year (international individuals), $1075.00 per year (international institutions), $100.00 per year (Canadian Students), and $230.00 per year (International Students). International air speed delivery is included in all Clinics subscription prices. All prices are subject to change without notice. **POSTMASTER:** Send address changes to Clinics in Chest Medicine, Elsevier Health Sciences Division, Subscription Customer Service, 3251 Riverport Lane, Maryland Heights, MO 63043. **Customer Service: Telephone: 1-800-654-2452** (U.S. and Canada); **1-314-447-8871** (outside U.S. and Canada). **Fax: 1-314-447-8029.** E-mail: **journalscustomerservice-usa@elsevier.com (for print support); journalsonlinesupport-usa@elsevier.com (for online support).**

Reprints. For copies of 100 or more of articles in this publication, please contact the Commercial Reprints Department, Elsevier Inc., 360 Park Avenue South, New York, NY 10010-1710. Tel.: 212-633-3874; Fax: 212-633-3820; E-mail: reprints@elsevier.com.

Clinics in Chest Medicine is covered in *MEDLINE/PubMed (Index Medicus), Current Contents/Clinical Medicine, EMBASE/ Excerpta Medica, Science Citation Index,* and *ISI/BIOMED.*

Contributors

EDITOR

MARGARET A. PISANI, MD, MPH
Professor, Division of Pulmonary, Critical Care
and Sleep
Medicine, Department of Medicine, Yale
University School of Medicine, New Haven,
Connecticut, USA

AUTHORS

MOIRA L. AITKEN, MD, FRCP
Department of Medicine, Professor, University
of Washington, Seattle, Washington

ABDULLAH AL-ABCHA, MD
Department of Internal Medicine, Michigan
State University, East Lansing, Michigan, USA

DANUZIA AMBROZIO-MARQUES, PhD
Department of Pediatrics, Université Laval,
Centre de Recherche de l'Institut Universitaire
de Cardiologie et Pneumologie de Québec,
Québec, Québec, Canada

ANDREEA ANTON, MD, FCCP
Associate Professor of Medicine, Department
of Pulmonary, Critical Care and Sleep
Medicine, Medical College of Wisconsin, Chief
of Medicine, Zablocki VA Medical Center,
Milwaukee, Wisconsin, USA

VIBEKE BACKER, MD, DMSci
Centre for Physical Activity Research,
Rigshospitalet, Copenhagen University
Hospital, Copenhagen, Denmark

GHADA BOURJEILY, MD
Professor, Department of Medicine,
Department of Medicine, Divisions of
Pulmonary, Critical Care and Sleep Medicine,
and Obstetric Medicine, Lifespan Hospitals,
Warren Alpert Medical School of Brown
University, Providence, Rhode Island, USA

KUBRA M. BOZKANAT, MD
Department of Pediatrics, Pulmonary Fellow,
University of Texas Southwestern, Dallas,
Texas

RACHEL N. CRINER, MD
Division of Pulmonary, Allergy and Critical
Care, University of Pennsylvania, Philadelphia,
Pennsylvania, USA

CAROLYN M. D'AMBROSIO, MD, MS, FCCP
Director, Harvard-Brigham and Women's
Hospital, Fellowship in Pulmonary and Critical
Care Medicine, Brigham and Women's
Hospital, Associate Professor of Medicine,
Harvard Medical School, Boston,
Massachusetts, USA

CLAIRE DEBOLT, MD
Fellow, Division of Pulmonary and Critical Care,
Department of Medicine, University of Virginia,
Charlottesville, Virginia, USA

CLAIRE C. ENG, PharmD, BCPS, BCCCP
Critical Care, Clinical Pharmacy Specialist,
Memorial Hermann Katy Hospital, Department
of Pharmacy, Katy, Texas, USA

MARIANNE GAGNON, BSc
Department of Pediatrics, Université Laval,
Centre de Recherche de l'Institut Universitaire
de Cardiologie et Pneumologie de Québec,
Québec, Québec, Canada

ERIK SOEREN HALVARD HANSEN, MD
Centre for Physical Activity Research,
Rigshospitalet, Copenhagen University
Hospital, Copenhagen, Denmark

MEILAN K. HAN, MD, MS
Division of Pulmonary and Critical Care
Medicine, University of Michigan, Ann Arbor,
Michigan, USA

DREW HARRIS, MD
Assistant Professor, Division of Pulmonary and
Critical Care, Department of Medicine,
University of Virginia, Charlottesville, Virginia,
USA

**MOJDEH S. HEAVNER, PharmD, BCPS,
BCCCP, FCCM**
Associate Professor and Vice Chair for
Clinical Services, Department of Pharmacy
Practice & Science, University of Maryland
School of Pharmacy, Baltimore, Maryland,
USA

RAKSHA JAIN, MD, MSCI
Department of Medicine, Associate Professor
of Medicine, University of Texas Southwestern,
Dallas, Texas

**CHRISTINE JENKINS, AM, MD, FRACP,
FThorSoc**
Professor, Respiratory Medicine, UNSW
Medicine and Health, UNSW Sydney, Clinical
Professor, Concord Clinical School, University
of Sydney, NSW Australia

PHILLIP JOSEPH, MD
Assistant Professor of Medicine, Pulmonary,
Critical Care, and Sleep Medicine, Yale New
Haven Hospital/Yale School of Medicine, New
Haven, Connecticut, USA

VINCENT JOSEPH, PhD
Department of Pediatrics, Université Laval,
Centre de Recherche de l'Institut Universitaire
de Cardiologie et Pneumologie de Québec,
Québec, Québec, Canada

THEODOROS KARAMPITSAKOS, MD, MSc
Department of Respiratory Medicine,
University Hospital of Patras, Greece

MATTHAIOS KATSARAS, MD
Department of Respiratory Medicine,
University Hospital of Patras, Greece

SHANNON KAY, MD
Department of Medicine, Yale University
School of Medicine, New Haven,
Connecticut, USA

TRACI M. KAZMERSKI, MD, MS
Department of Pediatrics, Assistant Professor,
University of Pittsburgh School of Medicine,
Pittsburgh, Pennsylvania

RICHARD KINKEAD, PhD
Professor, Department of Pediatrics, Faculté
de Médecine, Université Laval, Centre de
Recherche de l'Institut Universitaire de
Cardiologie et Pneumologie de Québec,
Québec, Québec, Canada

SUNITA KUMAR, MD, FCCP
Professor of Medicine, Department of
Pulmonary, Critical Care and Sleep, Loyola
University Medical Center and Stritch School of
Medicine, Maywood, Illinois, USA

ALLISON A. LAMBERT, MD, MHS
Department of Pulmonary and Critical Care
Medicine, University of Washington, Seattle,
Washington, USA; Providence Medical
Research Center, Spokane, Washington, USA

TASNIM I. LAT, DO
Clinical Assistant Professor, Division of
Pulmonary, Critical Care & Sleep Medicine,
Baylor Scott & White Health, Temple, Texas,
USA

ISABELLE MALHAMÉ, MD, MSc
Assistant Professor, Department of Medicine,
Obstetric Medicine Division, McGill University
Health Center and Research Institute of the
McGill University Health Center, Montreal,
Quebec, Canada

MEGHAN K. McGRAW, MD
Fellow, Division of Pulmonary, Critical Care &
Sleep Medicine, Baylor Scott & White Health,
Temple, Texas, USA

MARGARET MILLER, MD
Associate Professor, Department of Medicine,
Division of Obstetric Medicine, Lifespan
Hospitals, Alpert Medical School of Brown
University, Providence, Rhode Island, USA

KRISTINA MONTEMAYOR, MD, MHS
Department of Medicine, Instructor, Johns
Hopkins University, Baltimore, Maryland

NICHOLAS NASSIKAS, MD
Department of Medicine, Pulmonary and
Critical Care Medicine Fellowship, Lifespan
Hospitals, Alpert Medical School of Brown
University, Providence, Rhode Island, USA

HANNAH TAKAHASHI OAKLAND, MD
Fellow in Medicine, Pulmonary, Critical Care,
and Sleep Medicine, Yale New Haven Hospital/
Yale School of Medicine, New Haven,
Connecticut, USA

OURANIA PAPAIOANNOU, MD
Department of Respiratory Medicine,
University Hospital of Patras, Greece

MARGARET A. PISANI, MD, MPH
Professor, Division of Pulmonary, Critical Care
and Sleep Medicine, Department of Medicine,
Yale University School of Medicine, New
Haven, Connecticut, USA

MADDIE PORANSKI
Adult with Cystic Fibrosis, St Paul, Minnesota

SOEREN MALTE RASMUSSEN, MD
Centre for Physical Activity Research,
Rigshospitalet, Copenhagen University
Hospital, Copenhagen, Denmark

FRÉDÉRIC SÉRIÉS, MD
Department of Medicine, Université Laval,
Centre de Recherche de l'Institut Universitaire
de Cardiologie et Pneumologie de Québec,
Québec, Québec, Canada

FOTIOS SAMPSONAS, MD, PhD
Department of Respiratory Medicine,
University Hospital of Patras, Greece

JACQUI SJOBERG
Adult with Cystic Fibrosis, Oceanside,
California

LYNN T. TANOUE, MD, MBA
Professor of Medicine, Yale School of
Medicine, New Haven, Connecticut, USA

JENNIFER L. TAYLOR-COUSAR, MD, MSCS
Departments of Medicine, and Pediatrics,
Professor, National Jewish Health, Denver,
Colorado

SRITIKA THAPA, MD
Clinical Instructor in Medicine, Department of
Internal Medicine, Section of Pulmonary,

Critical Care and Sleep Medicine, Yale
University School of Medicine, New Haven,
Connecticut, USA

CASPER TIDEMANDSEN, MD
Department of Respiratory Medicine, Hvidovre
University Hospital, Denmark

LAUREN TOBIAS, MD
Assistant Professor of Medicine, Veterans
Affairs Connecticut Healthcare System, West
Haven, Connecticut, USA; Department of
Internal Medicine, Section of Pulmonary,
Critical Care and Sleep Medicine, Yale
University School of Medicine, New Haven,
Connecticut, USA

ARGYRIS TZOUVELEKIS, MD, MSc, PhD
Associate Professor of Internal and
Respiratory Medicine, Head, Department of
Respiratory Medicine, University Hospital of
Patras, Greece

CHARLOTTE SUPPLI ULRIK, MD, DMSci
Department of Respiratory Medicine, Hvidovre
University Hospital, Denmark

KAREN VON BERG, PT, DPT
Department of Physical Medicine and
Rehabilitation, Physical Therapist II, Johns
Hopkins Hospital, Baltimore, Maryland

NATALIE WEST, MD, MHS
Department of Medicine, Assistant Professor,
Johns Hopkins University, Baltimore, Maryland

HEATH D. WHITE, DO, MS, FCCP
Clinical Assistant Professor, Division of
Pulmonary, Critical Care & Sleep Medicine,
Baylor Scott & White Health, Temple, Texas,
USA

ALEXANDRA WILSON, MS, RDN, CDE
Department of Medicine, Manager, Cystic
Fibrosis Clinical Research, National Jewish
Health, Denver, Colorado

CHRISTINE H.J. WON, MD, MS
Associate Professor of Medicine, Veterans
Affairs Connecticut Healthcare System, West
Haven, Connecticut, USA; Department of
Internal Medicine, Section of Pulmonary,
Critical Care and Sleep Medicine, Yale
University School of Medicine, New Haven,
Connecticut, USA

Contents

Disparities in health care have risen to the forefront of medicine in the past several years. One of the most notable disparities in the research and delivery of health care relates to sex and gender. Sex and gender affect the epidemiology, pathophysiology, and outcomes of disease and social determinants of health and access to medical care. This article discusses some of the history of considering sex as a biologic variable in medical research and clinical care. It also clarifies the definitions and terminology necessary for understanding the biologic and social underpinnings of sex and gender.

The respiratory system of women and men develops and functions in distinct neuroendocrine milieus. Despite differences in anatomy and neural control, homeostasis of arterial blood gases is ensured in healthy individuals regardless of sex. This convergence in function differs from the sex-based differences observed in many respiratory diseases. Sleep-disordered breathing (SDB) results mainly from episodes of upper airway closure. This complex and multifactorial respiratory disorder shows significant sexual dimorphism in its clinical manifestations and comorbidities. Guided by recent progress from basic research, this review discusses the hypothesis that stress is necessary to reveal the sexual dimorphism of SDB.

Gender is the centerpiece to an individual's understanding of self and encompasses many behavioral, social, and cultural arenas; its broad scope means that it also intersects many social determinants of health. Multiple examples of social determinants highlighted in this article, including income, education, occupation, domestic exposures, and cultural norms such as sexual identity, are critical factors that contribute to ongoing respiratory disparities between genders. Each of these social factors can have disparate impact on patients of differing genders. Understanding and addressing social determinants of health between genders is an essential first step toward achieving respiratory health equity.

CLINICS IN CHEST MEDICINE

SERIES OF RELATED INTEREST

Cardiology Clinics
Available at: https://www.cardiology.theclinics.com/

THE CLINICS ARE AVAILABLE ONLINE!
Access your subscription at:
www.theclinics.com

CLINICS IN CHEST MEDICINE

FORTHCOMING ISSUES

December 2021
Pleural Disease
David Feller-Kooman and Fabien Maldonado,
Editors

March 2022
Bronchiectasis
James D. Chalmers, Editor

June 2022
Sleep Deficiency and Health
Melissa P. Knauert, Editor

RECENT ISSUES

June 2021
Interstitial Lung Disease
Harold Collard, Luca Richeldi, Kerri A.
Johannson, Editors

March 2021
Pulmonary Hypertension
Inderjit Singh and Aaron B. Waxman, Editors

December 2020
**Advances in Occupational and Environmental
Lung Diseases**
Carrie A. Redlich, Kristin Cummings, and Peggy
Lai, Editors

SERIES OF RELATED INTEREST

Cardiology Clinic
Available at: https://www.theclinics.com/

Preface
Gender and Respiratory Disease

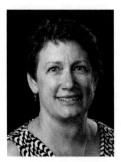

Margaret A. Pisani, MD, MPH
Editor

There is increasing evidence that sex and gender impact the incidence, susceptibility, and severity of lung diseases. Sex has been shown to influence lung development and physiology. The 3 most common lung diseases in women are asthma, chronic obstructive pulmonary disease (COPD), and lung cancer. In addition to the biological differences attributed to sex, there are gender differences in rates of diagnosis of lung disease and treatments prescribed.

In this issue of *Clinics in Chest Medicine*, diverse experts in the field of pulmonary, critical care, and sleep medicine address the most up-to-date research on the impact of sex and gender in a variety of pulmonary and sleep disorders as well as critical care. These articles offer insights on the current state of knowledge, ongoing research, and where the field of sex and gender medicine needs to advance in the future.

Kay and Pisani give a general overview of the definitions of sex and gender, the history of research incorporating these important factors, and a discussion of the biology. The underpinnings of sex-based differences of respiratory control are reviewed by Kinkead and colleagues, where they use sleep-disordered breathing as a model for understanding sexual dimorphism. They go on to review the impact of sex on respiratory control from neonates to adults. Debolt and Harris discuss intersectionality of gender and other important social determinants of health as they relate to lung diseases. They include gender differences seen in both occupational and domestics exposures that lead to disparities

in lung diseases and review the impact of cultural norms.

Sleep disorders, including insomnia and obstructive sleep apnea (OSA), are responsible for much morbidity and can negatively impact quality of life. Sex differences in OSA have garnered attention in recent years, and Kumar and colleagues review the impact of sex on pathogenesis, presentation, and treatment of OSA. Tobias and colleagues examine the impact of sex on sleep disorders across the lifespan, including the impact of pregnancy and menopause.

Women now account for 58% of the 14.7 million people living with COPD in the United States, and more women than men are currently dying of COPD. Jenkins highlights the sex and gender differences, prevalence, pathogenesis, diagnosis, treatment, and outcomes in COPD. Asthma is one of the most common chronic conditions affecting women in Western society. Tidemandsen and colleagues discuss sex and gender differences in asthma and asthma phenotypes and associated comorbidities, including vocal cord dysfunction.

Oakland and Joseph review the literature on the pathophysiology of sex differences in pulmonary hypertension, the role sex hormones play in the disease, and the female paradox whereby data suggest that despite higher disease prevalence and greater pulmonary vascular resistance, women have better survival rates. There is substantial evidence that both sex and gender impact the prevalence, susceptibility, and severity of interstitial lung disease (ILD). Karampitsakos and

Clin Chest Med 42 (2021) xiii–xiv
https://doi.org/10.1016/j.ccm.2021.06.002
0272-5231/21/© 2021 Published by Elsevier Inc.

colleagues summarize the experimental and clinical data on the impact of sex hormones and gender on ILDs.

There is a global epidemic of lung cancer in women, and it is the leading cause of cancer deaths in industrialized countries. While tobacco use is the most important risk factor for lung cancer development, it is more common in never-smoking women compared with men. Tanoue reviews the impact of sex and gender on lung cancer pathogenesis, incidence, and response to treatment.

Pregnant women are often excluded from research studies, including research on disease diagnosis, drug trials, and therapeutic intervention studies. Respiratory disorders are common in pregnancy, and Nassikas and colleagues discuss important pulmonary considerations in pregnant women. There are several diseases that are seen predominately in women, including lymphangioleiomyomatosis and thoracic endometriosis. These disorders and the role of sex hormones in their pathogenesis are reviewed by Criner and colleagues.

Cystic fibrosis (CF), an autosomal recessive inherited disease, has an equal prevalence between men and women, but the data suggest that women have worse outcomes across several domains. As people with CF are living longer, women are living through their reproductive years and facing issues related to pregnancy and menopause. Jain and colleagues discuss the unique challenges that women with CF encounter.

Many studies of critical illness suggest reduced admission rates to the intensive care unit for women despite similar severity of illness compared with men. There are limited data on sex and gender outcomes in critical illness, but Lat discusses what is known about specific diseases, including acute respiratory distress syndrome, sepsis, and obstetric critical illness. Woman, and especially women of childbearing age, have long been excluded from clinical drug trials. There is a body of research that demonstrates differences between men and women in drug-specific pharmacokinetics and pharmacodynamics. These differences are often not appreciated, or they are underestimated. Eng and Heavner review pharmacologic issues related to women with lung disease and in critical illness.

The articles included in this issue of *Clinics in Chest Medicine* are intended to update the reader on the important aspects of sex and gender in lung disease and in critical illness. Future research in pulmonary and critical care medicine should include the variables of sex and gender to further our understanding of disease and allow for more personalized treatment of both women and men.

Margaret A. Pisani, MD, MPH
Division of Pulmonary, Critical Care
and Sleep Medicine
Department of Medicine
Yale University School of Medicine
P.O. Box 208057
New Haven, CT 06501, USA

E-mail address:
margaret.pisani@yale.edu

An Overview of Sex and Gender in Pulmonary and Critical Care Medicine

Shannon Kay, MD, Margaret A. Pisani, MD, MPH*

KEYWORDS

• Gender-based biology • Genetic differences • Sex differences • Gender differences

KEY POINTS

- Sex is defined as the biologic and physiologic characteristics, ranging from genetic makeup to physical features, that distinguish males from females.
- Gender is a social construct of roles, relationships, behaviors, and traits ascribed to men and women.
- Sex and gender are distinct concepts and should not be confused nor used interchangeably.
- Precise terminology is key, because sex and gender have significant but distinct roles in human health and disease.
- Future studies, including basic, animal, and human research, should incorporate sex and genders as variables and address their impact in causal pathways, response to treatment, and outcomes.

DEFINITIONS

Sex and gender affect the epidemiology, pathophysiology, and outcomes of disease and social determinants of health and access to medical care. Recently, there has been an evolution in the terminology related to sex- and gender-based medicine and several groups and organizations have advocated for precise standard terminology as knowledge of sex and gender differences progresses.[1] Dr Florence Haseltine coined the term "gender-based biology" in the mid-1990s and was influential in establishing the Society for Women's Health Research. The Society for Women's Health Research began to change the terminology to "sex-based biology."[2]

The definitions of the terms sex and gender need to be understood to appreciate their role in the study of medicine. Although often inaccurately used interchangeably in society and the medical literature, sex and gender are distinct concepts and should not be confused nor used interchangeably. In humans, sex is defined as the biologic and physiologic characteristics, ranging from genetic makeup to physical features, that distinguish males from females.[3] However, gender is a social construct of roles, relationships, behaviors, and traits ascribed to men and women.[3] In general, the terms male and female refer to biologic sex, whereas boy, girl, man, and woman typically refer to gender and are not synonymous with biologic sex. For example, an individual born biologically male may identify with the female gender, and vice versa, whereas other individuals may identify with both or neither gender. Precise terminology is key, because sex and gender have significant but distinct roles in human health and disease. The terms sex and gender as defined here are limited to humans, because there are some organisms that exhibit both male and female characteristics, and others that change their biologic sex during their lifetime.[4]

Recent data estimate that 1.4 million adults identify as transgender in the United States, so ensuring that sex- and gender-based terms are inclusive of all individuals is important to reducing

Department of Medicine, Yale University School of Medicine, 333 Cedar Street, PO Box 208057, New Haven, CT 06519, USA
* Corresponding author.
E-mail address: Margaret.pisani@yale.edu

Clin Chest Med 42 (2021) 385–390
https://doi.org/10.1016/j.ccm.2021.04.001

chestmed.theclinics.com

stigma and improving health care outside the binary categories of sex and gender.[5]

Sex is often categorized as female or male based on the assumption that external genitalia and reproductive organs match chromosomal sex of XX or XY. Sexual dimorphism is the concept that males and females exhibit biologic differences beyond the sex organs.[4] Sexual dimorphism has been applied to many animal species and several plants. One illustrative example of sexual dimorphism in the animal kingdom is the striking physical differences between peacocks and peahens, among many other bird species.[6] The idea of sexual dimorphism is central to the discussion of the role of sex and gender in medicine.

HISTORY

The role of sex and gender differences in medicine in physiology and pathophysiology were understudied until modern times, especially in the realm of pulmonary and critical care medicine. The first study of sex differences in respiratory physiology was attributed to a prominent figure in pulmonary medicine, John Hutchinson, a London surgeon credited with the development of the spirometer.[7] Hutchinson used his invention to measure the vital capacity of more than 2000 men and 26 young women and noted an apparent divergence in the mechanism of breathing between the sexes. In his 1846 report to the Royal Medical and Chirurgical Society, he postulated "in men these are chiefly by the diaphragm; in women chiefly by the ribs," which he attributed to a potential "provision against those periods when the abdomen contains the gravid uterus" rather than "their peculiar costume."[7]

Another important figure in the study of sex and gender in medicine is Henry Havelock Ellis, an English physician and progressive social reformist who wrote "Man and Woman: A Study of Secondary and Tertiary Sexual Characters."[8] Since its publication in 1894, this work has been extensively cited in more recent studies of sex and gender differences. In his book, Ellis noted differences in respiratory physiology, including "vital capacity is decidedly less in women than in men," which he explained by "women have less need of air than men," referring to lower metabolic rates, and social factors, such as "artificial constriction of the dress." Hutchinson and Ellis were both ahead of their time by drawing attention to sex differences in medicine, because the role of sex and gender remain understudied.

Historically, clinical research was based predominantly on male subjects in the United States until Congress passed the National Institutes of Health (NIH) Revitalization Act, which mandated the inclusion of women and minorities in NIH-funded clinical research.[9] Before this law was passed in 1993, clinical research almost exclusively focused on human male health and disease, and the results of these investigations have been generalized to the female population with uncertain and sometimes disputed appropriateness.

In the past 3 decades, more efforts have been devoted to sex-specific research efforts. The National Academy of Medicine (the Institute of Medicine at the time) published "Exploring the Biological Contributions to Human Health: Does Sex Matter" in 2001.[10] In this report, they emphasized sex as a biologic variable, rather than an observable feature, and urged researchers to focus their efforts on exploring the role of sex and gender in medicine.

Cardiology has been at the forefront of studying sex and gender and their role in disease. Former NIH director Dr Bernadine Healy was one of the first to highlight the problem of excluding women and females from clinical research. In her 1991 *New England Journal of Medicine* publication, Dr Healy described "The Yentyl syndrome," highlighting the sex bias in the identification and management of coronary disease in the United States.[11] Since that time, important efforts have been made to study the causes and effects of sex differences in cardiovascular medicine.

The implications of sex and gender have begun to gain attention in the realm of respiratory medicine. The role of sex steroids on health and pulmonary disease is one area of research, although it is clear that male and female hormones paint an incomplete picture in explaining the entirety of the observed differences seen clinically.[12] Socially defined gender roles, including participation in physical activity and patterns of substance use, have also been considered in this discussion.[13]

GENETIC DIFFERENCES

Traditionally, the major genetic distinction between males and females is defined within the sex chromosomes, XX for females and XY in males. X-linked disorders have been recognized for many centuries, with high index of disease severity in affected males and variable phenotypic expression in carrier females because of complex genetic architecture including skewed X-inactivation and somatic mosaicism.[14] The Y chromosome is one of the smallest chromosomes and is almost entirely made up by the male-specific region that is inherited intact from father to son,[15] and has generally been overlooked in most genetic analysis. However, accumulating evidence has linked the Y chromosome to disease, such as coronary artery disease and autoimmunity.[16,17]

Although sex chromosomes account for a significant portion of the genetic divergence between males and females, recent studies suggest that variation in the autosomal genome also leads to differing anatomic, physiologic, and behavioral traits in many species.[18] Sex has even been proposed as an "environmental" variable that interacts with genes and gene expression in a comparable manner to other environmental influences leading to sex-specific differences in the prevalence and severity of disease.[19] For example, three studies have shown that polymorphisms in the angiotensin-converting enzyme (ACE) locus have been shown to increase the risk for hypertension in men, but not in women in populations across the world.[20–22] Future investigation in the regulatory genome is necessary to better understand the genetic contributions to sexual dimorphism in human health and disease.

HORMONES

Much of the work regarding sex differences has focused on sex steroid hormones. The impact of sex hormones begins during prenatal development and these hormones have effects on genomic activation, receptors, and neurochemical pathways over the lifespan. These hormones are regulated by the hypothalamic-pituitary-gonadal axis and dysregulation of this axis results in a host of disorders in women and men including polycystic ovarian disease in women and increased risks of cancer and cardiovascular disease based on time of menarche. There are also sex differences in osteoporosis risk with more than 70% of osteoporotic fractures occurring in females.[23] In examining transgender individuals, we see a strong interplay of sex hormones and gender evidenced by lower bone density in transgender women compared with cisgender men and a higher bone mass in transgender men than in cisgender women.[24]

Sex differences in human lung structure and function are present even in utero and manifest during the lifespan.[25] The modulatory role of sex steroids (estrogen, progesterone, testosterone) and their metabolites on lung structure and function is suggested by sex differences seen at puberty, pregnancy, menopause, and with aging. In addition, there are sex differences in susceptibility, incidence, and severity of several lung diseases including asthma, chronic obstructive pulmonary disease, pulmonary fibrosis, pulmonary hypertension, and lung cancer. Understanding the role of sex steroid signaling in the lung could lead to the

development of novel biomarkers and targeted treatments for lung disease.[26]

IMMUNE FUNCTION

Sex and gender play a role in immune function as evidenced by the preponderance of autoimmune disease in females compared with males. In addition, fluctuating sex hormones may affect the risk for autoimmune disease evidenced by the changes in autoimmune disease prevalence during pregnancy and the reproductive years. There is growing evidence that sex and gender impact baseline immune function. Studies on vaccine efficacy demonstrate stronger innate and adaptive immune responses in women compared with men.[27]

CLINICAL MEDICINE

Sex- and gender-based medicine is a new paradigm of clinical practice that considers the association of sex and gender in all aspects of health and disease. This includes considering sex and gender in disease risk, presentation, response to treatment, access to health care, and impact on quality of life. Although sex and gender each can independently affect health it is far more common for them to interact to affect disease. In general, sex likely plays a larger role in disease cause, onset, and progression but gender can impact disease risk, symptom recognition, disease manifestations, access to care, quality of life, and adherence to treatment. Ultimately health is influenced by the interactions between sex and gender.

A recent review addresses the clinical advances of sex- and gender-informed medicine.[24] They present evidence on clinical conditions that highlights the importance of considering sex and gender when caring for patients. We briefly highlight a few areas that impact clinical care and where sex and gender are important to consider.

One area that deserves further investigation is the impact of sex and gender on tobacco use and subsequent lung disease. Over the last 50 years the risk of disease from tobacco use in women has risen sharply and is now equal to men.[28] Current smoking prevalence for teenage boys and girls is similar and most adults who smoke began before the age of 18. Early age of onset of tobacco use has been associated with delayed puberty in boys and girls. It is unclear whether sex and gender differences impact smoking cessation efforts, the impact of reduced nicotine cigarettes on disease, and the prevalence of use of e-cigarettes and their impact on adverse lung outcomes.

Circadian rhythms are endogenous, self-sustaining oscillations in physiology that follow a 24-hour cycle. They are generated by a biologic pacemaker located in the suprachiasmatic nucleus in the anterior hypothalamus.[29] The hypothalamus receives light/dark information, synchronizes this system to the 24-hour solar day, and transmits information to the rest of the body via autonomic and endocrine signals. In addition to light, circadian timing information is also sent to the cells, tissues, and organ via other inputs, such as feeding, social cues, and activity. These rhythms control several biologic processes, such as sleep-wake cycle, body temperature, feeding, hormone secretion, glucose homeostasis, and cell-cycle regulation. When synchronized and optimally timed, the circadian system allows the body to respond to physiologic challenges.[30] Alterations in the timing of these physiologic rhythms can cause internal desynchronization, which can have negative consequences on rest-activity cycles and other physiologic and behavioral functions. Irregular sleep schedules, travel across time zones, exposure to artificial light especially at night, and shift work can desynchronize these rhythms resulting in suboptimal functioning and over time increase the risk for diseases, such as diabetes, cancer, depression, cardiovascular disease, and reproductive problems. Sex differences in the circadian system may result in differential susceptibility to circadian misalignment, sleep disorders, and pathophysiology between males and females.[31] A study examining sex differences in circadian regulation of sleep demonstrated that females experience more cognitive impairment than males with the implication that women may be more susceptible to the effects of shift work and jet lag.[32]

Although data are currently limited one needs to consider the impact of sex and gender on pharmacokinetics and pharmacodynamics of medications. Biologic variables including age, race, and sex have significant influence on pharmaceutical effects in the body. Differences in drug response between males and females may be explained by variable pharmacokinetics and pharmacodynamics, including rates of absorption, drug distribution, metabolism, and excretion. However, these differences are mostly explained by differences in body weight.[33] This becomes especially important in the adult population, in whom most drugs are prescribed at a fixed dose, because females may experience higher levels of drug exposure than males. As an example, the antinausea medication ondansetron has 1.5- to 2-times the peak drug plasma concentrations and lower oral clearance compared with men, although no dosage adjustment based on weight or sex is recommended.[33]

Females are more vulnerable to potentially fatal drug-induced torsades de pointes (TdP) because of a longer baseline QTc interval than males.[34] This risk is compounded in certain QTc-prolonging medications, such as dofetilide, in which drug concentrations are significantly higher in females even after correcting for bodyweight and creatinine clearance.[33] Similarly, the increased risk of TdP has also been demonstrated with other antiarrhythmic medications including sotalol and quinidine.[33] Furthermore, women treated with antiplatelet and antithrombotic medications have higher rates of major and minor bleeding events in addition to higher fracture risk in women with diabetes with thiazolidinedione drugs.[35,36]

The US Government Accountability Office published a report in 2001 examining the 10 drugs withdrawn from the US market between 1997 and 2000 and found that eight of those drugs were associated with greater health risk for women compared with men. In four cases, the pharmaceuticals were prescribed more often to women and in the remaining four, there were more adverse events in women, despite similar prescribing patterns for male patients, including higher risk of TdP.[37] Although the implementation of sex-specific analysis in evaluating the safety of pharmaceuticals has improved since this report in 2001, many experts agree that this area remains a work in progress.[38]

RESEARCH DIRECTIONS

In 2017 the National Heart, Lung, and Blood Institute in partnership with the NIH Office of Research on Women's Health and the Office of Rare Diseases Research convened a workshop to review the current understanding of the biologic, behavioral, and clinical implications of female sex and gender on lung and sleep health and disease to formulate recommendations to address research gaps.[39] This group identified several areas for basic science and clinical research. Their key recommendations included establishing guidelines and standardization that include sex for reporting of cellular and animal models for in vitro experiments. They suggest developing multidisciplinary platforms for understanding sex steroid expression and signaling for basic science and clinical research. In addition, they recommend the reporting of sex-stratified analysis to allow for future meta-analyses of sex differences.

There are many animal models that have been developed to study lung diseases and these models have helped us understand pathobiology.[40] Often times sex variables are not reported in animal studies, especially when modeling changes across the lifespan. In asthma future research should focus on better understanding the effect of female sex, obesity, menstrual cycle, and menopause on disease severity and outcomes.[41] Animal models are frequently used to examine the impact of smoke exposure on lung disease but there is a scarcity of data on sex differences.[39] A review article found that in studies using cell lines 20% of cell lines were male origin, 5% were female origin, and 75% of studies did not report the sex.[42]

One area of research where there are minimal data, but which is likely important, is the microbiome. The human microbiome plays a role in several diseases and differences in anatomy, environmental exposures, hormones, and medications may alter the microbiome and also point to the possibility of sex and gender influences. In addition, the microbiome can change over the lifespan and across reproductive phases. Although the gut is where most microbiome studies have occurred, investigators are exploring the microbiome in lung diseases, such as chronic obstructive pulmonary disease, asthma, and cystic fibrosis, but the data about the impact of sex and gender are limited. Future studies should incorporate sex as a variable and address causal pathways examining the importance of sex and gender influences on the structure and function of the microbiome.

SUMMARY

Treating all adults as equivalent and not considering sex, gender, race, and environment is imprecise, and focusing basic and clinical research only on one sex or gender to the exclusion of the other is no longer acceptable.[43]

DISCLOSURE

Dr S. Kay and Dr M.A. Pisani have no commercial or financial conflicts of interest with this article.

REFERENCES

1. Madsen TE, Bourjeily G, Hasnain M, et al. Sex- and gender-based medicine: the need for precise terminology. Gend Genome 2017;1(3):122–8.
2. Haseltine F. Gender-based biology. The Scientist 1988. Available at: https://www.the-scientist.com/commentary/gender-based-biology-56753.
3. Coen S, Banister E. What a difference sex and gender make: a gender, sex and health research casebook. Vancouver, British Columbia: Canadian Institutes of Health; 2012.
4. Klymkowsky MW, Cooper MM. 4.9: sexual dimorphism. Biol LibreTexts 2016;p. 4120.
5. Flores AR, Herman JL, Gates GJ, et al. How many adults identify as transgender in the United States? Los Angeles, CA: The Williams Institute; 2016.
6. Zi J, Yu X, Li Y, et al. Coloration strategies in peacock feathers. Proc Natl Acad Sci U S A Oct 2003; 100(22):12576–8.
7. Hutchinson J. On the capacity of the lungs, and on the respiratory functions, with a view of establishing a precise and easy method of detecting disease by the spirometer. Med Chir Trans 1846;29: 137–252.
8. Ellis H. Man and woman: a study of human secondary and tertiary sexual characteristics. New York: Charles Scribner's Sons; 1894.
9. Women and Health Research. Ethical and legal issues of including women in clinical studies, vol. I. Washington, DC: Institute of Medicine (US) Committee on Ethical and Legal Issues Relating to the Inclusion of Women in Clinical Studies. National Academies Press (US); 1984.
10. The Committee on Understanding the Biology of Sex and Gender Differences. Exploring the biologic contribtions to human health: does sex matter? Washington, DC: Institute of Medicine (US) Committee on Understanding the Biology of Sex and Gender Differences. National Acadamies Press; 2001.
11. Healy B. The Yentl syndrome. N Engl J Med 1991; 325(4):274–6.
12. Townsend EA, Miller VM, Prakash YS. Sex differences and sex steroids in lung health and disease. Endocr Rev 2012;33(1):1–47.
13. Becklake MR, Kauffmann F. Gender differences in airway behaviour over the human life span. Thorax Dec 1999;54(12):1119–38.
14. Dobyns WB, Filauro A, Tomson BN, et al. Inheritance of most X-linked traits is not dominant or recessive, just X linked. Am J Med Genet A 2004;129A(2): 136–43.
15. Skaletsky H, Kuroda-Kawaguchi T, Minx PJ, et al. The male-specific region of the human Y chromosome is a mosaic of discrete sequence classes. Nature 2003;423(6942):825–37.
16. Bloomer LD, Nelson CP, Eales J, et al. Male-specific region of the Y chromosome and cardiovascular risk: phylogenetic analysis and gene expression studies. Arterioscler Thromb Vasc Biol 2013;33(7): 1722–7.
17. Case LK, Wall EH, Dragon JA, et al. The Y chromosome as a regulatory element shaping immune cell transcriptomes and susceptibility to autoimmune disease. Genome Res 2013;23(9):1474–85.
18. Korstanje R, Li R, Howard T, et al. Influence of sex and diet on quantitative trait loci for HDL cholesterol levels in an SM/J by NZB/BlNJ intercross population. J Lipid Res 2004;45(5):881–8.

19. Ober C, Loisel DA, Gilad Y. Sex-specific genetic architecture of human disease. Nat Rev Genet 2008; 9(12):911–22.

20. Higaki J, Baba S, Katsuya T, et al. Deletion allele of angiotensin-converting enzyme gene increases risk of essential hypertension in Japanese men: the Suita Study. Circulation 2000;101(17):2060–5.

21. O'Donnell CJ, Lindpaintner K, Larson MG, et al. Evidence for association and genetic linkage of the angiotensin-converting enzyme locus with hypertension and blood pressure in men but not women in the Framingham Heart Study. Circulation 1998; 97(18):1766–72.

22. Stanković A, Zivković M, Alavantić D. Angiotensin I-converting enzyme gene polymorphism in a Serbian population: a gender-specific association with hypertension. Scand J Clin Lab Invest 2002; 62(6):469–75.

23. Burge R, Dawson-Hughes B, Solomon DH, et al. Incidence and economic burden of osteoporosis-related fractures in the United States, 2005-2025. J Bone Miner Res 2007;22(3):465–75.

24. Bartz D, Chitnis T, Kaiser UB, et al. Clinical advances in sex- and gender-informed medicine to improve the health of all: a review. JAMA Intern Med 2020;180(4):574–83.

25. Seaborn T, Simard M, Provost PR, et al. Sex hormone metabolism in lung development and maturation. Trends Endocrinol Metab Dec 2010;21(12): 729–38.

26. Sathish V, Martin YN, Prakash YS. Sex steroid signaling: implications for lung diseases. Pharmacol Ther 2015;150:94–108.

27. Klein SL, Flanagan KL. Sex differences in immune responses. Nat Rev Immunol 2016;16(10):626–38.

28. National Center for Chronic Disease Prevention and Health Promotion (US) Office on Smoking and Health. The Health Consequences of Smoking—50 Years of Progress: A Report of the Surgeon General. Atlanta (GA): Centers for Disease Control and Prevention (US); 2014. PMID: 24455788.

29. Golombek DA, Rosenstein RE. Physiology of circadian entrainment. Physiol Rev 2010;90(3):1063–102.

30. Hastings MH, Reddy AB, Maywood ES. A clockwork web: circadian timing in brain and periphery, in health and disease. Nat Rev Neurosci 2003;4(8): 649–61.

31. Duffy JF, Wright KP Jr. Entrainment of the human circadian system by light. J Biol Rhythms 2005; 20(4):326–38.

32. Santhi N, Lazar AS, McCabe PJ, et al. Sex differences in the circadian regulation of sleep and waking cognition in humans. Proc Natl Acad Sci U S A 2016;113(19):E2730–9.

33. Parekh A, Fadiran EO, Uhl K, et al. Adverse effects in women: implications for drug development and regulatory policies. Expert Rev Clin Pharmacol 2011;4(4):453–66.

34. Drici MD, Clément N. Is gender a risk factor for adverse drug reactions? The example of drug-induced long QT syndrome. Drug Saf 2001;24(8): 575–85.

35. Cho L, Topol EJ, Balog C, et al. Clinical benefit of glycoprotein IIb/IIIa blockade with abciximab is independent of gender: pooled analysis from EPIC, EPILOG and EPISTENT trials. Evaluation of 7E3 for the prevention of ischemic complications. Evaluation in percutaneous transluminal coronary angioplasty to improve long-term outcome with abciximab GP IIb/IIIa blockade. Evaluation of platelet IIb/IIIa inhibitor for stent. J Am Coll Cardiol 2000;36(2):381–6.

36. Kahn SE, Zinman B, Lachin JM, et al. Rosiglitazone-associated fractures in type 2 diabetes: an analysis from A Diabetes Outcome Progression Trial (ADOPT). Diabetes Care May 2008;31(5):845–51.

37. Drug Safety. Most drugs withdrawn in recent years had greater health risks for women. Available: https://www.gao.gov/products/gao-01-286r. Accessed October 20, 2020.

38. Accounting for sex and gender makes for better science. Nature 2020;588(7837):196.

39. Han MK, Arteaga-Solis E, Blenis J, et al. Female sex and gender in lung/sleep health and disease. Increased understanding of basic biological, pathophysiological, and behavioral mechanisms leading to better health for female patients with lung disease. Am J Respir Crit Care Med 2018;198(7): 850–8.

40. Mercer PF, Abbott-Banner K, Adcock IM, et al. Translational models of lung disease. Clin Sci (Lond) 2015;128(4):235–56.

41. Zein JG, Erzurum SC. Asthma is different in women. Curr Allergy Asthma Rep 2015;15(6):28.

42. Shah K, McCormack CE, Bradbury NA. Do you know the sex of your cells? Am J Physiol, Cell Physiol 2014;306(1):C3–18.

43. Mauvais-Jarvis F, Arnold AP, Reue K. A guide for the design of pre-clinical studies on sex differences in metabolism. Cell Metab 2017;25(6):1216–30.

Stress and Loss of Ovarian Function

Novel Insights into the Origins of Sex-Based Differences in the Manifestations of Respiratory Control Disorders During Sleep

Richard Kinkead, PhD[a,*], Marianne Gagnon, BSc[a], Vincent Joseph, PhD[a],
Frédéric Sériès, MD[b], Danuzia Ambrozio-Marques, PhD[a]

KEYWORDS

- Control of breathing • Sleep apnea • Sex-based differences • Intermittent hypoxia
- Maternal separation

KEY POINTS

- The respiratory system of women and men develops and functions in distinct neuroendocrine milieus. This leads to sex-based differences in anatomy and neural control.
- In healthy individuals, homeostasis of arterial blood gases is ensured, regardless of sex. This convergence in function differs from the sex-based differences observed in many respiratory diseases.
- Sleep disordered breathing (SDB) is complex and multifactorial respiratory disorder that shows significant sexual dimorphism in its clinical manifestations and comorbidities.
- Menopause is a normal part of life but for a subgroup of women, this process is associated with the onset of SDB.
- Guided by recent progress from basic research, this review discusses the hypothesis that stress is necessary to reveal the sexual dimorphism of SDB.

SEX-BASED DIFFERENCES IN RESPIRATORY FUNCTION: CURRENT STATE OF KNOWLEDGE

There is growing interest in and appreciation for sex-based differences in respiratory physiology by comparison with other fields (eg, cardiovascular and neuroscience);respiratory research is lagging, because current literature is mainly descriptive.[1–3] There is limited comprehension of the mechanisms underlying the dimorphisms and this limitation reflects in part an important lack of basic knowledge from both female humans and female animals. The other challenge that the community faces is that sex-based differences in respiratory function are apparent at various life stages, the phenotypes are highly variable, and the distinction of the sex-specific traits not always is obvious.[1] At this stage, the origins of sex-based differences in respiratory disorders still are unknown, but a basic principle developed in sex-based research[4] can offer a novel approach to this problem.

[a] Department of Pediatrics, Université Laval, Centre de Recherche de l'Institut Universitaire de Cardiologie et Pneumologie de Québec, 2725 Chemin Ste-Foy, Québec, Québec G1V 4G5, Canada; [b] Department of Medicine, Université Laval, Centre de Recherche de l'Institut Universitaire de Cardiologie et Pneumologie de Québec, Québec, Québec, Canada
* Corresponding author. Department of Pediatrics, Université Laval, Centre de Recherche de l'Institut Universitaire de Cardiologie et Pneumologie de Québec, 2725 Chemin Ste-Foy, Québec, Québec G1V 4G5, Canada.
E-mail address: Richard.Kinkead@fmed.ulaval.ca

Clin Chest Med 42 (2021) 391–405
https://doi.org/10.1016/j.ccm.2021.04.002

The notion of sexual divergence and convergence in biological systems states that although men and women use different strategies to perform a given task, they converge on a similar endpoint.[4] In that regard, spatial orientation and immunologic responses are well-documented examples. The male/female differences in respiratory control observed in healthy animals or humans is another excellent example of sexual convergence in physiologic function (**Fig. 1**). For instance, it is known that sex hormones have profound (and distinct) stimulatory effects on the peripheral (carotid body) and central components of the respiratory control system.[1–3] The neuroendocrine milieu in which the respiratory control network of men and women develop and perform differ substantially; yet, despite those differences in regulatory strategies, the respiratory control system of healthy men and women ensures effective gas exchange that meets metabolic demands.

This convergence contrasts with sex divergence in which a challenging condition (ie, stressor) reveals male/female differences that otherwise were latent and inconsequential.[4] Excessive or chronic stress often leads to abnormal phenotypes, but because regulation of the sex-specific neuroendocrine axis differs between men and women,[5] the impacts often are sex-specific.[4] This form of sexual dimorphism exists in respiratory control, and there is growing appreciation for the fact that the clinical manifestations of sleep-disordered breathing (SDB) and related comorbidities show significant sex-based differences (see **Fig. 1**). The pathophysiology of SDB in men is well described. This review focuses on differences between men and women; the main traits found in the clinical literature are summarized in **Table 1** and discussed in the following section. This then raises the following question: Is stress sufficient to cause sexual divergence in respiratory control and, if so, how does it work? This review puts forward a rationale linking stress to sex-specific respiratory control disturbances. In the process, observations from basic research are highlighted that, hopefully, will spark stimulating exchanges on this topic. First is a brief overview of SDB and the sex-based differences of its prevalence and manifestations.

SLEEP-DISORDERED BREATHING: A SEXUALLY DIMORPHIC RESPIRATORY DISORDER

SDB is a complex and highly heterogeneous respiratory disorder. It is characterized by prolonged

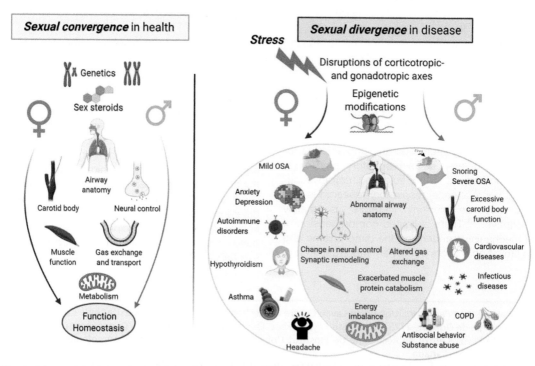

Fig. 1. Schematic representation of sex-based differences in respiratory control that allow either convergence in function (health [*left*]) or divergent responses to stressors that lead to sex-specific manifestations of respiratory dysfunction and comorbidities (disease [*right*]). Created with BioRender.com. OSA, obstructive sleep apnea; COPD, chronic obstructive pulmonary disease.

Table 1
Sex-based differences in clinical manifestations of sleep-disordered breathing and related comorbidities

Symptoms	Sex Prevalence (Increased Risk)	Relative Occurrence and Manifestations	Age Range (Years)	References
AHI ≥5: mild-to-severe	Men (1.8×)	Men: 59%; women: 33%	20–81	154
AHI ≥15–30: moderate-to-severe	Men (2.2×)	Men: 29%; women: 13%	20–81	154
AHI >30: severe	Men (1.5×)	Men: 8%–11%; women: 4%–7%	20–81	14,154
Obstructive events	Men (1.1×)		47–56	155
Central events	Men (not reported)		47–56	155
Mixed events	Similar		47–56	155
Increased AHI during REM	Women (4.9×)	During REM, AHI in women doubles from 17.3–20 to 36–42. AHI in men increases in 30%: from 21–31 to 30–40	46–56	155,156
Inflammatory signals (tumor necrosis factor α)	Women (not reported)		47–56	155
Craniofacial abnormalities (1)	Men (not reported)		29–33	157
Sleeping disturbances (2)	Women (1.3×–2×)		30–62	14,158–161
Snoring	Men (1.05×–2.2×)		40–62	14,159,162–165
Respiratory comorbidity (3)*	Women (1.3×–6.5×)		46–62	14,160,166,167
Chronic obstructive pulmonary disease	Men (2.1××9×)		48–52	160,168
Collapsibility of the airway	Men (not reported)		27–32	162,169
Hypertension	Men (1.05×–3.2×) Women (1.07×–1.6×)		40–63 40–63	14,158,159,163,166 160,161,168,170
Cardiovascular disease (4)	Men (1.5×–3 ×) Women (not reported)	Coronary heart disease	21–80 48–56	14,166,170 171
Diabetes mellitus	Men (1.25×) Women (1.8×)		21–80 24–74	170 166,171
High-density lipoprotein cholesterol (<40 mg/dL)	Women (not reported)		47–55	155
Morning headache	Women (1.2×–2.1×)		48–59	159–161,166,168
Hypothyroidism	Women (5.0×–5.5×)		48–52	166,168
Psychiatric disorders (5)	Women (2×–3×)		46–56	161,166–168
Elevated BMI <30.0	Similar		47–63	155,158,168,172
Alcohol consumption	Men (2.1×–17×)		43–63	155,160,161,163

Abbreviation: AHI, apnea-hypopnea index.

and repeated episodes of partial or complete upper airway closure leading to decreases or cessations of breathing during sleep that often are resolved by arousals. Each apneic/hypopneic event is associated with a drop in blood O_2 levels that, over time, disrupts vital physiologic and cellular processes. SDB also causes sleep fragmentation, which, besides its detrimental effects on vigilance, disrupts neurologic function. Together, these deleterious consequences of SDB augment the risk of metabolic syndrome, depression, neurodegenerative diseases, and cancer.[6–9] Cardiovascular disease is the most important associated comorbidity because moderate to severe sleep apnea increases the risk for hypertension and cardiac infarction by 2-fold to 4-fold.[9–11]

A recent study estimates that nearly 1 billion adults worldwide suffer from SDB.[12] In North America, SDB affects approximately 26% of the population but up to 80% of those with the disorder are undiagnosed.[7,13] Because its occurrence is 2.5 times more frequent in men, SDB is considered "a men's disease" and women are less likely to be diagnosed.[14,15] This is a problem because as women age, the prevalence of SDB rises, and studies estimate that 47% of postmenopausal women suffer from moderate to severe SDB[13,16–18] (**Fig. 2**). Understanding of the origins and pathophysiology of SDB in women is limited because women are systematically underrepresented in clinical research[14] and female animals still are underused in animal research.

During the night, SDB patients show transient decreases or complete cessations of airflow to the lungs (hypopneas or apneas, respectively) due to upper airway obstruction with persisting inspiratory efforts. Besides obstructive events that represent the majority of SDB, central (no respiratory effort) or mixed[6] events also may be observed. A narrow or collapsible upper airway is a main cause of obstructive SDB; obesity is an aggravating factor because the body mass index (BMI) is positively correlated with the severity of SDB.[6,19] In women, BMI often increases at menopause but the severity of SDB between premenopausal and postmenopausal persists after adjusting for BMI and neck circumference.[18,20] Thus, by comparison with men, the causes of SDB in postmenopausal women may reside more in functional rather than anatomic differences in the upper airways.[18,20]

The fact that sleep apnea patients breathe normally during daytime indicates that SDB is more than an anatomic problem.[21–23] Abnormalities in respiratory control become apparent when the respiratory drive associated with wakefulness is lost. Recent studies estimate that nonanatomic traits (ie, arousal threshold, loop gain, and upper airway gain) play an important role in 56% of SDB patients.[21,22] The key distinctions in the manifestations of SDB between men and women reported in the clinical literature are summarized in **Table 1**. The intensity, absence, or combination of these traits contributes to the heterogeneity of sleep apnea clinical presentation between individuals.[21,22]

Excessive Ventilatory Responses to Respiratory Stimuli (High Loop Gain)

During an obstructive SDB, stimulation of the carotid bodies and/or upper airway receptors trigger progressive recruitment of compensatory reflexes that restore normal blood gases and relieve the obstruction without affecting sleep.[24–26] These responses to respiratory disturbances are regulated by the respiratory control network but, in some subjects, this system is oversensitive. Patients with this trait, therefore, generate excessive ventilatory responses that lead to transient and cyclical loss of CO_2-related respiratory drive. This, in turn, promotes further respiratory instability and SDB.[6,19]

Abnormal Motor Control of the Airway

Skeletal muscle tone decreases during sleep. The uvula, soft palate, and tongue are common sites of airway collapse and, in some SDB patients, a greater loss of genioglossus motor tone during

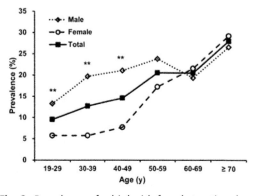

Fig. 2. Prevalence of a high risk for obstructive sleep apnea according to age and sex in a South Korean population. High risk for obstructive sleep apnea was defined as positive symptom categories of 2 on the Berlin questionnaire. ** *P*<.01 for comparisons between men and women in each age group, n = 1368 in men and n = 1372 in women. (*From* Sunwoo J-S, Hwangbo Y, Kim W-J, Chu MK, Yun C-H, Yang KI (2018) Prevalence, sleep characteristics, and comorbidities in a population at high risk for obstructive sleep apnea: A nationwide questionnaire study in South Korea. PLoS ONE 13(2): e0193549.)

sleep contributes to airway obstruction.[19,27] During such events, stimulation of the carotid bodies and/or upper airway receptors triggers progressive recruitment of airway muscles but, in some patients, this increase in neural drive fails to translate into an effective airway dilation.[22]

Respiratory Arousal Threshold

In another group of apneic patients, the level of respiratory stimuli required to recruit pharyngeal dilator muscles is very close to the level that triggers arousal.[23,28] Having a low arousal threshold implies that the termination of an apnea often is accompanied by an arousal, which prevents the orderly recruitment of upper airway muscles. If arousals are associated with an excessive increase in breathing, this then promotes the recurrence of apneas and arousals.[19] A low arousal threshold therefore contributes to sleep fragmentation, which is an important consequence of sleep apnea. Apneic women report sleep-related problems more frequently than men[29] (see **Table 1**).

LOSS OF OVARIAN FUNCTION: THE TRIGGER OF SLEEP-DISORDERED BREATHING IN WOMEN

A review of the current knowledge points to menopause as a key factor in the onset of SDB and related complications in women.[18,30–35] Ovarian hormones promote sleep[36] and stimulate respiratory reflexes and motor tone of the upper airways.[2,3,37–39] At first, withdrawal of these "endogenous respiratory stimulants" provides a simple explanation for the rise of respiratory disorders and sleep problems in menopausal women. The effectiveness of hormone replacement therapy at alleviating south apnea in some women supports this view[17,40–42]; however, there is no clear explanation for the heterogeneity in treatment efficacy or the fact that not all menopausal women develop SDB. Female SDB patients have lower levels of 17β-estradiol (E_2) and progesterone than those measured in age-matched healthy subjects,[41,43] but the origins of this trait are unknown. These observations indicate that female SDB patients are a distinct population in which menopause and its impact on physiology and health are different. Elucidating the different phenotypes of SDB and their origins is key to proper treatment,[21,22] yet comprehension of the different aging trajectories in women remains limited. Based on the rationale, discussed previously, stress plays a crucial role in the emergence of sex-specific manifestations of SDB and in that regard, Sapolsky and colleagues' "glucocorticoid cascade hypothesis of aging"[44] provides a valuable perspective on the problem.

Aging is associated with an impairment of the negative feedback control of the neuroendocrine response to stress (corticotropic axis).[45–47] This results in prolonged elevation of stress hormones following stress exposure, thereby increasing the risks of adverse effects. The cortisol response to stress of older women (69 y ± 6 y) is almost 3-fold stronger than for men of similar age.[48] Because the sex-based differences in the stress axis become more pronounced following menopause, it was proposed that ovarian steroids (estradiol and/or progesterone) could be involved, but again, studies investigating the effects of estrogen treatment on basal cortisol levels have led to mixed findings.[49] These observations provide evidence (albeit indirect) that an age-dependent and sex-dependent dependent increase in corticotropic function contributes to sex-based differences in SDB.

THE LINK BETWEEN STRESS AND RESPIRATORY CONTROL DISORDERS

There now is a strong scientific consensus acknowledging that stress experienced chronically or during a critical period of development is a major cause of disease in adult.[50–53] Stress has persistent and sex-specific effects on health and the brain is a major target.[54] Clearly, one neural system of considerable interest is the respiratory control network because pathology in this homeostatic system underlies is key to SDB.[6,19,21] The role of stress, however, either during development or as adults, in the etiology of SDB has been virtually ignored. For clinical and basic researchers in respiratory physiology, the link between stress and psychiatric conditions, such as depression or anxiety disorders, is far more intuitive than with SDB.

The paraventricular nucleus of the hypothalamus (PVH) is the main structure that orchestrates the release of peptides and hormones in response to stress.[55–58] From a respiratory perspective, it is important to highlight that the PVH sends direct projections onto structures generating the respiratory rhythm, integrating respiratory stimuli, and motoneurons controlling the diaphragm and upper airways.[2] Thus, the PVH exerts a top-down influence on the medullary structures that generate and regulate breathing and consequently, stressful conditions that affect PVH function likely will influence respiratory control. Clinical studies repeatedly have documented the link between stress and respiratory control dysfunction (including SDB) in both children and adults.[59–62] The fact that psychiatric patients are 2 times to 3 times more likely to suffer from SDB than the normal population supports this relationship[63–66]; the coexistence of anxiety and SDB is most notable in women.[67] Finally, stress in itself is an acknowledged risk factor for the main comorbidities of SDB, including obesity, depression, and hypertension.[68–71] Clearly, these evidences are circumstantial because stress is a multifaceted physiologic, sociologic, and emotional condition. Establishing causality in clinical studies is challenging and mechanistic investigations are virtually impossible. It is not surprising therefore, that human studies that have addressed the link between chronic stress, dysfunction of the hypothalamic-pituitary-adrenal (HPA) axis, and SDB have yielded conflicting results.[72–75] Experiments performed on animal models, however, now offer valuable insights and further our understanding of the basic neurobiological principles underlying the role of stress in the emergence of sex-specific manifestations of respiratory control disorders. How 2 distinct yet complementary approaches have furthered comprehension of the problem is discussed.

EARLY LIFE STRESS AND SEX-BASED DIFFERENCES IN THE PROGRAMMING OF THE STRESS NEUROENDOCRINE PATHWAYS AND RESPIRATORY CONTROL

The perinatal period is critical to healthy development.[50,52,53] In mammals (including humans), the tactile, olfactory, and auditory stimuli that the mother provides to her offspring are among the most potent stimuli affecting brain development of the newborn.[76–78] Consequently, adverse conditions, such as unstable/inadequate parental environment and specialized medical care that interferes with mother-infant interactions, compromise neurologic outcomes.[50,76,79–82] Inadequate maternal care augments basal activity of the HPA axis and potentiates the responsiveness to stress throughout life.[56,83–85] Much like chronic stress, this condition, therefore, augments the risk for a broad range of health issues, including anxiety, diabetes, and cardiovascular diseases,[50,62,70,86] which are significant comorbidities associated with SDB.[6]

Neonatal maternal separation (NMS) is a well-established and clinically relevant form of stress. Although it poses no direct threat to respiratory homeostasis, inadequate maternal care disrupts brain function by weakening inhibition of the stress pathways.[57,58,84,87,88] The authors previously demonstrated that exposure of rat pups to NMS (3 h/d, postnatal days 3–12) elicits sex-specific dysfunction in respiratory control that persist well into adulthood. Furthermore, NMS male pups (but not female pups) are hypertensive by comparison with controls.[85] Studies in neuroscience and

psychiatry show that puberty often reveals latent conditions resulting from exposure to adverse conditions during early life and several of these manifestations can be sex-specific.[89–91] Excessive ventilatory responses to respiratory stimuli (high loop gain) is an important trait in SDB and, prior to puberty, the hypoxic ventilatory response (HVR) of pups generally is similar in male pups and female pups, and NMS does not affect this chemoreflex.[92] When rats reach sexual maturity, the HVR of male rats previously subjected to NMS is 25% to 30% greater than controls due to an augmented tidal volume response. In female rats, however, the HVR of NMS rats is 31% less than controls, owing to a decrease in the frequency response.[57,85] The authors then questioned the physiologic (and clinical) relevance of the NMS phenotype reported in male rats. Instrumentation of male rats to monitor sleep/wake states allowed the authors to demonstrate that NMS augments the HVR in male rats during non–rapid eye movement (REM) sleep and that the intensity of the response correlated positively with respiratory variability during non-REM sleep[93] (**Fig. 3**).

NEONATAL STRESS AND SEX-SPECIFIC INCREASE IN NEURAL CONTROL OF THE O_2 CHEMOREFLEX

Evidence gathered to date indicates that NMS increases carotid body function.[94–96] For instance, in anesthetized or awake animals, the immediate rise in breathing frequency observed at the onset of hypoxia, is more important in NMS that controls.[57,85,97] To address this issue, Soliz and colleagues[98] utilized an ex vivo carotid body preparation from adult rats to record the carotid sinus nerve activity and compare the responses to hypoxia and hypercapnia. Hypoxia increased carotid sinus nerve activity in all animals and this response was reversible upon return to baseline O_2 conditions. The response observed in control animals did not differ between male rats and female rats. In male rats, however, NMS augmented the carotid sinus firing frequency in response to hypoxia 1.5-fold above that recorded for controls. In contrast, female rats subjected to NMS showed carotid sinus nerve response that was blunted significantly during hypoxia (3-fold reduction). Exposing carotid preparations to an increase in CO_2/H^+ stimulated firing rate also; however, this response was not influenced by stress or sex. Taken together, these data support the assertion that the alteration of carotid body O_2 sensing contributes to the phenotype observed in NMS animals exposed to hypoxia. The origins of these sex-specific effects of stress on carotid body function remain unaddressed. Current data indicate, however, that

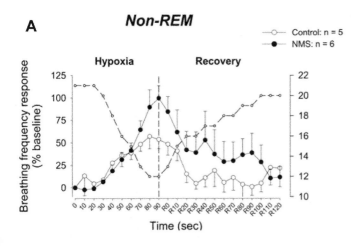

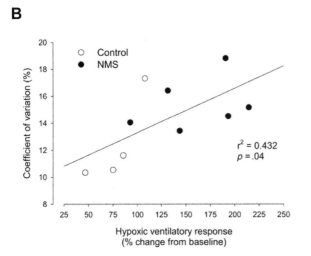

Fig. 3. NMS augments the hyperventilatory response to a brief hypoxic episode and promotes respiratory instability during non-REM sleep. (*A*) Comparison of the breathing frequency response to hypoxia (90 s) between controls (*white circles*) and rats previously subjected to NMS (*black circles*) during non-REM sleep. The figure also shows the change in frequency during the return to normoxia (recovery: 120 s). The small circles show the fraction of inspired O_2 measured in the chamber during the experiment (right axis). In this panel, data were obtained every 10 seconds. (*B*) Correlation between the minute ventilation response to hypoxia (last 20 s of hypoxia expressed as a percentage change from baseline and the coefficient of variation for this variable during the 2.5 hours of recording under normoxia. These measurements were obtained during non-REM sleep. Open circles: control rats (n = 4); black circles: rats previously subjected to NMS (n = 6). (*Adapted from* Kinkead R, Montandon G, Bairam A, Lajeunesse Y, Horner RL. Neonatal maternal separation disrupts regulation of sleep and breathing in adult male rats. Sleep. 2009;32(12):1611-1620.)

estrogen, progesterone, and testosterone stimulate the carotid body[3,38,99,100] and that stress interferes with the secretion of these hormones during acute respiratory challenge.

The authors then investigated the neural mechanisms underlying the physiologic phenotype of male NMS rats. To do so, the authors used electrical stimulation of the carotid sinus nerve to activate the neural pathways involved in the hypoxic chemoreflex without the confounding effects of brain hypoxia or treatment related differences in carotid body function. Although the frequency response to carotid sinus nerve stimulation was similar between groups, the rise in phrenic burst amplitude was greater in NMS than in control rats. Therefore, in addition to the enhancement of the carotid body's response to hypoxia, a more efficient central integration of the chemoafferent signal contributes to the augmented O_2 chemoreflex gain in male rats subjected to NMS than control animals.[97]

Results from subsequent studies showed that in adults, disruption of the delicate balance between inhibitory and excitatory neurotransmission contributes to the elevated HVR in NMS rats. On the one hand, auto-radiographic and pharmacologic studies show that NMS potentiates GABAergic regulation of the PVH and the caudal region of the medulla that receives chemosensory afferent.[57,101] On the other hand, results from in vivo experiments demonstrated that inactivation of AMPA/kainate receptors attenuated the HVR to a greater degree in NMS male rats versus controls; the latter result is consistent with a greater level of AMPA receptor expression in the PVH and cervical spinal cord.[58] Based on the functional outcomes, it is clear that stress-related potentiation of glutamatergic neurotransmission overcomes increases in GABAergic modulation. As discussed previously, the PVH has significant anatomic and functional interactions with key structures of the brainstem and spinal cord that regulate breathing. As a whole, these data show that NMS-related increase in PVH function augments the O_2 chemoreflex. Conversely, PVH inhibition returns the HVR of stressed rats to a normal (control) levels and reduces it below normal in control rats.[57,102] Thus, it is now clear that, in addition to its role in regulation of the stress response, the PVH sets the gain of the O_2 chemoreflex, a concept that has significant clinical implications regarding the etiology of respiratory control disorders.

ROLE OF SEX HORMONES

Sex steroids are potent ventilatory stimulants and, in healthy women, menopause is associated with a relative alveolar hypoventilation and arterial hypercapnia by comparison with a premenopausal population that are alleviated with hormone replacement therapy.[2,103] Because the intensity of O_2 chemoreflex measured in premenopausal versus postmenopausal women was similar, the hypoventilation was explained (in part) by a reduced central but not peripheral chemoreflex drive to breathe.[103] Similar changes in baseline ventilation have been reported in control (unstressed) rats, but, unlike in humans, the HVR decreased significantly.[104–106]

In a subpopulation of women, menopause is associated with the onset of significant neurologic problems, including cognitive decline, hypertension, and SDB.[18,33,34,36,42,107] The emergence of these problems is due partly to the loss of ovarian hormones (especially E_2), which have neuroprotective effects against various stressors, such as intermittent hypoxia (IH) (discussed later). Because loss of ovarian function is a normal part of aging, why do some women develop problems whereas others do not? The authors hypothesize that in women, early life stress creates a latent vulnerability and that loss of ovarian function reveals its deleterious impacts on respiratory control. Unlike controls rats, NMS women show no age-related decline in their HVR and, consequently, their response becomes greater than controls. Because ovariectomy has similar effects, these stress-related differences in aging trajectory are due mainly to the drop in ovarian hormones[106] (**Fig. 4**).

CHRONIC INTERMITTENT HYPOXIA AND ITS SEX-SPECIFIC IMPACTS ON RESPIRATORY CONTROL IN ADULT ANIMALS

Over the past 20 years, there has been an explosion of studies using chronic IH (CIH) to mimic the repeated drops in O_2 saturation experienced by SDB patients. The amount of data obtained with

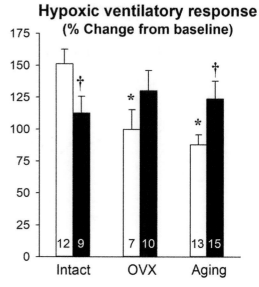

Fig. 4. Comparison of the ventilatory response to hypoxia (fraction of inspired oxygen = 0.12; 20 min) between stressed rats (NMS [*black bars*]) and control female rats (*open bars*). Female rats were measured at adulthood with intact gonads or following decline in ovarian function by aging or ovariectomy (OVX). Data reported as means ± SEM. Aging = 57 weeks. Number of rats/group appears in the histograms. * Different from intact at $P<.05$; † different from control at $P<.05$. (*Adapted from* Fournier S, Gulemetova R, Baldy C, Joseph V, Kinkead R. Neonatal stress affects the aging trajectory of female rats on the endocrine, temperature, and ventilatory responses to hypoxia. Am J Physiol Regul Integr Comp Physiol. 2015;308(7):R659-R667. Copyright © 2015 the American Physiological Society.)

this model is impressive and is not reviewed here (see Johnson and colleagues,[108] Prabhakar and colleagues,[109] and Dewan and colleagues[110]). Although CIH is a consequence, not a cause, of SDB,[22] it is a valuable experimental approach to evaluate how this form of systemic stress affects the organism at multiple levels and reveal sex-based differences in respiratory control. Its effects on the organism range from therapeutic to toxic, depending on the intensity and duration of the protocol used.[111–113] The carotid bodies are necessary for those processes because CIH does not affect the organism if the carotid bodies are denervated.[114–116] When sufficiently severe, CIH can activate the stress pathways, sensitize stress reactivity, and increase plasma corticosterone levels.[74,117–120] It is now firmly established that CIH reproduces key respiratory control anomalies observed in SDB patients, including a greater number of apneas during sleep,[121–123] an increased HVR due excessive carotid body sensitivity, and abnormal integration of chemosensory stimuli.[109,124] CIH also can cause diverse systemic dysfunctions commonly observed as comorbidities in SDB patients, including hypertension, cognitive decline, and metabolic disorder.[11,115,123,125,126] Inflammation and oxidative stress appear as key elements contributing to those deleterious effects,[123,127] and recent data provide valuable insights into the role of ovarian hormones in the manifestations of these disturbances.

17-β ESTRADIOL AND PROGESTERONE PREVENT OXIDATIVE STRESS IN ANIMAL MODELS OF SLEEP APNEA

Oxidative stress is an imbalance between the production of reactive oxygen species (ROS) and antioxidant defenses, leading to tissue injury.[128,129] Ovarian hormones are well known for their protective roles against oxidative stress, being able to down-regulate the expression of key pro-oxidant enzymes[130] and up-regulate the expression of antioxidant enzymes.[131] Moreover, by increasing mitochondrial respiratory activity, estradiol also reduces the production of reactive oxygen by the complexes of the electron transport chain.[132,133] Increased production of ROS is a key element involved in the cardiorespiratory disorders observed in sleep apnea patients.

In apneic patients, there are clear-cut signs of oxidative stress, such as excessive release of ROS by leukocytes, increased lipid peroxidation and reduced antioxidant capacity in the plasma, and oxidative stress correlates with high blood pressure and endothelial dysfunction.[134] One of the most largely acknowledged mechanisms underlying the effects of IH on arterial pressure in humans[135,136] and animals[116] is an increased activity of the sympathetic system triggered by oxidative stress at the level of the peripheral chemoreceptors.[109,137] Exposure to IH in rats increases the expression of the NADPH oxidase family members Nox1, Nox2, and Nox3 in the peripheral chemoreceptors,[109,138] and the activity of complex I of the mitochondrial electron transport chain is reduced,[139] leading to enhanced cytosolic and mitochondrial ROS production. IH also induces oxidative stress in adipose tissue,[140–142] and in the liver.[143] In rats, MnTMPyP, a membrane-permeable antioxidant, prevents the effects of IH on the sensory activity of the peripheral chemoreceptors.[137] Other antioxidant molecules (ibuprofen or vitamin C) also reduce these effects and efficiently prevent the development of hypertension in rats exposed to IH.[127] Clinical studies are consistent with these data, and it has been shown that vascular dysfunction is reduced

in apneic patients who received treatment with the antioxidant vitamin C[144,145] or with a xanthine oxidase inhibitor (allopurinol[146]).

To better understand the role of E_2 on exaggerated chemoreflex activity, hypertension, and oxidative stress, the authors established an animal model by using ovariectomized female rats exposed to IH.[123,147,148] The classic E_2 receptors (ERα and ERβ) are expressed in peripheral chemoreceptors[149] and in central areas controlling breathing and the sympathetic nervous system.[150] ERα reduces sympathetic activity,[151] thereby protecting women against hypertension.[152] Over the past few years, the authors have conducted a series of studies showing that E_2 and progesterone protect against cardiorespiratory disturbances, oxidative stress, and mitochondrial dysfunction in ovariectomized female rats exposed to IH. Exposure to IH-enhanced arterial blood pressure and the ventilatory response to hypoxia,[123] while also increasing respiratory variability and frequency of apnea during sleep, supplying direct evidence of increased activity of the peripheral chemoreceptors. In the brain cortex, IH decreased antioxidant enzyme activities and increased the activity of pro-oxidant enzyme and markers of oxidative stress.[123] Female rats exposed to IH and treated with E_2 had normal blood pressure and a normal ventilatory response to hypoxia. In the brain cortex, E_2 treatment also prevented the effects of IH on pro-oxidant and antioxidant enzyme activities.[123] A major source of oxidative stress is linked to mitochondrial oxidative phosphorylation. In the brain cortex, the authors' results show that IH reduces mitochondrial O_2 consumption and increases mitochondrial ROS production[148] and selective agonists of ERα and ERβ given during the exposure to IH restored mitochondrial respiration and ROS production to normal levels. Progesterone is able to prevent the excessive HVR induced by IH and reduced the frequency of apnea during sleep.[153] In the brain cortex of female rats exposed to IH, progesterone reduced the activity of prooxidant enzymes while increasing the activity of glutathione peroxidase (and cytosolic and mitochondrial superoxide dismutase).[153]

SUMMARY

There is growing appreciation for the phenotypic diversity in the pathophysiology and clinical manifestations of SDB. Data from basic research support clinical observations indicating that regardless of its form, stress is an important factor in the etiology of the disorder and the sex-based differences in the manifestations. Future research elucidating the mechanisms by which stress leads to respiratory control dysfunction in men and women is an important step toward developing novel therapeutic targeted interventions.

CLINICS CARE POINTS

- Manifestations of sleep disordered breathing (SDB) differ between men and women.
- Following menopause, the prevalence of SDB observed in women reaches that of men.
- In aging women, SDB is underdiagnosed; this respiratory disorder can be confused with other sleep problems.

DISCLOSURE

The authors have no financial or commercial conflict to declare.

REFERENCES

1. Gargaglioni LH, Marques DA, Patrone LGA. Sex differences in breathing. Comp Biochem Physiol A Mol Integr Physiol 2019;238:110543.
2. Behan M, Kinkead R. Neuronal control of breathing: sex and stress hormones. Compr Physiol 2011;1:2101–39.
3. Joseph V, Behan M, Kinkead R. Sex, hormones, and stress: how they impact development and function of the carotid bodies and related reflexes. Respir Physiol Neurobiol 2013;185:75–86.
4. McCarthy MM, Arnold AP, Ball GF, et al. Sex differences in the brain: the not so inconvenient truth. J Neurosci 2012;32(7):2241–7.
5. Goel N, Workman JL, Lee TT, et al. Sex differences in the HPA axis. Compr Physiol 2014;4:1121–55.
6. Dempsey JA, Veasey SC, Morgan BJ, et al. Pathophysiology of sleep apnea. Physiol Rev 2010;90(1):47–112.
7. Snyder B, Cunningham RL. Sex differences in sleep apnea and comorbid neurodegenerative diseases. Steroids 2018;133:28–33.
8. Gozal D, Ham SA, Mokhlesi B. Sleep apnea and cancer: analysis of a nationwide population sample. Sleep 2016;39(8):1493–500.
9. Lim DC, Pack AI. Obstructive sleep apnea: update and future. Annu Rev Med 2017;68(1):99–112.
10. Gopalakrishnan P, Tak T. Obstructive sleep apnea and cardiovascular disease. Cardiol Rev 2011;19(6):279–90.
11. Floras JS. Hypertension and sleep apnea. Can J Cardiol 2015;31(7):889–97.
12. Benjafield AV, Ayas NT, Eastwood PR, et al. Estimation of the global prevalence and burden of obstructive sleep apnoea: a literature-based analysis. Lancet Respir Med 2019;7(8):687–98.
13. Mirer AG, Young T, Palta M, et al. Sleep-disordered breathing and the menopausal transition among participants in the Sleep in Midlife Women Study. Menopause 2017;24(2):157–62.
14. Lindberg E, Benediktsdottir B, Franklin KA, et al. Women with symptoms of sleep-disordered breathing are less likely to be diagnosed and treated for sleep apnea than men. Sleep Med 2017;35:17–22.
15. Jordan AS, McSharry DG, Malhotra A. Adult obstructive sleep apnoea. Lancet 2014;383(9918):736–47.
16. Heinzer R, Vat S, Marques-Vidal P, et al. Prevalence of sleep-disordered breathing in the general population: the HypnoLaus study. Lancet Respir Med 2015;3(4):310–8.
17. Valipour A. Gender-related differences in the obstructive sleep apnea syndrome. Pneumologie 2012;66(10):584–8.
18. Dancey DR, Hanly PJ, Soong C, et al. Impact of menopause on the prevalence and severity of sleep apnea. Chest 2001;120(1):151–5.
19. White D, Younes M. Obstructive sleep apnea. Compr Physiol 2012;2:2541–94.
20. Dancey DR, Hanly PJ, Soong C, et al. Gender differences in sleep apnea: the role of neck circumference. Chest 2003;123(5):1544–50.
21. Eckert DJ, White DP, Jordan AS, et al. Defining phenotypic causes of obstructive sleep apnea. Identification of novel therapeutic targets. Am J Respir Crit Care Med 2013;188(8):996–1004.
22. Eckert DJ. Phenotypic approaches to positional therapy for obstructive sleep apnoea. Sleep Med Rev 2018;37:175–6.
23. Eckert DJ, Younes MK. Arousal from sleep: implications for obstructive sleep apnea pathogenesis and treatment. J Appl Physiol (1985) 2014;116(3):302–13.
24. Younes M. Contributions of upper airway mechanics and control mechanisms to severity of obstructive apnea. Am J Respir Crit Care Med 2003;168(6):645–58.
25. Younes M. Role of arousals in the pathogenesis of obstructive sleep apnea. Am J Respir Crit Care Med 2004;169(5):623–33.
26. Younes M, Loewen AHS, Ostrowski M, et al. Genioglossus activity available via non-arousal mechanisms vs. that required for opening the airway in obstructive apnea patients. J Appl Physiol (1985) 2012;112(2):249–58.
27. Mezzanotte WS, Tangel DJ, White DP. Waking genioglossal electromyogram in sleep apnea patients versus normal controls (a neuromuscular compensatory mechanism). J Clin Invest 1992;89(5):1571–9.

28. Younes M, Ostrowski M, Atkar R, et al. Mechanisms of breathing instability in patients with obstructive sleep apnea. J Appl Physiol (1985) 2007;103(6): 1929–41.

29. Theorell-Haglöw J, Miller CB, Bartlett DJ, et al. Gender differences in obstructive sleep apnoea, insomnia and restless legs syndrome in adults – what do we know? A clinical update. Sleep Med Rev 2018;38:28–38.

30. Anttalainen U, Polo O, Saaresranta T. Is 'MILD' sleep-disordered breathing in women really mild? Acta Obstet Gynecol Scand 2010;89(5):605–11.

31. Galvan T, Camuso J, Sullivan K, et al. Association of estradiol with sleep apnea in depressed perimenopausal and postmenopausal women: a preliminary study. Menopause 2017;24(1):112–7.

32. Heinzer R, Marti-Soler H, Marques-Vidal P, et al. Impact of sex and menopausal status on the prevalence, clinical presentation, and comorbidities of sleep-disordered breathing. Sleep Med 2018;51: 29–36.

33. Huang T, Hu FB, Lin BM, et al. Type of menopause, age at menopause, and risk of developing obstructive sleep apnea in postmenopausal women. Am J Epidemiol 2018;187(7):1370–9.

34. Young T, Finn L, Austin D, et al. Menopausal status and sleep-disordered breathing in the Wisconsin sleep cohort study. Am J Respir Crit Care Med 2003;167(9):1181–5.

35. Sunwoo J-S, Hwangbo Y, Kim W-J, et al. Prevalence, sleep characteristics, and comorbidities in a population at high risk for obstructive sleep apnea: a nationwide questionnaire study in South Korea. PLoS One 2018;13(2):e0193549.

36. Gervais NJ, Mong JA, Lacreuse A. Ovarian hormones, sleep and cognition across the adult female lifespan: an integrated perspective. Front Neuroendocrinol 2017;47:134–53.

37. Popovic RM, White DP. Upper airway muscle activity in normal women: influence of hormonal status. J Appl Physiol (1985) 1998;84(3):1055–62.

38. Hannhart B, Pickett CK, Moore LG. Effects of estrogen and progesterone on carotid body neural output responsiveness to hypoxia. J Appl Physiol (1985) 1990;68(5):1909–16.

39. Tatsumi K, Pickett CK, Jacoby CR, et al. Role of endogenous female hormones in hypoxic chemosensitivity. J Appl Physiol (1985) 1997;83(5):1706–10.

40. Wesström J, Ulfberg J, Nilsson S. Sleep apnea and hormone replacement therapy: a pilot study and a literature review. Acta Obstet Gynecol Scand 2005; 84(1):54–7.

41. Lozo T, Komnenov D, Badr MS, et al. Sex differences in sleep disordered breathing in adults. Respir Physiol Neurobiol 2017;245:65–75.

42. Bixler EO, Vgontzas AN, Lin HM, et al. Prevalence of sleep-disordered breathing in women: effects of gender. Am J Respir Crit Care Med 2001;163(3 Pt 1):608–13.

43. Netzer NC, Eliasson AH, Strohl KP. Women with sleep apnea have lower levels of sex hormones. Sleep Breath 2003;7(1):25–9.

44. Sapolsky RM, Krey LC, McEwen BS. The neuroendocrinology of stress and aging: the glucocorticoid cascade hypothesis. Endocr Rev 1986;7(3): 284–301.

45. Traustadóttir T, Bosch PR, Matt KS. The HPA axis response to stress in women: effects of aging and fitness. Psychoneuroendocrinology 2005; 30(4):392–402.

46. Gaffey AE, Bergeman CS, Clark LA, et al. Aging and the HPA axis: stress and resilience in older adults. Neurosci Biobehav Rev 2016;68:928–45.

47. Aguilera G. HPA axis responsiveness to stress: implications for healthy aging. Exp Gerontol 2011; 46(2–3):90–5.

48. Otte C, Hart S, Neylan TC, et al. A meta-analysis of cortisol response to challenge in human aging: importance of gender. Psychoneuroendocrinology 2005;30(1):80–91.

49. Wolf OT, Kudielka BM. Stress, health and ageing: a focus on postmenopausal women. Menopause Int 2008;14(3):129–33.

50. Shonkoff JP, Boyce WT, McEwen BS. Neuroscience, molecular biology, and the childhood roots of health disparities: building a new framework for health promotion and disease prevention. JAMA 2009;301(21):2252–9.

51. Kivimäki M, Steptoe A. Effects of stress on the development and progression of cardiovascular disease. Nat Rev Cardiol 2018;15(4):215–29.

52. Nelson CA III, Gabard-Durnam LJ. Early adversity and critical periods: neurodevelopmental consequences of violating the expectable environment. Trends Neurosci 2020;43(3):133–43.

53. Shonkoff JP. Capitalizing on advances in science to reduce the health consequences of early childhood adversity: reducing the health consequences of early adversityreducing the health consequences of early adversity. JAMA Pediatr 2016; 170(10):1003–7.

54. McEwen BS, Bowles NP, Gray JD, et al. Mechanisms of stress in the brain. Nat Neurosci 2015; 18(10):1353–63.

55. Ulrich-Lai YM, Herman JP. Neural regulation of endocrine and autonomic stress responses. Nat Rev Neurosci 2009;10(6):397–409.

56. Liu D, Diorio J, Tannenbaum B, et al. Maternal care, hippocampal glucocorticoid receptors, and hypothalamic- pituitary-adrenal responses to stress. Science 1997;277(5332):1659–62.

57. Genest SE, Balon N, Gulemetova R, et al. Neonatal maternal separation and enhancement of the hypoxic ventilatory response: the role of GABAergic

neurotransmission within the paraventricular nucleus of the hypothalamus. J Physiol 2007;583(1):299–314.

58. Gulemetova R, Drolet G, Kinkead R. Neonatal stress augments the hypoxic chemoreflex of adult male rats by increasing AMPA-receptor mediated modulation. Exp Physiol 2013;98(8):1312–24.

59. Ursache A, Merz EC, Melvin S, et al. Socioeconomic status, hair cortisol and internalizing symptoms in parents and children. Psychoneuroendocrinology 2017;78:142–50.

60. Kristenson M, Eriksen HR, Sluiter JK, et al. Psychobiological mechanisms of socioeconomic differences in health. Soc Sci Med 2004;58(8):1511–22.

61. Kunz-Ebrecht SR, Kirschbaum C, Steptoe A. Work stress, socioeconomic status and neuroendocrine activation over the working day. Soc Sci Med 2004;58(8):1523–30.

62. McEwen BS, Gianaros PJ. Central role of the brain in stress and adaptation: links to socioeconomic status, health, and disease. Ann N Y Acad Sci 2010;1186(1):190–222.

63. Abelson JL, Weg JG, Nesse RM, et al. Persistent respiratory irregularity in patients with panic disorder. Biol Psychiatry 2001;49(7):588–95.

64. Bystritsky A, Craske M, Maidenberg E, et al. Autonomic reactivity of panic patients during a CO_2 inhalation procedure. Depress Anxiety 2000;11(1):15–26.

65. Nardi AE, Freire RC, Zin WA. Panic disorder and control of breathing. Respir Physiol Neurobiol 2009;167:133–43.

66. Stein MB, Millar TW, Larsen DK, et al. Irregular breathing during sleep in patients with panic disorder. Am J Psychiatry 1995;152(8):1168–73.

67. Diaz SV, Brown LK. Relationships between obstructive sleep apnea and anxiety. Curr Opin Pulm Med 2016;22(6):563–9.

68. Reiche EMV, Nunes SOV, Morimoto HK. Stress, depression, the immune system, and cancer. Lancet Oncol 2004;5(10):617–25.

69. Slavich GM, Irwin MR. From stress to inflammation and major depressive disorder: a social signal transduction theory of depression. Psychol Bull 2014;140(3):774–815.

70. Lombard JH. Depression, psychological stress, vascular dysfunction, and cardiovascular disease: thinking outside the barrel. J Appl Physiol (1985) 2010;108(5):1025–6.

71. Bornstein SR, Schuppenies A, Wong ML, et al. Approaching the shared biology of obesity and depression: the stress axis as the locus of gene-environment interactions. Mol Psychiatry 2006; 11(10):892–902.

72. Bratel T, Wennlund A, Carlstrom K. Pituitary reactivity, androgens and catecholamines in obstructive sleep apnoea. Effects of continuous positive airway pressure treatment (CPAP). Respir Med 1999; 93(1):1–7.

73. Vgontzas AN, Fernandez-Mendoza J. Is there a link between mild sleep disordered breathing and psychiatric and psychosomatic disorders? Sleep Med Rev 2011;15(6):403–5.

74. Schmoller A, Eberhardt F, Jauch-Chara K, et al. Continuous positive airway pressure therapy decreases evening cortisol concentrations in patients with severe obstructive sleep apnea. Metabolism 2009;58(6):848–53.

75. Lattova Z, Keckeis M, Maurovich-Horvat E, et al. The stress hormone system in various sleep disorders. J Psychiatr Res 2011;45(9):1223–8.

76. Gunnar MR. Integrating neuroscience and psychological approaches in the study of early experiences. Ann N Y Acad Sci 2003;1008:238–47.

77. Nicolson NA. Childhood parental loss and cortisol levels in adult men. Psychoneuroendocrinology 2004;29(8):1012–8.

78. Parker KJ, Buckmaster CL, Sundlass K, et al. Maternal mediation, stress inoculation, and the development of neuroendocrine stress resistance in primates. Proc Natl Acad Sci U S A 2006;103(8):3000–5.

79. Battaglia M, Pesenti-Gritti P, Medland SE, et al. A genetically informed study of the association between childhood separation anxiety, sensitivity to co2, panic disorder, and the effect of childhood parental loss. Arch Gen Psychiatry 2009;66(1):64–71.

80. D'Amato FR, Zanettini C, Lampis V, et al. Unstable maternal environment, separation anxiety, and heightened CO_2 sensitivity induced by gene-by-environment interplay. PLoS One 2011;6(4):e18637.

81. Marco EM, Llorente R, López-Gallardo M, et al. The maternal deprivation animal model revisited. Neurosci Biobehav Rev 2015;51(0):151–63.

82. Lehmann J, Feldon J. Long-term biobehavioral effects of maternal separation in the rat: consistent or confusing? Rev Neurosci 2000;11(4):383–408.

83. Caldji C, Tannenbaum B, Sharma S, et al. Maternal care during infancy regulates the development of neural systems mediating the expression of fearfulness in the rat. Proc Natl Acad Sci U S A 1998; 95(9):5335–40.

84. Francis DD, Meaney MJ. Maternal care and the development of stress responses. Curr Opin Neurobiol 1999;9(1):128–34.

85. Genest SE, Gulemetova R, Laforest S, et al. Neonatal maternal separation and sex-specific plasticity of the hypoxic ventilatory response in awake rat. J Physiol 2004;554(Pt 2):543–57.

86. Pietrobon CB, Miranda RA, Bertasso IM, et al. Early weaning induces short- and long-term effects on pancreatic islets in Wistar rats of both sexes. J Physiol 2020;598(3):489–502.

87. Enthoven L, de Kloet ER, Oitzl MS. Differential development of stress system (re)activity at weaning dependent on time of disruption of maternal care. Brain Res 2008;1217:62–9.

88. Francis DD, Diorio J, Plotsky PM, et al. Environmental enrichment reverses the effects of maternal separation on stress reactivity. J Neurosci 2002; 22(18):7840–3.

89. Reardon LE, Leen-Feldner EW, Hayward C. A critical review of the empirical literature on the relation between anxiety and puberty. Clin Psychol Rev 2009;29(1):1–23.

90. Gunnar MR, Wewerka S, Frenn K, et al. Developmental changes in hypothalamus–pituitary–adrenal activity over the transition to adolescence: normative changes and associations with puberty. Dev Psychopathol 2009;21(1):69–85.

91. Foilb AR, Lui P, Romeo RD. The transformation of hormonal stress responses throughout puberty and adolescence. J Endocrinol 2011;210(3):391–8.

92. Gulemetova R, Kinkead R. Neonatal stress increases respiratory instability in rat pups. Respir Physiol Neurobiol 2011;176(3):103–9.

93. Kinkead R, Montandon G, Bairam A, et al. Neonatal maternal separation disrupts regulation of sleep and breathing in adult male rats. Sleep 2009; 32(12):1611–20.

94. Kinkead R, Genest SE, Gulemetova R, et al. Neonatal maternal separation and early life programming of the hypoxic ventilatory response in rats. Respir Physiol Neurobiol 2005;149:313–24.

95. Bairam A, Kinkead R, Joseph V. Neonatal environment and neuroendocrine programming of the peripheral respiratory control system current. Pediatr Rev 2006;2(3):199–208.

96. Kinkead R, Guertin P, Gulemetova R. Sex, stress and their influence on respiratory regulation. Curr Pharm Des 2013;19(24):4471–84.

97. Kinkead R, Gulemetova R, Bairam A. Neonatal maternal separation enhances phrenic responses to hypoxia and carotid sinus nerve stimulation in the adult anesthetised rat. J Appl Physiol (1985) 2005;99(1):189–96.

98. Soliz J, Tam R, Kinkead R. Neonatal maternal separation augments carotid body response to hypoxia in adult males but not female rats. Front Physiol 2016;7:432.

99. Tatsumi K, Hannhart B, Pickett CK, et al. Effects of testosterone on hypoxic ventilatory and carotid body neural responsiveness. Am J Respir Crit Care Med 1994;149(5):1248–53.

100. Joseph V, Niane LM, Bairam A. Antagonism of progesterone receptor suppresses carotid body responses to hypoxia and nicotine in rat pups. Neuroscience 2012;207:103–9.

101. Kinkead R, Balon N, Genest SE, et al. Neonatal maternal separation and enhancement of the inspiratory (phrenic) response to hypoxia in adult rats: disruption of GABAergic neurotransmission in the nucleus tractus solitarius. Eur J Neurosci 2008; 27(5):1174–88.

102. Ruyle BC, Martinez D, Heesch CM, et al. The PVN enhances cardiorespiratory responses to acute hypoxia via input to the nTS. Am J Physiol Regul Integr Comp Physiol 2019;317(6):R818–33.

103. Preston ME, Jensen D, Janssen I, et al. Effect of menopause on the chemical control of breathing and its relationship with acid-base status. Am J Physiol Regul Integr Comp Physiol 2009;296(3): R722–7.

104. Marques DA, de Carvalho D, da Silva GSF, et al. Influence of estrous cycle hormonal fluctuations and gonadal hormones on the ventilatory response to hypoxia in female rats. Pflugers Archiv 2017; 469(10):1277–86.

105. Joseph V, Soliz J, Soria R, et al. Dopaminergic metabolism in carotid bodies and high-altitude acclimatization in female rats. Am J Physiol Regul Integr Comp Physiol 2002;282(3):R765–73.

106. Fournier S, Gulemetova R, Baldy C, et al. Neonatal stress affects the aging trajectory of female rats on the endocrine, temperature, and ventilatory responses to hypoxia. Am J Physiol Regul Integr Comp Physiol 2015;308(7):R659–67.

107. Maric-Bilkan C, Gilbert EL, Ryan MJ. Impact of ovarian function on cardiovascular health in women: focus on hypertension. Int J Womens Health 2014;6:131–9.

108. Johnson SM, Randhawa KS, Epstein JJ, et al. Gestational intermittent hypoxia increases susceptibility to neuroinflammation and alters respiratory motor control in neonatal rats. Respir Physiol Neurobiol 2018;256:128–42.

109. Prabhakar NR, Peng YJ, Kumar GK, et al. Peripheral chemoreception and arterial pressure responses to intermittent hypoxia. Compr Physiol 2015;5(2):561–77.

110. Dewan NA, Nieto FJ, Somers VK. Intermittent hypoxemia and OSA: implications for comorbidities. Chest 2015;147(1):266–74.

111. Navarrete-Opazo A, Mitchell GS. Therapeutic potential of intermittent hypoxia: a matter of dose. Am J Physiol Regul Integr Comp Physiol 2014; 307(10):R1181–97.

112. Prabhakar NR, Kline DD. Ventilatory changes during intermittent hypoxia: importance of pattern and duration. High Alt Med Biol 2002;3(2):195–204.

113. Farré R, Montserrat JM, Gozal D, et al. Intermittent hypoxia severity in animal models of sleep apnea. Front Physiol 2018;9:1556.

114. Shin M-K, Yao Q, Jun JC, et al. Carotid body denervation prevents fasting hyperglycemia during chronic intermittent hypoxia. J Appl Physiol (1985) 2014;117(7):765–76.

115. Lesske J, Fletcher EC, Bao G, et al. Hypertension caused by chronic intermittent hypoxia–influence of chemoreceptors and sympathetic nervous system. J Hypertens 1997;15(12 Pt 2):1593–603.

116. Fletcher EC. Invited review: physiological consequences of intermittent hypoxia: systemic blood pressure. J Appl Physiol (1985) 2001;90(4):1600–5.

117. Ma S, Mifflin SW, Cunningham JT, et al. Chronic intermittent hypoxia sensitizes acute hypothalamic-pituitary-adrenal stress reactivity and Fos induction in the rat locus coeruleus in response to subsequent immobilization stress. Neuroscience 2008;154(4):1639–47.

118. Liguori C, Mercuri NB, Nuccetelli M, et al. Obstructive sleep apnea may induce orexinergic system and cerebral β-amyloid metabolism dysregulation: is it a further proof for Alzheimer's disease risk? Sleep Med 2019;56:171–6.

119. Zoccal DB, Bonagamba LGH, Antunes-Rodrigues J, et al. Plasma corticosterone levels is elevated in rats submitted to chronic intermittent hypoxia. Auton Neurosci 2007;134(1–2):115–7.

120. Maruyama NO, Mitchell NC, Truong TT, et al. Activation of the hypothalamic paraventricular nucleus by acute intermittent hypoxia: implications for sympathetic long-term facilitation neuroplasticity. Exp Neurol 2019;314:1–8.

121. Peng Y-J, Zhang X, Gridina A, et al. Complementary roles of gasotransmitters CO and H_2S in sleep apnea. Proc Natl Acad Sci U S A 2017;114(6):1413–8.

122. Julien C, Bairam A, Joseph V. Chronic intermittent hypoxia reduces ventilatory long-term facilitation and enhances apnea frequency in newborn rats. Am J Physiol Regul Integr Comp Physiol 2008; 294(4):R1356–66.

123. Laouafa S, Ribon-Demars A, Marcouiller F, et al. Estradiol protects against cardiorespiratory dysfunctions and oxidative stress in intermittent hypoxia. Sleep 2017;40(8):1–13.

124. Kline DD. Chronic intermittent hypoxia affects integration of sensory input by neurons in the nucleus tractus solitarii. Respir Physiol Neurobiol 2010; 174(1–2):29–36.

125. Del Rio R, Andrade DC, Lucero C, et al. Carotid body ablation abrogates hypertension and autonomic alterations induced by intermittent hypoxia in rats. Hypertension 2016;68(2):436–45.

126. Weiss JW, Tamisier R, Liu Y. Sympathoexcitation and arterial hypertension associated with obstructive sleep apnea and cyclic intermittent hypoxia. J Appl Physiol (1985) 2015;119(12):1449–54.

127. Iturriaga R, Moya EA, Del Rio R. Inflammation and oxidative stress during intermittent hypoxia: the impact on chemoreception. Exp Physiol 2015; 100(2):149–55.

128. Betteridge DJ. What is oxidative stress? Metabolism 2000;49(2 Suppl 1):3–8.

129. Lavie L. Oxidative stress in obstructive sleep apnea and intermittent hypoxia–revisited–the bad ugly and good: implications to the heart and brain. Sleep Med Rev 2015;20:27–45.

130. Brann D, Raz L, Wang R, et al. Oestrogen signalling and neuroprotection in cerebral ischaemia. J Neuroendocrinol 2012;24(1):34–47.

131. Moorthy K, Sharma D, Basir SF, et al. Administration of estradiol and progesterone modulate the activities of antioxidant enzyme and aminotransferases in naturally menopausal rats. Exp Gerontol 2005;40(4):295–302.

132. Razmara A, Sunday L, Stirone C, et al. Mitochondrial effects of estrogen are mediated by estrogen receptor alpha in brain endothelial cells. J Pharmacol Exp Ther 2008;325(3):782–90.

133. Borrás C, Gambini J, López-Grueso R, et al. Direct antioxidant and protective effect of estradiol on isolated mitochondria. Biochim Biophys Acta 2010; 1802(1):205–11.

134. Eisele HJ, Markart P, Schulz R. Obstructive sleep apnea, oxidative stress, and cardiovascular disease: evidence from human studies. Oxid Med Cell Longev 2015;2015:608438.

135. Foster GE, Brugniaux JV, Pialoux V, et al. Cardiovascular and cerebrovascular responses to acute hypoxia following exposure to intermittent hypoxia in healthy humans. J Physiol 2009;587(Pt 13):3287–99.

136. Tamisier R, Pépin JL, Rémy J, et al. 14 nights of intermittent hypoxia elevate daytime blood pressure and sympathetic activity in healthy humans. Eur Respir J 2011;37(1):119–28.

137. Peng YJ, Nanduri J, Raghuraman G, et al. Role of oxidative stress-induced endothelin-converting enzyme activity in the alteration of carotid body function by chronic intermittent hypoxia. Exp Physiol 2013;98(11):1620–30.

138. Peng YJ, Nanduri J, Yuan G, et al. NADPH oxidase is required for the sensory plasticity of the carotid body by chronic intermittent hypoxia. J Neurosci 2009;29(15):4903–10.

139. Peng YJ, Overholt JL, Kline D, et al. Induction of sensory long-term facilitation in the carotid body by intermittent hypoxia: implications for recurrent apneas. Proc Natl Acad Sci U S A 2003;100(17):10073–8.

140. Gileles-Hillel A, Almendros I, Khalyfa A, et al. Prolonged exposures to intermittent hypoxia promote visceral white adipose tissue inflammation in a murine model of severe sleep apnea: effect of normoxic recovery. Sleep 2017;40(3):1–10.

141. Carreras A, Zhang SX, Almendros I, et al. Resveratrol attenuates intermittent hypoxia-induced macrophage migration to visceral white adipose tissue and insulin resistance in male mice. Endocrinology 2015;156(2):437–43.

142. Gozal D, Gileles-Hillel A, Cortese R, et al. Visceral white adipose tissue after chronic intermittent and sustained hypoxia in mice. Am J Respir Cell Mol Biol 2017;56(4):477–87.

143. Quintero M, Gonzalez-Martin MDC, Vega-Agapito V, et al. The effects of intermittent hypoxia on redox status, NF-κB activation, and plasma lipid

levels are dependent on the lowest oxygen satura-tion. Free Radic Biol Med 2013;65:1143–54.

144. Grebe M, Eisele HJ, Weissmann N, et al. Antioxi-dant vitamin C improves endothelial function in obstructive sleep apnea. Am J Respir Crit Care Med 2006;173(8):897–901.

145. Büchner NJ, Quack I, Woznowski M, et al. Micro-vascular endothelial dysfunction in obstructive sleep apnea is caused by oxidative stress and improved by continuous positive airway pressure therapy. Respiration 2011;82(5):409–17.

146. El Solh AA, Saliba R, Bosinski T, et al. Allopurinol improves endothelial function in sleep apnoea: a randomised controlled study. Eur Respir J 2006;27(5):997–1002.

147. Ribon-Demars A, Pialoux V, Boreau A, et al. Protec-tive roles of estradiol against vascular oxidative stress in ovariectomized female rats exposed to normoxia or intermittent hypoxia. Acta Physiol (Oxf) 2019;225(2):e13159.

148. Laouafa S, Roussel D, Marcouiller F, et al. Roles of oestradiol receptor alpha and beta against hyper-tension and brain mitochondrial dysfunction under intermittent hypoxia in female rats. Acta Physiol (Oxf) 2019;226(2):e13255.

149. Joseph V, Doan VD, Morency C-E, et al. Expression of sex-steroid receptors and steroidogenic en-zymes in the carotid body of adult and newborn male rats. Brain Res 2006;1073-1074:71–82.

150. Hay M, Xue B, Johnson AK. Yes! Sex matters: sex, the brain and blood pressure. Curr Hypertens Rep 2014;16(8):458.

151. Xue B, Pamidimukkala J, Lubahn DB, et al. Estro-gen receptor-alpha mediates estrogen protection from angiotensin II-induced hypertension in conscious female mice. Am J Physiol Heart Circ Physiol 2007;292(4):H1770–6.

152. Leuzzi C, Modena MG. Hypertension in postmeno-pausal women: pathophysiology and treatment. High Blood Press Cardiovasc Prev 2011;18(1):13–8.

153. Joseph V, Laouafa S, Marcouiller F, et al. Progester-one decreases apnoea and reduces oxidative stress induced by chronic intermittent hypoxia in ovariecto-mized female rats. Exp Physiol 2020;105(6):1025–34.

154. Fietze I, Laharnar N, Obst A, et al. Prevalence and association analysis of obstructive sleep apnea with gender and age differences - results of SHIP-Trend. J Sleep Res 2019;28(5):e12770.

155. Hirotsu C, Albuquerque RG, Nogueira H, et al. The relationship between sleep apnea, metabolic dysfunction and inflammation: the gender influ-ence. Brain Behav Immun 2017;59:211–8.

156. O'Connor C, Thornley KS, Hanly PJ. Gender differ-ences in the polysomnographic features of obstructive sleep apnea. Am J Respir Crit Care Med 2000;161(5):1465–72.

157. Lee JJ, Ramirez SG, Will MJ. Gender and racial variations in cephalometric analysis. Otolaryngol Head Neck Surg 1997;117(4):326–9.

158. Baldwin CM, Kapur VK, Holberg CJ, et al. Associ-ations between gender and measures of daytime somnolence in the sleep heart health study. Sleep 2004;27(2):305–11.

159. Ambrogetti A, Olson LG, Saunders NA. Differences in the symptoms of men and women with obstructive sleep apnoea. Aust N Z J Med 1991;21(6):863–6.

160. Basoglu OK, Tasbakan MS. Gender differences in clinical and polysomnographic features of obstruc-tive sleep apnea: a clinical study of 2827 patients. Sleep Breath 2018;22(1):241–9.

161. Quintana-Gallego E, Carmona-Bernal C, Capote F, et al. Gender differences in obstructive sleep ap-nea syndrome: a clinical study of 1166 patients. Respir Med 2004;98(10):984–9.

162. Brooks LJ, Strohl KP. Size and mechanical proper-ties of the pharynx in healthy men and women. Am Rev Respir Dis 1992;146(6):1394–7.

163. Cano-Pumarega I, Barbé F, Esteban A, et al. Sleep apnea and hypertension: are there sex differ-ences? The vitoria sleep cohort. Chest 2017; 152(4):742–50.

164. Durán J, Esnaola S, Rubio R, et al. Obstructive sleep apnea-hypopnea and related clinical fea-tures in a population-based sample of subjects aged 30 to 70 yr. Am J Respir Crit Care Med 2001;163(3 Pt 1):685–9.

165. Young T, Palta M, Dempsey J, et al. The occurrence of sleep-disordered breathing among middle-aged adults. N Engl J Med 1993;328(17):1230–5.

166. Shepertycky MR, Banno K, Kryger MH. Differences between men and women in the clinical presenta-tion of patients diagnosed with obstructive sleep apnea syndrome. Sleep 2005;28(3):309–14.

167. Smith R, Ronald J, Delaive K, et al. What are obstructive sleep apnea patients being treated for prior to this diagnosis? Chest 2002;121(1):164–72.

168. Dursunoglu N, Ozkurt S, Sarikaya S. Is the clinical presentation different between men and women admitting to the sleep laboratory? Sleep Breath 2009;13(3):295–8.

169. Pillar G, Malhotra A, Fogel R, et al. Airway me-chanics and ventilation in response to resistive loading during sleep: influence of gender. Am J Re-spir Crit Care Med 2000;162(5):1627–32.

170. Gabbay IE, Lavie P. Age- and gender-related char-acteristics of obstructive sleep apnea. Sleep Breath 2012;16(2):453–60.

171. Strausz S, Havulinna AS, Tuomi T, et al. Obstructive sleep apnoea and the risk for coronary heart dis-ease and type 2 diabetes: a longitudinal population-based study in Finland. BMJ Open 2018;8(10):e022752.

172. Redline S, Kump K, Tishler PV, et al. Gender differ-ences in sleep disordered breathing in a community-based sample. Am J Respir Crit Care Med 1994;149(3 Pt 1):722–6.

The Impact of Social Determinants of Health on Gender Disparities Within Respiratory Medicine

Claire DeBolt, MD, Drew Harris, MD*

KEYWORDS

- Health disparities • Health equity • Social determinants of health • Environmental health
- Occupational health • Intersectionality

KEY POINTS

- Many social determinants of health contribute to gender disparities within respiratory diseases.
- When intersectionality is used, understanding of health inequities between genders can be fully realized.
- Several risk factors for pulmonary disparities are highlighted in this article and include poverty, education, occupational exposures, cultural norms (such as gender identity), and domestic factors, such as exposure to violence.

INTRODUCTION

Despite well-documented improvements in health and disease outcomes for many Americans, there are concerning disparities among marginalized groups. Increasing awareness of how social determinants of health impact individual and population health has not yet translated to improved outcomes for all, including between genders. Sex, as a biological variable, is often discussed in medical research because it can cause differences in respiratory disease with regard to underlying pathology of disease. For example, there are diseases that occur almost exclusively in female sex, such as lymphangioleiomyomatosis or pleural/parenchymal endometriosis. Yet, it is gender that directly interacts with other social determinants of health and cumulatively impacts risk for respiratory disease and outcomes. In this article, we describe how social determinants of health impact gender disparities within respiratory disease.

In a discussion of gender as a social determinant of health, it is important to acknowledge that the term itself describes a nonbinary and fluid identification of self. Gender describes how a person may see oneself as a man or woman, with traditional pronouns of her or she, or may identify as other, with pronouns of they/them. Gender references behavioral, social, and cultural domains and thus can be a dynamic product of changes in an individual's environment. The influence of gender has not been significantly considered through history or medical research, perhaps because the terms "sex" and "gender" have often been used interchangeably. For the purposes of this article, we will generally be discussing binary terms for gender, although it is certain that more work must be done to identify how best to evaluate transgender patients for respiratory disease and the consequences of that disease they may develop.

INTERSECTIONALITY

Intersectionality is a framework for understanding the ways in which multiple social identities and

Department of Medicine, Division of Pulmonary and Critical Care Medicine, University of Virginia, PO Box 800546, Charlottesville, VA 22908, USA
* Corresponding author.
E-mail address: drew.harris@virginia.edu

Clin Chest Med 42 (2021) 407–415
https://doi.org/10.1016/j.ccm.2021.04.003
0272-5231/21/© 2021 Elsevier Inc. All rights reserved.

conditions converge to produce a broad range of unequal outcomes among both individuals and populations, resulting in interdependent forms of privilege and oppression.[1-3] Studies often parse demographic characteristics as a method to identify the relationship of one factor with an outcome, independent from all other demographics. However, an understanding based on intersectionality would likely describe this approach as unrealistic. It may be impossible to ascribe a health outcome to a single demographic variable for the patient who identifies as a transgender, lesbian, or black woman of low socioeconomic status (SES), as any one of these demographics may increase the risk for disease and likely compound risk when they intersect. When research takes an approach that is informed by intersectionality, it transcends the description and categorization of health inequities and instead takes a more holistic view.[2,3] When care providers integrate intersectionality, it adjusts and widens the clinician's view, to then consider social determinants of care and improve medical outcomes (**Fig. 1**). Gender is a critical risk factor for respiratory illness. Understanding respiratory disease as it is affected by gender and the intersectionality of other social determinants of health is a foundational step toward eliminating health disparities.[1-3] In the following sections, we highlight the intersectionality of gender and other important social determinants of health as they relate to disparities in lung disease.

SOCIOECONOMIC AND EDUCATIONAL DETERMINANTS OF GENDER DISPARITIES

SES is a measure of social standing and is represented by the combination of occupation, educational level, and income.[4] Women in the United States generally live in greater poverty and with lower earnings than men, despite achieving higher educational attainment.[5] In 2019, 17.7% of women in the United States lived on an income less than 125% below the poverty level (compared with 14.9% of men).[5] Education improves public health

and promotes health equity. Although increasing levels of education are protective for life expectancy, benefit does not translate to equal degrees between gender.[6] Regardless of their level of completed education, women in the United States live longer than men at every age.[6] The impact of educational attainment can be seen specifically within respiratory disease given its contribution in determining occupation, dependence on employment (or potential mobility between types of work), income and financial resources, and access to health care. Although no single indicator can illustrate the entire complexity of SES, differences between genders are reflected in differences in income, poverty, and educational attainment, and all 3 indicators change the risk for pulmonary disease. Income and education both represent unique points of potential interventions to reduce disparities, and both will be explored here. Given the significance of occupational determinants of gender disparities in lung diseases, this will be discussed later in the article.

Asthma

Associations of SES and asthma are not consistent worldwide. In some regions, urban children of higher SES have a greater incidence of asthma; in other regions, asthma prevalence is greater among children of poor urban communities.[7-9] It is unclear what drives these differences, because urbanization is often associated with increased sedentarism but poverty is generally associated with overcrowding, poor-quality housing, and limited access to health care with decreased diagnoses.[8-11] The complexity of the relationship between SES and asthma is even greater when gender is considered. Boys born into low-income households or who have higher parental stress seem to have higher rates of asthma.[12] However, the relationship changes around puberty; by age 14 years, low income is strongly associated with asthma among girls, but not boys.[12] The interactions between gender, SES, and asthma is not

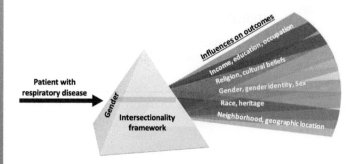

Fig. 1. Applying an Intersectional Framework: Considering only the patient's gender is an insufficient initial step in evaluation and treatment. We advocate for clinicians to apply a framework of intersectionality to each interaction with a patient, which acts as a prism in adjusting and widening a clinician's view; this invites the consideration of other social determinants of health and improves outcomes in medical care.

well reported in adults. After puberty, asthma prevalence, severity, and morbidity disproportionately impact women.[13] Given the previously described patterns that women live in greater poverty and with lower earnings, it may be that lower SES is associated with increased risk for asthma. Women of lower SES may have greater financial pressure to continue employment, which then could result in continued exposure to high-risk occupational triggers. Interaction analyses based on sex and income of Swedish citizens have demonstrated that compared with those with high income, women with lower SES have significantly increased risk for current asthma, allergic asthma, and asthmatic wheeze.[14] However, there have not been investigations that have identified statistically significant sex differences on the effects of educational level specifically to the incidence of asthma and respiratory symptoms.[15] Please refer to the article that discusses the impact of sex on asthma.

Chronic Obstructive Pulmonary Disease

Census-level poverty is associated with chronic obstructive pulmonary disease (COPD), even among never smokers.[16] Women with household incomes less than 100% of the poverty level are more than twice as likely to report a COPD diagnosis compared with those with incomes of 400% or more of poverty level (10.1% vs 4.6%).[17] Women living in poverty, especially in developing countries, have higher exposure to household air pollution via biomass fuels, which is then associated with greater COPD prevalence among women (further discussed in a later section).[18] Lower educational attainment has been linked to increased COPD morbidity including lower lung function, greater disease severity, and higher risk of hospitalization for COPD.[19] It is unknown if greater educational attainment confers equal protective benefit between men and women.

Lung Cancer

Age-adjusted incidence and mortality rates associated with lung cancer remain lower in women than in men, largely due to lower historical rates of smoking among women.[20] However, among those born since the mid-1960s, incidence rates of lung cancer have become higher among young women than among young men.[21] Compared with men, women are (1) more likely to be diagnosed with lung cancer at an early age,[22] (2) more likely to be diagnosed at earlier stages,[23] and (3) more likely to be diagnosed with lung cancer if a nonsmoker.[24] Despite these differences, many studies have shown more favorable survival for women with lung cancer regardless of age,

histologic subtype, or stage of disease at presentation.[23,24] There is a social gradient between genders in lung cancer. Men who have lower occupational SES carry greater risk for lung cancer, which persists after adjusting for smoking habits, when compared with women and the impact of occupational SES.[25] There is also a relationship between unemployment periods greater than 5 years and lung cancer, among men but not women.[25] Education has been observed to have a larger (protective) effect on men's mortality from lung cancer compared with women's.[26] Please refer to the article that discusses the impact of sex on lung cancer.

OCCUPATIONAL DETERMINANTS OF GENDER DISPARITIES IN LUNG DISEASE
Asthma

Gender differences in asthma prevalence, morbidity, and mortality are widely reported in epidemiologic studies. Women with asthma have increased risk for life-threatening asthma and emergency room visitations for asthma exacerbations, and in the United States, asthma mortality rates are significantly higher in females than in males.[27,28] Occupational factors are important to consider as upstream causes of gender disparities in asthma. Multiple studies in the United States suggest a higher incidence of work-related asthma in women.[29–31] Although the gender distribution of work-related asthma may reflect the gender distribution of adult asthma, other potential contributing factors include differences in job tasks, inadequate fit testing in females who use respirators, and sex differences in lung size/structure impacting lung deposition of toxic inhaled agents.[31] It should be noted that the incidence of work-related asthma may be higher in males than in females for those working outside of the United States.[32,33] In a population-based study of Swedish adults, occupational exposures to vapors, gas, dust, and fumes (that may exacerbate asthma) were more common in males.[34]

Chronic Obstructive Pulmonary Disease

The development of COPD is linked to occupational exposure to air pollutants including inorganic and organic particulate matter as well as vapors, gases, and fumes. Most studies of occupational exposures in COPD have been focused on jobs held predominantly by men.[35] As one example, there is abundant evidence that in the male-dominated coal mining industry, exposure to occupational dusts is an independent risk factor for the development of COPD including chronic bronchitis and emphysema.[36] However, multiple recent studies suggest that women may be more susceptible than men to develop COPD after a wide array of occupational exposures. Women employed in protective service, food preparation and serving, production, and transportation and material moving demonstrate prevalence estimates of COPD that were 2 to 4 times higher than in males.[37] Another study has shown that occupations with exposure to biological dust was a significant risk factor for COPD and emphysema in women (7-fold increase in risk), but an increased risk was not present in men. Health care professions, food and textile workers, artists, and cleaners were occupations that were associated with increased risk of COPD in women in this study.[38] An analysis of the National Health and Nutrition Examination Survey (NHANES III) participants demonstrated that COPD was associated with employment in agriculture, textiles, rubber and plastic industries, and sales-related jobs; these associations were higher in woman than in men.[39] Not all studies have reached similar conclusions, however; a recent analysis of patients with occupational exposures to dust and fumes noted similar associations with airflow obstruction, respiratory symptoms, radiographic emphysema, and air trapping in both men and women.[40]

Pneumoconiosis

There are limited data examining the prevalence, severity, or causation of gender disparities in pneumoconiosis. These diagnoses are largely seen in men because of cultural norms within at-risk occupations. In recent descriptions, nearly 100% of those with advanced coal worker's pneumoconiosis are men.[41,42] Similarly, in large epidemiologic surveillance programs for silicosis across multiple states in the United States, greater than 95% of cases occurred in men[43] including in the recent resurgence of silicosis in artificial stone manufacturing.[44] Although asbestos exposures can occur due to both occupational and nonoccupational exposures, asbestosis predominantly impacts males, which is largely due to the occupational risk factors. Construction work was the most frequently recorded industry on death certificates with asbestosis as the cause of death,[45] and women comprise less than 10% of the US construction workforce.[46] However, women have been found to have paraoccupational exposure to asbestosis via household contamination from asbestos fibers brought home on workers' clothing and the handling and washing of contaminated clothing, which then increases the risk for mesothelioma.[47] Two cohort studies have described increased relative risk among household members of workers, with standardized incidence ratio of 25.19 (95% confidence interval [CI], 12.57–45.07) for the wives of Italian cement workers and a nonstatistically significant hazard ratio of 2.61 (95% CI, 0.85–7.99) among household members of workers of the Australian Blue Asbestos Company.[48,49] These studies should prompt physicians to consider family and household member occupations as an exposure risk for patients.

Lung Cancer

Age-adjusted incidence and mortality rates associated with lung cancer remain lower in women than in men, largely due to lower historical rates of smoking among women.[20] However, among those born since the mid-1960s, incidence rates of lung cancer have become higher among young women than among young men.[21] Additional causative factors outside smoking and susceptibility to tobacco smoke are unclear.[21,25–27,50,51] Other possible explanations for gender disparities in lung cancer incidence include a reduction in occupational and environmental carcinogens (eg, asbestos) in recent decades that has resulted in a decrease in lung cancers in males (and not females) due to gender differences within occupations associated with increased exposures.[52]

DOMESTIC EXPOSURES LEADING TO GENDER DISPARITIES IN LUNG DISEASE
Chronic Obstructive Pulmonary Disease

In addition to cigarette smoke, environmental exposures within individual homes are important in the development of COPD. Smoke generated from the burning of biomass fuel (wood, charcoal, animal dung) is a major risk factor for the development of COPD around the world. Worldwide, 50% of all households and 90% of rural households around the world rely on biomass fuels and coal as their primary source of domestic energy.[53] This risk is not limited to low- and middle-income countries: more than 11 million US homes use a wood stove as their primary source of heat.[54] Although exposure to smoke from biomass fuels is associated with COPD in both men and women,[55] the risk of COPD due to biomass fuels disproportionately burdens women owing to sociocultural norms and domestic responsibilities, including a greater amount of time spent cooking.[56,57] This risk has been shown in both rural- and urban-dwelling women.[57] Compared with women who are exposed to tobacco smoke, never-smoking women exposed to biomass smoke had worse perceived dyspnea, more air trapping, but less radiographic emphysema.[58]

Households burning biomass fuels for cooking and heating are more likely to be living in poverty; however, the ill health effects of burning biomass fuels are not limited to those in poverty.[59] Non-low-income families often use biomass fuels as a secondary or seasonal source of heating. Furthermore, a "neighborhood effect" of biomass fuel burning contributing to ambient particulate matter levels in the United States suggests that the impact of biomass fuel burning extends beyond each individual household.[60]

Asthma

Multiple overlapping social and environmental factors within homes or neighborhoods are important drivers of ongoing asthma disparities.[61] Many of these health determinants have disparate impacts on women. Exposure to violence is one such example. Recent observational studies have shown that exposure to violence can lead to new-onset or worsening asthma in exposed individuals.[62] This violence includes direct exposure (eg, experiencing intimate partner violence) or indirect exposure (eg, violence within communities). Chronic maternal interpersonal trauma is associated with worsened asthma control during pregnancy, as well as the development of asthma in children of affected mothers.[63] Experiencing abuse during childhood has been linked to adult asthma in a study of African American Women in the United States.[64] In US women with asthma, those who experienced sexual violence were 2 times more likely to report an acute exacerbation of asthma compared with women who did not experience this violence.[65] Many studies highlight the importance of intersectionality between experiencing violence and other social and environmental determinants of health, such as air pollution,[66] poverty, experiencing racial/ethnic discrimination, and heightened psychosocial stress.[62] Mechanistically, these intersecting factors lead to psychosocial stress-related changes in epigenetics, gene expression, and immune responses.[67]

CULTURAL NORMS LEADING TO GENDER DISPARITIES IN LUNG DISEASE
Asthma

Gender differences in asthma prevalence, morbidity, and mortality are widely recognized, but understanding of intersectional effects with sexual orientation are not. Disparities in respiratory risk and disease are well documented among sexual minorities. Sexual minority women (SMW) describes women who identify with a lesbian or bisexual identity, as well as women who participate in sex with other women without identifying as lesbian or bisexual.[68] SMW are more likely than heterosexual women to be diagnosed with asthma.[69] Sexual orientation may contribute to gender disparities in asthma prevalence through increased psychosocial stress, smoking exposure, obesity rates, and cultural competency among providers.[69] Other factors including deficiencies in cultural competency among providers of sexual minority women can lead to health care avoidance and worsened health outcomes.[68]

Transgender status is also associated with significantly higher risk of lifetime asthma. In analyzing a large dataset of 56 million unique patients, with approximately 7000 patients diagnosed with gender identity disorder and/or who had gender-affirming surgery, Morales-Estrella et al.[70] in 2019 found that asthma prevalence is higher in transgender individuals and those with gender-affirming surgery compared with nontransgender individuals of their original birth sex. The investigators also reported that asthma risk is the highest in male-to-female transgender individuals (odds ratio [OR], 3.49; 3.18–3.84; $P<.001$) but is also high among female-to-male transgender individuals (OR, 2.62; 2.40–2.85; $P<.001$).[70] Very little is known about the impact of transgender sex hormone therapy on respiratory health, and this may certainly be a contributor. However, transgender status is associated with increased minority stress (stress of being part of a stigmatized minority)[71] and low cultural competency among providers, which may then impact health beliefs and behaviors that then affect asthma management.[72]

Chronic Obstructive Pulmonary Disease

Traditional gender roles may also contribute to gender disparities in COPD outcomes. In many cultures, men are traditionally expected to be physically strong and robust and women are expected to be beautiful and remain youthful appearing. COPD impacts these expectations. For example, individuals may be perceived as weaker if they are on oxygen. These individuals may develop weight loss and increased chest size (barrel chest),[73] and this results in perceived or experienced stigmatization[74] and could contribute to the differences in quality of life (QOL) scores observed between women with COPD and men with COPD.[75]

Cystic Fibrosis

Women with cystic fibrosis (CF) have shorter life expectancy than men, despite accounting for CF-related comorbidities. Women are also colonized earlier and have worse outcomes with common pathogens, such as *Pseudomonas aeruginosa*.[76] On the Cystic Fibrosis Quality of

Life Questionnaire, there are gender differences in scores for chest symptoms, emotional functioning, concerns for the future, body image, and career. Women have worse health-related QOL than men in all areas except for body image; men have poorer body image than females.[77] When comparing with non-CF controls, females with CF were happier with their body image, whereas males with CF desired to be heavier[78]; this potentially could reflect cultural stereotypes and gender norms, which encourage women to desire thin bodies, whereas cause males to desire heavier and more muscular bodies.[77] Data also suggest that there is reduced adherence to nutritional support among women, which then contributes to worsened survival.[79]

DEVELOPMENTS IN CULTURAL COMPETENCY

Health care organizations and governmental agencies are increasingly directing resources to develop programs to increase cultural competency among health care providers for racial, ethnic, and sexual minorities.[80–82] It is theorized that effective implementation of cultural competency education increases appropriate services for minority group members, which then improves outcomes in health status, functioning, and satisfaction.[83] There are many ways that this goal is being targeted, including increased recruitment and retention of minority group members in health systems, greater coordination with community health workers, and increased education during medical training. For example, American and Canadian medical schools have allotted more time for teaching lesbian, gay, bisexual, and transgender (LGBT)-related topics (increasing from a median of 2–5 hours), although the quantity, content, and perceived quality vary substantially.[84] Emerging evidence shows that educational curricula for health care students and professionals on racial and LGBT health care issues does, in the short-term, improve knowledge, attitudes, and medical practice.[82,83,85] Given the heterogeneity of interventions designed to improve cultural competency among health care providers, assessment of practitioner behavioral outcomes and measures of intervention impact on health care and health outcomes are needed to build a stronger evidence base.[82,86]

SUMMARY

Gender is a centerpiece to an individual's understanding of self and encompasses many behavioral, social, and cultural arenas; its broad scope means that it also intersects many social determinants of health. Multiple examples of social determinants highlighted in this article, including income, education, occupation, domestic exposures, and cultural norms such as sexual identity, are critical factors that contribute to ongoing respiratory disparities between genders.

We recommend that clinicians take an intersectional approach when considering how gender interacts with other important social factors while caring for patients with lung disease. This intersectional approach will provide a context in which modifiable risk factors can be optimized to create innovative, individualized care plans for vulnerable patients. Understanding and addressing social determinants of health between genders is an essential first step toward achieving respiratory health equity. Using an intersectional approach to inform health and public health policies holds promise to reduce social gradients that contribute to gender differences in respiratory diseases.

DISCLOSURE

The authors have nothing to disclose.

REFERENCES

1. Bowleg L. The problem with the phrase women and minorities: intersectionality-an important theoretical framework for public health. Am J Public Health 2012;102(7):1267–73.
2. Eckstrand KL, Eliason J, St Cloud T, et al. The priority of intersectionality in academic medicine. Acad Med 2016;91(7):904–7.
3. Wilson Y, White A, Jefferson A, et al. Intersectionality in clinical medicine: the need for a conceptual framework. Am J Bioeth 2019;19(2):8–19.
4. APA. Socioeconomic status. Available at: https://www.apa.org/topics/socioeconomic-status/index. Accessed September 27, 2020.
5. U.S. Census Bureau. American community survey. Available at: https://data.census.gov/cedsci/table?q=education&tid=ACSST1Y2019.S1501&hidePreview=false. Accessed September 27, 2020.
6. Olshansky SJ, Antonucci T, Berkman L, et al. Differences in life expectancy due to race and educational differences are widening, and many may not catch up. Health Aff (Millwood) 2012;31(8):1803–13.
7. Thakur N, Oh SS, Nguyen EA, et al. Socioeconomic status and childhood asthma in urban minority youths. The GALA II and SAGE II studies. Am J Respir Crit Care Med 2013;188(10):1202–9.
8. Bacon SL, Bouchard A, Loucks EB, et al. Individual-level socioeconomic status is associated with worse asthma morbidity in patients with asthma. Respir Res 2009;10:125.
9. Estrada RD, Ownby DR. Rural asthma: current understanding of prevalence, patterns, and

interventions for children and adolescents. Curr Allergy Asthma Rep 2017;17(6):37.

10. Lautenbacher L, Perzanowski MS. Global asthma burden and poverty in the twenty-first century. Int J Tuberc Lung Dis 2017;21(11):1093.

11. Cardet JC, Louisias M, King TS, et al. Income is an independent risk factor for worse asthma outcomes. J Allergy Clin Immunol 2018;141(2):754–760 e3.

12. Kozyrskyj AL, Kendall GE, Jacoby P, et al. Association between socioeconomic status and the development of asthma: analyses of income trajectories. Am J Public Health 2010;100(3):540–6.

13. de Marco R, Locatelli F, Synyer J, et al. Differences in incidence of reported asthma related to age in men and women. A retrospective analysis of the data of the European Respiratory Health Survey. Am J Respir Crit Care Med 2000;162(1):68–74.

14. Schyllert C, Lindberg A, Hedman L, et al. Low socioeconomic status relates to asthma and wheeze, especially in women. ERJ Open Res 2020;6(3).

15. Eagan TM, Gulsvik A, Eide GE, et al. The effect of educational level on the incidence of asthma and respiratory symptoms. Respir Med 2004;98(8):730–6.

16. Raju S, Keet CA, Paulin LM, et al. Rural residence and poverty are independent risk factors for chronic obstructive pulmonary disease in the United States. Am J Respir Crit Care Med 2019;199(8):961–9.

17. USDHHS. Women's health USA 2013. Rockville, Maryland. Available at: https://mchb.hrsa.gov/whusa13/. Accessed September 27, 2020.

18. Siddharthan T, Grigsby MR, Goodman D, et al. Association between household air pollution exposure and chronic obstructive pulmonary disease outcomes in 13 low- and middle-income country settings. Am J Respir Crit Care Med 2018;197(5):611–20.

19. Eisner MD, Blanc PD, Omachi TA, et al. Socioeconomic status, race and COPD health outcomes. J Epidemiol Community Health 2011;65(1):26–34.

20. Holford TR, Levy DT, McKay LA, et al. Patterns of birth cohort-specific smoking histories, 1965-2009. Am J Prev Med 2014;46(2):e31–7.

21. Jemal A, Miller KD, Ma J, et al. Higher lung cancer incidence in young women than young men in the United States. N Engl J Med 2018;378(21):1999–2009.

22. Harichand-Herdt S, Ramalingam SS. Gender-associated differences in lung cancer: clinical characteristics and treatment outcomes in women. Semin Oncol 2009;36(6):572–80.

23. Sagerup CM, Smastuen M, Johannesen TB, et al. Sex-specific trends in lung cancer incidence and survival: a population study of 40,118 cases. Thorax 2011;66(4):301–7.

24. Wakelee HA, Chang ET, Gomez SL, et al. Lung cancer incidence in never smokers. J Clin Oncol 2007;25(5):472–8.

25. Hovanec J, Siemiatycki J, Conway DI, et al. Lung cancer and socioeconomic status in a pooled analysis of case-control studies. PLoS One 2018;13(2):e0192999.

26. Ross CE, Masters RK, Hummer RA. Education and the gender gaps in health and mortality. Demography 2012;49(4):1157–83.

27. van der Merwe L, de Klerk A, Kidd M, et al. Case-control study of severe life threatening asthma (SLTA) in a developing community. Thorax 2006;61(9):756–60.

28. Kodadhala V, Obi J, Wessly P, et al. Asthma-related mortality in the United States, 1999 to 2015: a multiple causes of death analysis. Ann Allergy Asthma Immunol 2018;120(6):614–9.

29. Fletcher AM, London MA, Gelberg KH, et al. Characteristics of patients with work-related asthma seen in the New York state occupational health Clinics. J Occup Environ Med 2006;48(11):1203–11.

30. White GE, Seaman C, Filios MS, et al. Gender differences in work-related asthma: surveillance data from California, Massachusetts, Michigan, and New Jersey, 1993-2008. J Asthma 2014;51(7):691–702.

31. Anderson NJ, Reeb-Whitaker CK, Bonauto DK, et al. Work-related asthma in Washington State. J Asthma 2011;48(8):773–82.

32. McDonald JC, Chen Y, Zekveld C, et al. Incidence by occupation and industry of acute work related respiratory diseases in the UK, 1992-2001. Occup Environ Med 2005;62(12):836–42.

33. Ameille J, Pauli G, Calastreng-Crinquand A, et al. Reported incidence of occupational asthma in France, 1996-99: the ONAP programme. Occup Environ Med 2003;60(2):136–41.

34. Schyllert C, Ronmark E, Andersson M, et al. Occupational exposure to chemicals drives the increased risk of asthma and rhinitis observed for exposure to vapours, gas, dust and fumes: a cross-sectional population-based study. Occup Environ Med 2016;73(10):663–9.

35. Kennedy SM, Chambers R, Weiwei D, et al. Environmental and occupational exposures: do they affect chronic obstructive pulmonary disease differently in women and men? Proc Am Thorac Soc 2007;4(8):692–4.

36. Kuempel ED, Wheeler MW, Smith RJ, et al. Contributions of dust exposure and cigarette smoking to emphysema severity in coal miners in the United States. Am J Respir Crit Care Med 2009;180(3):257–64.

37. Doney B, Hnizdo E, Syamlal G, et al. Prevalence of chronic obstructive pulmonary disease among US working adults aged 40 to 70 years. National Health Interview Survey data 2004 to 2011. J Occup Environ Med 2014;56(10):1088–93.

38. Matheson MC, Benke G, Raven J, et al. Biological dust exposure in the workplace is a risk factor for chronic obstructive pulmonary disease. Thorax 2005;60(8):645–51.

39. Hnizdo E, Sullivan PA, Bang KM, et al. Association between chronic obstructive pulmonary disease and employment by industry and occupation in the US population: a study of data from the Third National Health and Nutrition Examination Survey. Am J Epidemiol 2002;156(8):738–46.

40. Marchetti N, Garshick E, Kinney GL, et al. Association between occupational exposure and lung function, respiratory symptoms, and high-resolution computed tomography imaging in COPDGene. Am J Respir Crit Care Med 2014;190(7):756–62.

41. Laney AS, Blackley DJ, Halldin CN. Radiographic disease progression in contemporary US coal miners with progressive massive fibrosis. Occup Environ Med 2017;74(7):517–20.

42. Blackley DJ, Reynolds LE, Short C, et al. Progressive massive fibrosis in coal miners from 3 Clinics in Virginia. JAMA 2018;319(5):500–1.

43. Maxfield R, Alo C, Reilly MJ, et al. Surveillance for silicosis, 1993–Illinois, Michigan, New Jersey, North Carolina, Ohio, Texas, and Wisconsin. MMWR CDC Surveill Summ 1997;46(1):13–28.

44. Rose C, Heinzerling A, Patel K, et al. Severe silicosis in Engineered stone fabrication workers - California, Colorado, Texas, and Washington, 2017-2019. MMWR Morb Mortal Wkly Rep 2019;68(38):813–8.

45. Center for Disease Control and Prevention. Asbestosis. Available at: https://wwwn.cdc.gov/eWorld/Grouping/Asbestosis/92. Accessed September 27, 2020.

46. US Bureau of Labor Statistics. Labor force statistics from the current population survey. Available at: https://www.bls.gov/cps/cpsaat18.htm. Accessed September 27, 2020.

47. Goswami E, Craven V, Dahlstrom DL, et al. Domestic asbestos exposure: a review of epidemiologic and exposure data. Int J Environ Res Public Health 2013;10(11):5629–70.

48. Ferrante D, Bertolotti M, Todesco A, et al. Cancer mortality and incidence of mesothelioma in a cohort of wives of asbestos workers in Casale Monferrato, Italy. Environ Health Perspect 2007;115(10):1401–5.

49. Reid A, Heyworth J, De Klerk NH, et al. Cancer incidence among women and girls environmentally and occupationally exposed to blue asbestos at Wittenoom, Western Australia. Int J Cancer 2008; 122(10):2337–44.

50. Ramchandran K, Patel JD. Sex differences in susceptibility to carcinogens. Semin Oncol 2009;36(6): 516–23.

51. Risch HA, Howe GR, Jain M, et al. Are female smokers at higher risk for lung cancer than male smokers? A case-control analysis by histologic type. Am J Epidemiol 1993;138(5):281–93.

52. Hellyer JA, Patel MI. Sex disparities in lung cancer incidence: validation of a long-observed trend. Transl Lung Cancer Res 2019;8(4):543–5.

53. Salvi SS, Barnes PJ. Chronic obstructive pulmonary disease in non-smokers. Lancet 2009;374(9691): 733–43.

54. Rokoff LB, Koutrakis P, Garshick E, et al. Wood stove pollution in the developed world: a case to Raise awareness among pediatricians. Curr Probl Pediatr Adolesc Health Care 2017;47(6):123–41.

55. Hu G, Zhou T, Tian J, et al. Risk of COPD from exposure to biomass smoke: a metaanalysis. Chest 2010; 138(1):20–31.

56. Regalado J, Perez-Padilla R, Sansores R, et al. The effect of biomass burning on respiratory symptoms and lung function in rural Mexican women. Am J Respir Crit Care Med 2006;174(8):901–5.

57. Sana A, Somda SMA, Meda N, et al. Chronic obstructive pulmonary disease associated with biomass fuel use in women: a systematic review and meta-analysis. BMJ Open Respir Res 2018; 5(1):e000246.

58. Camp PG, Ramirez-Venegas A, Sansores RH, et al. COPD phenotypes in biomass smoke- versus tobacco smoke-exposed Mexican women. Eur Respir J 2014;43(3):725–34.

59. Rogalsky DK, Mendola P, Metts TA, et al. Estimating the number of low-income Americans exposed to household air pollution from burning solid fuels. Environ Health Perspect 2014;122(8):806–10.

60. Naeher LP, Brauer M, Lipset M, et al. Woodsmoke health effects: a review. Inhal Toxicol 2007;19(1): 67–106.

61. Forno E, Celedon JC. Health disparities in asthma. Am J Respir Crit Care Med 2012;185(10):1033–5.

62. Landeo-Gutierrez J, Forno E, Miller GE, et al. Exposure to violence, psychosocial stress, and asthma. Am J Respir Crit Care Med 2020;201(8):917–22.

63. Brunst KJ, Rosa MJ, Jara C, et al. Impact of maternal lifetime interpersonal trauma on children's asthma: mediation through maternal active asthma during pregnancy. Psychosom Med 2017;79(1): 91–100.

64. Coogan PF, Wise LA, O'Connor GT, et al. Abuse during childhood and adolescence and risk of adult-onset asthma in African American women. J Allergy Clin Immunol 2013;131(4):1058–63.

65. Bossarte RM, Swahn MH, Choudhary E. The associations between area of residence, sexual violence victimization, and asthma episodes among US adult women in 14 states and territories, 2005-2007. J Urban Health 2009;86(2):242–9.

66. Chiu YH, Coull BA, Sternthal M, et al. Effects of prenatal community violence and ambient air pollution

on childhood wheeze in an urban population. J Allergy Clin Immunol 2014;133(3):713–722 e4.

67. Rosenberg SL, Miller GE, Brehm JM, et al. Stress and asthma: novel insights on genetic, epigenetic, and immunologic mechanisms. J Allergy Clin Immunol 2014;134(5):1009–15.

68. Pinkerton KE, Harbaugh M, Han MK, et al. Women and lung disease. Sex differences and Global health disparities. Am J Respir Crit Care Med 2015;192(1):11–6.

69. Blosnich JR, Lee JGL, Bossarte R, et al. Asthma disparities and within-group differences in a national, probability sample of same-sex partnered adults. Am J Public Health 2013;103(9):e83–7.

70. Morales-Estrella JL, Boyle M, Zein JG. Transgender status is associated with higher risk of lifetime asthma. In: American Thoracic Society International conference. San Diego, California: American Thoracic Society; 2018.

71. Meyer IH. Prejudice, social stress, and mental health in lesbian, gay, and bisexual populations: conceptual issues and research evidence. Psychol Bull 2003;129(5):674–97.

72. Safer JD, Coleman E, Feldman J, et al. Barriers to healthcare for transgender individuals. Curr Opin Endocrinol Diabetes Obes 2016;23(2):168–71.

73. Johnson JL, Campbell AC, Bowers M, et al. Understanding the social consequences of chronic obstructive pulmonary disease: the effects of stigma and gender. Proc Am Thorac Soc 2007;4(8):680–2.

74. Earnest MA. Explaining adherence to supplemental oxygen therapy: the patient's perspective. J Gen Intern Med 2002;17(10):749–55.

75. de Torres JP, Casanova C, Hernandez C, et al. Gender associated differences in determinants of quality of life in patients with COPD: a case series study. Health Qual Life Outcomes 2006;4:72.

76. Harness-Brumley CL, Elliot AC, Rosenbluth DB, et al. Gender differences in outcomes of patients with cystic fibrosis. J Womens Health (Larchmt) 2014;23(12):1012–20.

77. Gee L, Abbott J, Conway SP, et al. Quality of life in cystic fibrosis: the impact of gender, general health perceptions and disease severity. J Cyst Fibros 2003;2(4):206–13.

78. Abbott J, Conway S, Etherington C, et al. Perceived body image and eating behavior in young adults with cystic fibrosis and their healthy peers. J Behav Med 2000;23(6):501–17.

79. Collins CE, O'Loughlin EV, Henry R. Discrepancies between males and females with cystic fibrosis in dietary intake and pancreatic enzyme use. J Pediatr Gastroenterol Nutr 1998;26(3):258–62.

80. Giroir BP. Providing Enhanced resources: cultural competency Training 2014. Available at: https://www.hhs.gov/programs/topic-sites/lgbt/enhanced-resources/competency-training/index.html. Accessed November 6, 2020.

81. Truong M, Paradies Y, Priest N. Interventions to improve cultural competency in healthcare: a systematic review of reviews. BMC Health Serv Res 2014;14:99.

82. Kripalani S, Bussey-Jones J, Katz MG, et al. A prescription for cultural competence in medical education. J Gen Intern Med 2006;21(10):1116–20.

83. Brach C, Fraser I. Can cultural competency reduce racial and ethnic health disparities? A review and conceptual model. Med Care Res Rev 2000;57(Suppl 1):181–217.

84. Obedin-Maliver J, Goldsmith ES, Sterwart L, et al. Lesbian, gay, bisexual, and transgender-related content in undergraduate medical education. JAMA 2011;306(9):971–7.

85. Sekoni AO, Gale NK, Manga-Atangana B, et al. The effects of educational curricula and training on LGBT-specific health issues for healthcare students and professionals: a mixed-method systematic review. J Int AIDS Soc 2017;20(1):21624.

86. Jongen C, McCalman J, Bainbridge R. Health workforce cultural competency interventions: a systematic scoping review. BMC Health Serv Res 2018;18(1):232.

Sex Differences in Obstructive Sleep Apnea

Sunita Kumar, MD, FCCP[a], Andreea Anton, MD, FCCP[b],
Carolyn M. D'Ambrosio, MD, MS, FCCP[c,*]

KEYWORDS

• Obstructive sleep apnea • Gender • CPAP • Polysomnogram • Phenotype • Endotype • Sex

KEY POINTS

- Prevalence of obstructive sleep apnea (OSA) increases with age and more so for women after menopause.
- OSA endotypes account for up to 30% of relative sex differences in the nonrapid eye movement (NREM) apnea hypopnea index. Women have lower loop gain, less airway collapsibility, and lower arousal threshold in NREM sleep.
- Presenting symptoms of OSA are different between men and women, with women having more vague symptoms and complaints of insomnia.
- Screening questionnaires and diagnostic studies are more biased toward men.
- Diagnostic criteria for OSA are more biased toward men.

INTRODUCTION

Obstructive sleep apnea (OSA) for many years has been thought to be a disease of men, but research performed more recently has revealed women are at significant risk for OSA as well as the morbidity associated with leaving it untreated. There are estimates that up to 90% of women with severe sleep apnea are not being diagnosed and that if diagnosed, they are less likely to be treated.[1,2] This article will explore the sex differences in OSA, specifically addressing areas of prevalence, phenotypes, diagnostic criteria, and treatment.

PREVALENCE

Our understanding on the prevalence of OSA evolved over time largely based on the changes related to diagnostic and scoring criteria, the type of sleep study (laboratory-based full polysomnogram [PSG] versus home sleep studies), and the impact of a rapidly growing obesity epidemic. As per the third edition of the International Classification of Sleep Disorders, the diagnosis of OSA is based on the presence of either suggestive signs or symptoms (ie, sleepiness, fatigue, insomnia, snoring) or associated medical or psychiatric comorbidities in addition to an apnea hypopnea index (AHI) $\geq$5 events per hour during a full PSG. An AHI $\geq$15 events per hour in the absence of symptoms or comorbidities also satisfies the diagnostic criteria.[3]

Large cohort studies conducted at the end of the 20th century in the United States reported a prevalence of OSA syndrome (AHI $\geq$5 or $\geq$10 and daytime hypersomnolence) of 1.2% to 2% in women and 3.9% to 4% in men,[4,5] resulting in an overall ratio of sleep apnea of 3.3:1 for men to women.[5] When defined by an AHI higher than 5,

[a] Department of Pulmonary, Critical Care and Sleep, Loyola University Medical Center and Stritch School of Medicine, 2160 South First Avenue, Building 54, Maywood, IL, USA; [b] Department of Pulmonary, Critical Care and Sleep Medicine, Medical College of Wisconsin, Zablocki VA Medical Center, 8500 West Wisconsin Avenue, Milwaukee, WI 53226, USA; [c] Harvard-Brigham and Women's Hospital, Fellowship in Pulmonary and Critical Care Medicine, Brigham and Women's Hospital, Harvard Medical School, 75 Francis Street PBB CA-3, Boston, MA 02115, USA
* Corresponding author.
E-mail address: cdambrosio@bwh.harvard.edu
Website: http://Brighamandwomens.org

Clin Chest Med 42 (2021) 417–425
https://doi.org/10.1016/j.ccm.2021.04.004
0272-5231/21/© 2021 Elsevier Inc. All rights reserved.

the prevalence of sleep-disordered breathing was 9% in women and 24% in men.[4] Disease prevalence was reported to be lower in premenopausal and menopausal women on hormone replacement therapy (HRT) than in postmenopausal women not on HRT (0.6% vs 2.7%).[5] In 2013, using updated data from the Wisconsin Sleep Cohort Study and extrapolating to the US population based on the body mass distribution, Peppard and colleagues[6] concluded that the estimated prevalence of moderate to severe sleep disordered breathing (SDB) (AHI ≥15) in the United States increased significantly in both men and women (relative increases between 14% and 55% depending on the age subgroup) in just two decades. A recent review on the epidemiology of sleep apnea concluded that the OSA (AHI ≥5) mean prevalence was 22% (range, 9%–37%) in men and 17% (range, 5%–40%) in women, and it is reported in 37% of men and 50% of women in studies from 2008 and 2013, respectively.[7,8] Prevalence increased with age from 24% in women between 20 and 44 years of age to 56% between age 45 and 54 years and up to 75% between age 55 and 70 years.[8] In the middle-aged to older population, sex and menopausal status greatly influence disease prevalence: the prevalence of OSA (AHI >15) was 50% in men, 9% in premenopausal women, and 30% in postmenopausal women.[9]

Two recent large population-based studies conducted in Europe (SHIP-Trend and HypnoLaus, respectively) further confirm the prevalence of OSA (defined as AHI ≥5) as 33% for women and 59% in men,[10] with an increased prevalence of moderate to severe OSA (AHI ≥15) up to 13% to 23.4% in women and 30% to 49.7% in men.[10,11] The higher reported prevalence is partly explained by changes in the scoring system and the diagnostic technology.

Overall, the current evidence consistently indicates that the prevalence of OSA is higher in men than in women and increases continuously with age in both genders; however, it does exhibit a later onset in women. In addition, in women, disease severity does not increase until the age of 50 years.[10] Central obesity and hormonal status impact the prevalence of sleep-disordered breathing in women.[11,12] The exact role and contributions of sex hormones in the pathophysiology of sleep apnea need to be further elucidated.

OBSTRUCTIVE SLEEP APNEA PATHOGENESIS: ENDOPHENOTYPES

OSA is a heterogeneous disorder with a complex disease mechanism. Four key physiologic traits have been identified to contribute to disease pathogenesis. These include the upper airway anatomy

(UA anatomic trait), the tone/responsiveness of the upper airway dilator muscles (upper airway gain), arousal in response to a respiratory event (arousal threshold), and the relative stability of the respiratory control system (loop gain).[13] In addition, decrease in lung volume during sleep and potential overnight rostral fluid shift from the legs to the neck area result in further decrease in the longitudinal traction of the pharynx and narrow the pharyngeal lumen, making it more collapsible. These different pathophysiological subtypes constitute distinct OSA endotypes, some of which can be identified by physical examination and/or via PSG.[13] A recent study by Won and colleagues[14] quantified sex differences in different pathophysiological endotypes. PSG data examination from 2057 participants in the Multi-Ethnic Study of Atherosclerosis (MESA) concluded that women exhibit lower loop gain, less airway collapsibility, and lower arousal threshold in non-rapid eye movement (NREM) sleep; overall endotypes accounted for 30% of relative sex differences in NREM-AHI4P.[14]

The classification of OSA into different phenotypes is based on the identification of a category of patients with OSA distinguished from others by a single disease feature or a combination of disease features, in relation to clinically meaningful attributes.[15] Sex, age, and menopause constitute different clinical phenotypes that are relevant to the current review. Individual OSA phenotype could be explained by one or more endotypes, which underline the disease mechanism (**Table 1**).

Obesity increases the risk and correlates with OSA disease severity (as measured by the AHI) in both sexes. Women seem to have better airway mechanics despite having a higher body mass index (BMI) and a significantly smaller oropharyngeal junction/pharynx than men.[16] The severity of OSA does not correlate with the upper airway size in women.[16] At a similar BMI, in patients with severe OSA (AHI ≥15), women have a lower neck circumference and waist/hip ratio than men.[11] The increased anatomic predisposition to OSA in men is related to increase in neck fat distribution, and a longer, therefore more vulnerable pharyngeal airway as well as android/central pattern of obesity.

Difference in prevalence between men and women diminishes in individuals older than 60 years, which has been attributed only in part to menopause.[10,11] Overall, upper airway anatomy/collapsibility plays a relatively greater pathogenic role in older adults with OSA, whereas a sensitive ventilatory control system is a more prominent trait in younger individuals.[17] Increase in parapharyngeal fat, independent of BMI,[18] lower lung volumes,

Table 1
OSA endophenotypes

OSA Phenotypes	OSA Endotypes		Gender Differences (Yes/No)

Sex	Women
	  Less collapsible upper airway
	  Lower loop gain
	  Lower arousal threshold in NREM
		Men
		Increased fat neck distribution
		Longer pharyngeal airway
			Yes

Aging (Older vs Young)	More collapsible upper airway Lower loop gain		No
Menopause	Central/android fat distribution Decrease in upper airway muscle tone		N/A
Fluid Overload	Rostral fluid distribution		No

and potential rostral fluid shift (augmented by a sedentary lifestyle) increase the susceptibility of the upper airway to collapse during sleep. Central obesity and hormonal status further increase the prevalence of sleep-disordered breathing in older women.[10,11]

Menopause, including type and age, affects the risk and severity of OSA in women. Young and colleagues[19] evaluated the association between menopausal transition and sleep-disordered breathing in the Wisconsin Sleep Cohort Study. Compared with premenopausal women, postmenopausal women were 2.6 times more likely to have an AHI ≥5 and 3.5 times more likely to have an AHI ≥15.[19] Recent data from the Nurses' Health Studies revealed that compared with natural menopause, surgical menopause (by hysterectomy/oophorectomy) resulted in a 27% increase risk of developing OSA[12] and risk was higher in women who were not obese and those who did not undergo HRTs. Aging, the stage of menopause (early vs late), changes in body fat, loss of female sex hormones, and pharyngeal dilator muscle activity have been proposed as potential contributing factors. Menopause has been associated with increased fat mass and an android-type fat distribution compared with premenopause.[20] Heinzer and colleagues[9] described no difference in waist circumference between premenopausal and postmenopausal women with OSA, whereas other investigators described waist circumference and postmenopausal stages (early and late) to be the main factors associated with moderate to severe OSA.[21] The role of sex hormones and impact of HRT need to be further elucidated; however, evidence suggests that abrupt withdrawal of reproductive hormones increases the OSA risk.[12] Genioglossus muscle activity seems to be impacted by sex hormone levels (progesterone) and may improve with HRT. Overall, the upper

dilator muscle activity was lower after menopause.[22] When examined via drug-induced sleep endoscopy, postmenopausal women showed a significant higher retrolingual and retropalatal collapse than premenopausal women.[23]

SYMPTOMS OF OBSTRUCTIVE SLEEP APNEAS

The prevalence of OSA in the general population and clinic-based samples indicate a male/female ratio anywhere between 3:1 and 8:1,[6,24] with women being underrepresented in sleep laboratory referrals.[24,25] The observed differences seem to be multifactorial and had been attributed to (1) underdiagnosis due to somewhat distinct clinical presentation in both sexes and/or failure to recognize by health-care providers, (2) underreporting because women are less likely to complain of OSA symptoms, and (3) potential differences in individual clinical presentation rather than sex differences (**Table 2**).

Men are more likely to complain of typical OSA symptoms of snoring and witnessed apnea, whereas women's presentation could be vague and nonspecific. It includes fatigue/tiredness, sleep-onset insomnia, and morning headaches, which can lead to alternative diagnosis initially.[26] In a recent large clinical cohort study of 6716 patients (24% women) evaluated for suspected SDB over a 10-year period, women were most likely to present with morning headaches, depressive symptoms, frequent awakenings, and nocturia, wherein men were most likely to report sleepiness (Epworth Sleepiness Scale [ESS] ≥16) and driving problems. There was no sex association with snoring, apneas, and insomnia symptoms.[27] Current evidence also indicates that even when men and women display similar symptoms suggestive of OSA (witnessed apnea, excessive daytime sleepiness [EDS], and/or snoring), women are less likely

Table 2
Symptoms and polysomnogram (PSG) findings in women and men

	Women	Men
Symptoms	Fatigue Insomnia Morning headaches Depression Nocturia	Snoring Witnessed apneas Excessive daytime sleepiness
Polysomnogram	Overall AHI is lower REM predominance More hypopneas than apneas Greater desaturation with hypopneas Longer hypopnea event duration	Overall AHI is higher Supine predominance More apneas than hypopneas Greater desaturation with apneas Shorter hypopnea event duration

to be referred for sleep laboratory evaluation.[2,25] The Respiratory Health in Northern Europe, a large prospective population study, provided information about snoring, EDS, and OSA diagnosis and treatment in 10,000 participants, including 5892 women. Women who were sleepy and snored were less likely to be diagnosed with sleep apnea and less likely to receive continuous positive airway pressure (CPAP) treatment than men. In men, but not in women, weight gain was significantly related to having both a diagnosis of and treatment for sleep apnea.[2]

Snoring could also be underobserved in women because they are less likely to be accompanied by their bed partner during the clinical evaluation, despite having similar frequency of snoring and daytime hypersomnolence.[28] A more recent analysis indicates that objective snoring (measured via the PSG) was less common in women.[29] Women were less likely to snore (8% vs 15%) and complain of sleepiness (when measured by the ESS) than men.[29,30] Age seems to further augment the discrepancy between genders. For patients younger than 30 years, the proportion of snorers among women was 55%, whereas the corresponding value for men was about 90%. In middle-aged and older women, frequency of snoring was similar between sexes.[29] Women complain of fatigue more frequently (53% vs 40%) and have higher fatigue scores, whereas men describe increased sleepiness (46% vs 38%, respectively).[30] This begs the question whether an appropriate tool to measure fatigue is needed and not to rely on the ESS to quantify fatigue.

Individual symptom heterogeneity regardless of the gender differences has been described and categorized by Ye and colleagues[31] in three distinct clusters: disturbed sleep group, minimally symptomatic group, and EDS group. The sleepy group represented less than 50% of the entire cohort of 822 patients, outlining the importance of detailed history and increased awareness regarding a diagnosis of OSA. The clusters did not differ significantly in terms of sex, BMI, and AHI; however, women represented only 19% of the study population.

A better understanding of the differences in clinical presentation between genders can lead to increased awareness and improve diagnosis, treatment, and outcomes in women with sleep apnea.

DIAGNOSIS
Screening Questionnaires

Screening questionnaires are commonly used to assess the likelihood of sleep-disordered breathing in the general population or specific cohorts such as those undergoing surgery. Most include classical symptoms of SDB such as snoring and daytime sleepiness. As noted previously, women are less likely to present with these symptoms and more likely to report insomnia and fatigue. This can result in underdiagnosis especially if referral for testing for SDB or to a sleep specialist is predicated on the meeting of the threshold cutoff values on such questionnaires. Likewise, the STOP-Bang (SB) questionnaire[32] is widely popular for its simplicity but inflates the scores for men. Although this takes into account the male predominance in SDB, it may oversimplify the gender discrepancies in diagnosis by making it more likely for men to be referred for testing. Pataka and colleagues[33] compared several questionnaires, STOP, SB,[32] ESS,[34] Berlin Questionnaire (BQ),[35] Athens Insomnia Scale (AIS),[36] and Fatigue Scale (FS),[37] in a group of 350 men and women matched for the severity of SDB. They found that the ESS was similar in both the groups with a respiratory event index higher than 15 events per hour. SB scores were higher in men, and STOP, AIS, and FS scores were higher in women. The BQ has the highest sensitivity in both genders. The STOP had the highest specificity in men, and the ESS showed the highest specificity in women. Women in this cohort were older (55 ± 13.2) and had a higher BMI (32.7 ± 10.7) than men (50 ± 14.5 years, 26.5 ± 5.55). Popular screening tools might need to incorporate gender-specific and not unified cutoff thresholds to improve their predictive accuracy. Mou and colleagues[38] studied the discriminative power of the SB questionnaire in 935 patients referred to a sleep clinic. They found the conventional cutoff value of ≥3 to have low specificity in men for detecting any severity of OSA. Instead, the score of ≥5 performed better in both genders with regard to sensitivity (66.7% in women and 71.7% in men) and specificity (69.4% in women and 61.9% in men). In women, using a BMI of >30 or >31 improved the utility of predicting any OSA, whereas incorporating a neck circumference of ≥17 inches improved the discriminative power in men.

Polysomnography

O'Connor and colleagues[39] were the first to describe the gender differences in the polysomnographic features of SDB. In a cohort of 830 patients, they found that women had similar severity of SDB, as determined by the AHI, in REM sleep but lower severity in NREM sleep than men. Women were also more likely to have exclusively REM-related OSA, whereas men were more likely to have supine-predominant OSA. Overall severity of OSA was milder in women than in men. These findings did not appear to be age or weight dependent. Similar findings have been reported in different racial and ethnic groups around the world.[40–43]

Women are more likely to have hypopneas than apneas.[44] Apnea event duration was longer in men than in women for all severity of OSA and associated with greater desaturation areas in moderate and severe OSA. In mild OSA, men had shorter hypopnea duration and desaturation areas than women.[44]

Koo and colleagues[45] studied the gender differences for REM-predominant OSA in patients referred to a sleep laboratory. They found that the prevalence of REM-OSA was higher in women than in men (24.5 vs 7.9%, respectively; P < .001). In both men and women, prevalence was higher in those younger than 55 years. Younger women with REM-OSA were more obese and more likely to suffer from depression than their older counterparts. Their study suggests that both age and gender differences play a role in REM-OSA. In contrast, Mano and colleagues[46] report in their study of Japanese patients with SDB that the prevalence of REM-OSA was higher in older women (age >50 years) than in younger women.

COMORBIDITIES

Sleep-disordered breathing is associated with cardiovascular morbidity including hypertension,[47] ischemic heart disease, arrhythmias,[48] stroke, insulin resistance, and diabetes mellitus.[49] Epidemiologic studies such as the Wisconsin Sleep Cohort Study reveal that people with OSA have a higher mortality than those without OSA.[50] Prevalence of these comorbidities shows gender-specific differences. Women with OSA are more likely to have comorbidities of hypothyroidism, asthma, diabetes, hypertension, and cardiac disease.[40,41] Mokhlesi and colleagues[51] reviewed a large nationwide insurance claims database and found a high prevalence of hypertension, type 2 diabetes, arrhythmias, depression, ischemic heart disease, and stroke in those with OSA than in a matched group without OSA. Women with OSA were more likely to have hypertension and depression, whereas ischemic heart disease and type 2 diabetes were more prevalent in men.[51]

OSA is associated with increased prevalence of acute coronary syndrome (ACS). Spanish investigators described that the severity of ACS showed sex-specific differences, with men showing a higher number of diseased vessels, a higher number of stents, and a lower ejection fraction than women.[52] In the Sleep Heart Health Study, a higher rate of cardiovascular events and mortality was observed in men and not in women.[53,54] These differences could be due to sex-specific differences in the intermediary mechanisms linking OSA with adverse cardiovascular outcomes such as endothelial function, which showed an impairment in women and not in men with OSA.[55] Subclinical markers of heart injury such as high-sensitivity troponin T showed a significant association with severity of OSA in women and not men although the overall levels were higher in men.[56] In addition, during a longitudinal follow-up of 13 years in a community-dwelling sample, OSA severity was associated with incident heart failure and left ventricular hypertrophy as seen on echocardiography, in women but not in men. In contrast, some other studies did not report gender-specific differences in severity of OSA and left ventricle mass using cardiac MRI.[57] In a large clinical cohort with suspected OSA, severity of OSA as assessed by the degree of nocturnal desaturation showed stronger association with composite cardiovascular outcomes in women than in men.[58]Use of CPAP mitigated the cardiovascular risk in women with OSA.[59] The MESA analysis of retinal vascular calibers showed that severe OSA was associated with retinal microaneurysms in women, whereas men with moderate to severe OSA were more likely to have retinal arterial narrowing and retinal venular widening.[60]

OSA is associated with poor quality of life. Women with SDB had significantly worse health-related quality of life scores than men, and women with insomnia had worse overall quality of life than all other groups.[40] Patients with untreated OSA were observed to have greater health-care utilization many years prior to diagnosis.[61] Health-care resource utilization was higher in women than in men with equivalent severity of SDB.[62]

TREATMENT

For many years, the diagnosis of OSA included not only the AHI but also the presence of symptoms such as sleepiness. The need to include sleepiness likely contributed to the undertreatment of women because some of the common questionnaires used to determine sleepiness such as the ESS are more sensitive in men than in women.[63,64] Additionally, women may offer complaints of insomnia or poor sleep rather than sleepiness, and this may be part of the reason why testing is often not performed.[65] However, once tested and diagnosed, OSA in women often is different than in men, with more apneas during REM sleep and more electroencephalogram arousals from sleep.[39,44] Studies on how men and women respond to treatment for OSA are quite limited. One study on autotitrating positive airway pressure (APAP) with an algorithm designed for women (increased sensitivity to airflow limitation and slower and lower pressure rise with airflow limitation) when compared with a standard APAP algorithm showed that the algorithm for women achieved superior control of airflow limited breaths.[66] Another study reveals that men with chronic insomnia symptoms and OSA are less likely to respond to CPAP treatment than women.[67] Overall, the few studies that have examined the response to CPAP between men and women have found minimal difference.

Other treatments for OSA such as mandibular repositioning splints (MRSs), hypoglossal nerve stimulation, and oral surgery have such a low percentage of women in the studies wherein difference in response to therapy is difficult to ascertain.[68,69] More women are treated with MRSs than men especially in mild OSA.[70] Weight loss, an important component to treatment of OSA in the patient with obesity, has a greater effect on AHI reduction in men than in women.[71]

SUMMARY

Sex differences and gender bias in OSA permeates the entire patient experience from the type of symptoms and diagnostic criteria all the way to the different treatment options that are available. Much more work is needed in this area to identify women at risk of OSA; improve diagnostic criteria; making them more appropriate for women; evaluate the impact of sex and gender on treatment options; and study women's response to various treatment modalities.

CLINICS CARE POINTS

- Up to 90% of women with severe OSA go undiagnosed or if diagnosed they are undertreated.
- Menopause affects the risk and severity of OSA.
- The symptoms of OSA are different between men and women with women using words like fatigue and depression more often.
- Screening questionnaires are not good at identifying OSA risk in women.
- Women are more likely to have apneas and hypopneas in Stage R and therefore an all night Apnea-Hypopnea Index may underestimate the degree of sleep disordered breathing in them.
- There is very limited data on how women respond to treatment of OSA.

DISCLOSURE

The authors have nothing to disclose.

REFERENCES

1. Young T, Evans L, Finn L, et al. Estimation of the clinically diagnosed proportion of sleep apnea syndrome in middle-aged men and women. Sleep 1997;20(9):705–6.
2. Lindberg E, Benediktsdottir B, Franklin KA, et al. Women with symptoms of sleep-disordered breathing are less likely to be diagnosed and treated for sleep apnea than men. Sleep Med 2017;35:17–22.

3. Sateia MJ. International classification of sleep disorders-third edition: highlights and modifications. Chest 2014;146(5):1387–94.

4. Young T, Palta M, Dempsey J, et al. The occurrence of sleep-disordered breathing among middle-aged adults. N Engl J Med 1993;328(17):1230–5.

5. Bixler EO, Vgontzas AN, Lin HM, et al. Prevalence of sleep-disordered breathing in women: effects of gender. Am J Respir Crit Care Med 2001;163(3 Pt 1):608–13.

6. Peppard PE, Young T, Barnet JH, et al. Increased prevalence of sleep-disordered breathing in adults. Am J Epidemiol 2013;177(9):1006–14.

7. Franklin KA, Lindberg E. Obstructive sleep apnea is a common disorder in the population-a review on the epidemiology of sleep apnea. J Thorac Dis 2015; 7(8):1311–22.

8. Franklin KA, Sahlin C, Stenlund H, et al. Sleep apnoea is a common occurrence in females. Eur Respir J 2013;41(3):610–5.

9. Heinzer R, Marti-Soler H, Marques-Vidal P, et al. Impact of sex and menopausal status on the prevalence, clinical presentation, and comorbidities of sleep-disordered breathing. Sleep Med 2018;51: 29–36.

10. Fietze I, Laharnar N, Obst A, et al. Prevalence and association analysis of obstructive sleep apnea with gender and age differences - results of SHIP-Trend. J Sleep Res 2019;28(5):e12770.

11. Heinzer R, Vat S, Marques-Vidal P, et al. Prevalence of sleep-disordered breathing in the general population: the HypnoLaus study. Lancet Respir Med 2015; 3(4):310–8.

12. Huang T, Lin BM, Redline S, et al. Type of menopause, age at menopause, and risk of developing obstructive sleep apnea in postmenopausal women. Am J Epidemiol 2018;187(7):1370–9.

13. Wellman A, Eckert DJ, Jordan AS, et al. A method for measuring and modeling the physiological traits causing obstructive sleep apnea. J Appl Physiol (1985) 2011;110(6):1627–37.

14. Won CHJ, Reid M, Sofer T, et al. Sex differences in obstructive sleep apnea phenotypes, the multi-ethnic study of atherosclerosis. Sleep 2020;43(5):zsz274.

15. Zinchuk AV, Gentry MJ, Concato J, et al. Phenotypes in obstructive sleep apnea: a definition, examples and evolution of approaches. Sleep Med Rev 2017;35:113–23.

16. Mohsenin V. Gender differences in the expression of sleep-disordered breathing : role of upper airway dimensions. Chest 2001;120(5):1442–7.

17. Edwards BA, Wellman A, Sands SA, et al. Obstructive sleep apnea in older adults is a distinctly different physiological phenotype. Sleep 2014; 37(7):1227–36.

18. Malhotra A, Huang Y, Fogel R, et al. Aging influences on pharyngeal anatomy and physiology: the predisposition to pharyngeal collapse. Am J Med 2006;119(1):72.e9–14.

19. Young T, Finn L, Austin D, et al. Menopausal status and sleep-disordered breathing in the Wisconsin sleep cohort study. Am J Respir Crit Care Med 2003;167(9):1181–5.

20. Ley CJ, Lees B, Stevenson JC. Sex- and menopause-associated changes in body-fat distribution. Am J Clin Nutr 1992;55(5):950–4.

21. Polesel DN, Hirotsu C, Nozoe KT, et al. Waist circumference and postmenopause stages as the main associated factors for sleep apnea in women: a cross-sectional population-based study. Menopause 2015;22(8):835–44.

22. Popovic RM, White DP. Upper airway muscle activity in normal women: influence of hormonal status. J Appl Physiol (1985) 1998;84(3):1055–62.

23. Koo SK, Ahn GY, Choi JW, et al. Obstructive sleep apnea in postmenopausal women: a comparative study using drug induced sleep endoscopy. Braz J Otorhinolaryngol 2017;83(3):285–91.

24. Redline S, Kump K, Tishler PV, et al. Gender differences in sleep disordered breathing in a community-based sample. Am J Respir Crit Care Med 1994;149(3 Pt 1):722–6.

25. Larsson LG, Lindberg A, Franklin KA, et al. Gender differences in symptoms related to sleep apnea in a general population and in relation to referral to sleep clinic. Chest 2003;124(1):204–11.

26. Nigro CA, Dibur E, Borsini E, et al. The influence of gender on symptoms associated with obstructive sleep apnea. Sleep Breath 2018;22(3):683–93.

27. Bouloukaki I, Mermigkis C, Markakis M, et al. Cardiovascular effect and symptom profile of obstructive sleep apnea: does sex matter? J Clin Sleep Med 2019;15(12):1737–45.

28. Quintana-Gallego E, Carmona-Bernal C, Capote F, et al. Gender differences in obstructive sleep apnea syndrome: a clinical study of 1166 patients. Respir Med 2004;98(10):984–9.

29. Forcelini CM, Buligon CM, Costa GJK, et al. Age-dependent influence of gender on symptoms of obstructive sleep apnea in adults. Sleep Sci 2019; 12(3):132–7.

30. Eliasson AH, Kashani MD, Howard RS, et al. Integrative cardiac health project registry. Fatigued on venus, sleepy on mars-gender and racial differences in symptoms of sleep apnea. Sleep Breath 2015;19(1):99–107.

31. Ye L, Pien GW, Ratcliffe SJ, et al. The different clinical faces of obstructive sleep apnoea: a cluster analysis. Eur Respir J 2014;44(6):1600–7.

32. Chung F, Yegneswaran B, Liao P. STOP questionnaire: a tool to screen patients for obstructive sleep apnea. Anesthesiology 2008;108:812–21.

33. Pataka A, Kotoulas S, Kalamaras G. Gender Differences in Obstructive Sleep Apnea: the value of

sleep questionnaires with a separate analysis of cardiovascular patients. J Clin Med 2020;9:130.

34. Johns MW. A new method for measuring daytime sleepiness: the Epworth Sleepiness Scale. Sleep 1991;14:540–5.

35. Netzer NC, Stoohs RA, Netzer CM. Using the Berlin Questionnaire to identify patients at risk for the sleep apnea syndrome. Ann Intern Med 1999;131:485–91.

36. Soldatos CR, Dikeos DG, Papparigopoulos TJ. Athens insomnia Scale: validation of an instrument based on ISD-10 criteria. J Psychosom Res 2000; 48:555–60.

37. Lorig KR, Ritter PL, Jacquez A. Outcomes of border health Spanish/English chronic disease self-management programs. Diabetes Educ 2005;31: 401–9.

38. Mou J, Pflugeisen BM, Crick BA. The discriminative power of STOP-Band as a screening tool for suspected obstructed sleep apnea in clinically referred patients: considering gender differences. Sleep and Breathing 2019;23:65–75.

39. O'Connor C, Thornley KS, Hanly PJ. Gender differences in the polysomnographic features of obstructive sleep apnea. Am J Respir Crit Care Med 2000; 161(5):1465–72.

40. Basoglu OK, Tasbakan MS. Gender differences in clinical and polysomnographic features of obstructive sleep apnea: a clinical study of 2827 patients. Sleep Breath 2018;22(1):241–9.

41. Alotair H, Bahammam A. Gender differences in Saudi patients with obstructive sleep apnea. Sleep Breath 2008;12(4):323–9.

42. Lim LL, Tham KW, Fook-Chong SM. Obstructive sleep apnoea in Singapore: polysomnography data from a tertiary sleep disorders unit. Ann Acad Med Singap 2008;37(8):629–36.

43. Vagiakis E, Kapsimalis F, Lagogianni I, et al. Gender differences on polysomnographic findings in Greek subjects with obstructive sleep apnea syndrome. Sleep Med 2006;7(5):424–30.

44. Leppänen T, Kulkas A, Duce B, et al. Severity of individual obstruction events is gender dependent in sleep apnea. Sleep Breath 2017;21(2):397–404.

45. Koo BB, Dostal J, Ioachimescu O, et al. The effects of gender and age on REM-related sleep-disordered breathing. Sleep Breath 2008;12(3):259–64.

46. Mano M, Hoshino T, Sasanabe R, et al. Impact of gender and age on rapid eye movement-related obstructive sleep apnea: a clinical study of 3234 Japanese OSA patients. Int J Environ Res Public Health 2019;16(6):1068.

47. Nieto FJ, Young TB, Lind BK, et al. Association of sleep-disordered breathing, sleep apnea, and hypertension in a large community-based study. Sleep Heart Health Study [published correction appears in JAMA 2002 Oct 23-30;288(16):1985]. JAMA 2000; 283(14):1829–36.

48. Shahar E, Whitney CW, Redline S, et al. Sleep-disordered breathing and cardiovascular disease: cross-sectional results of the Sleep Heart Health Study. Am J Respir Crit Care Med 2001;163(1):19–25.

49. Punjabi NM, Sorkin JD, Katzel LI, et al. Sleep-disordered breathing and insulin resistance in middle-aged and overweight men. Am J Respir Crit Care Med 2002;165(5):677–82.

50. Young T, Peppard PE, Gottlieb DJ. Epidemiology of obstructive sleep apnea: a population health perspective. Am J Respir Crit Care Med 2002; 165(9):1217–39.

51. Mokhlesi B, Ham SA, Gozal D. The effect of sex and age on the comorbidity burden of OSA: an observational analysis from a large nationwide US health claims database. Eur Respir J 2016;47(4):1162–9.

52. Sánchez-de-la-Torre A, Abad J, Durán-Cantolla J, et al. Effect of patient sex on the severity of coronary artery disease in patients with newly diagnosis of obstructive sleep apnoea admitted by an acute coronary syndrome. PLoS One 2016;11(7):e0159207.

53. Gottlieb DJ, Yenokyan G, Newman AB, et al. Prospective study of obstructive sleep apnea and incident coronary heart disease and heart failure: the sleep heart health study. Circulation 2010;122(4): 352–60.

54. Punjabi NM, Caffo BS, Goodwin JL, et al. Sleep-disordered breathing and mortality: a prospective cohort study. PLoS Med 2009;6(8):e1000132.

55. Faulx MD, Larkin EK, Hoit BD, et al. Sex influences endothelial function in sleep-disordered breathing. Sleep 2004;27(6):1113–20.

56. Roca GQ, Redline S, Claggett B, et al. Sex-specific association of sleep apnea severity with subclinical myocardial injury, ventricular hypertrophy, and heart failure risk in a community-dwelling cohort: the atherosclerosis risk in communities-sleep heart health study. Circulation 2015;132(14):1329–37.

57. Javaheri S, Sharma RK, Wang R, et al. Association between obstructive sleep apnea and left ventricular structure by age and gender: the multi-ethnic study of atherosclerosis. Sleep 2016;39(3):523–9.

58. Kendzerska T, Leung RS, Atzema CL, et al. Cardiovascular consequences of obstructive sleep apnea in women: a historical cohort study. Sleep Med 2020;68:71–9.

59. Campos-Rodriguez F, Martinez-Garcia MA, de la Cruz-Moron I, et al. Cardiovascular mortality in women with obstructive sleep apnea with or without continuous positive airway pressure treatment: a cohort study. Ann Intern Med 2012;156(2):115–22.

60. Lin GM, Redline S, Klein R, et al. Sex-specific association of obstructive sleep apnea with retinal microvascular signs: the multi-ethnic study of atherosclerosis. J Am Heart Assoc 2016;5(7):e003598.

61. Ronald J, Delaive K, Roos L, et al. Health care utilization in the 10 years prior to diagnosis in

obstructive sleep apnea syndrome patients. Sleep 1999;22(2):225–9.

62. Greenberg-Dotan S, Reuveni H, Simon-Tuval T, et al. Gender differences in morbidity and health care utilization among adult obstructive sleep apnea patients. Sleep 2007;30(9):1173–80.

63. Baldwin CM, Kapur VK, Holberg CJ, et al, Sleep Heart Health Study Group. Associations between gender and measures of daytime somnolence in the sleep heart health study. Sleep 2004;27(2): 305–11.

64. Lastra AC, Attarian HP. The persistent gender bias in the diagnosis of obstructive sleep apnea: a commentary. Gend Genome 2018;2(2):43–8.

65. Auer M, Frauscher B, Hochleitner M, et al. Gender-specific difference in access to polysomnography and prevalence of sleep disorders. J Womens Health 2018;27(4):525–30.

66. McArdle N, King S, Shepherd K, et al. Study of a novel APAP algorithm for the treatment of obstructive sleep apnea in women. Sleep 2015;38(11): 1775–81.

67. Loucao-de-Amoim I, Bentes C, Peralta AR. Men and women with chronic insomnia disorder and OSAS: different responses to CPAP. Sleep Sci 2019;1(3): 190–5.

68. Wray CM. Thaler ER Hypoglossal nerve stimulation for obstructive sleep apnea: a review of the literature. World J Otorhinolaryngol Head Neck Surg 2016;2:230–3.

69. Garg RK, Afifi AM, Sanchez R, et al. Obstructive sleep apnea in adults: the role of upper airway and facial skeletal surgery. Plast Reconstr Surg 2016; 138:889–98.

70. Vecchierini MF, Attali V, Collet JM, et al. Sex differences in mandibular repositioning device therapy effectiveness in patients with obstructive sleep apnea syndrome. Sleep Breath 2019;23:837–48.

71. Newman AB, Foster G, Givelber R, et al. Progression and regression of sleep-disordered breathing with changes in weight: the Sleep Heart Health Study. Arch Intern Med 2005;165:2408–13.

Impact of Sex on Sleep Disorders Across the Lifespan

Lauren Tobias, MD, Sritika Thapa, MD, Christine H.J. Won, MD, MS*

KEYWORDS

- Sleep • Gender/sex • Pregnancy • Menopause • Sleep-disordered breathing • Insomnia
- Restless legs syndrome • REM behavior disorder

KEY POINTS

- Sleep quality throughout a woman's life impacts her quality of life and medical comorbidities.
- The prevalence of sleep symptoms and disorders varies throughout a woman's life in association with the reproductive milestones of pregnancy and menopause.
- Studies have failed to identify a clear sex predominance of sleep disorders in childhood and adolescence other than nocturnal enuresis, which is 3 to 4 times more prevalent in males.
- Sleep disturbances in pregnancy are very common, likely underdiagnosed, and may be associated with increased risk for adverse maternal outcomes including pre-eclampsia, gestational diabetes, and preterm birth.
- Menopause is associated with sleep disruption owing to increased rates of sleep-disordered breathing, development of insomnia owing to vasomotor symptoms and hormonal changes, circadian derangements, and changes in sleep architecture.

INTRODUCTION

Sleep physiology and the prevalence of sleep disorders varies between woman and men. Paradoxically, although women generally exhibit objectively better sleep, they consistently report a greater burden of subjective sleep complaints. For example, although demonstrating shorter sleep latency and longer total sleep time than men of similar ages, women report poorer sleep quality, greater difficulties falling asleep, more frequent nocturnal awakenings, and longer periods spent awake during the night.[1] That many of the sex differences observed in sleep develop after puberty suggests that the gonadal hormones play an important role, although anatomic and psychological variables likely contribute as well. Studies have demonstrated a significant male predominance in referral to sleep centers, which may contribute to underdiagnosis of sleep disorders in women and disparities in sleep health.[2] A recently study found that female sex was associated with greater difficulty falling asleep and a higher likelihood of nonrestorative sleep in the setting of the coronavirus disease 2019 pandemic.[3]

This article highlights the sex differences in sleep across the lifespan, from childhood to the reproductive milestones of pregnancy and menopause. Changes in sleep architecture through a woman's life are shown in **Fig. 1**.[4]

CHILDHOOD AND ADOLESCENCE

The existence of sex-related sleep differences in neonates is controversial. Some studies show no difference, whereas others suggest longer active sleep in boys compared with girls.[4–6] In the first months of life, the change in sleep architecture is

Section of Pulmonary, Critical Care and Sleep Medicine, Yale University School of Medicine, 333 Cedar Street, New Haven, CT 06520, USA
* Corresponding author. Department of Internal Medicine, Section of Pulmonary, Critical Care and Sleep Medicine, Yale University School of Medicine, PO Box 208057, New Haven, CT 06520-8057.
E-mail address: Christine.won@yale.edu

Clin Chest Med 42 (2021) 427–442
https://doi.org/10.1016/j.ccm.2021.04.005
0272-5231/21/© 2021 Elsevier Inc. All rights reserved.

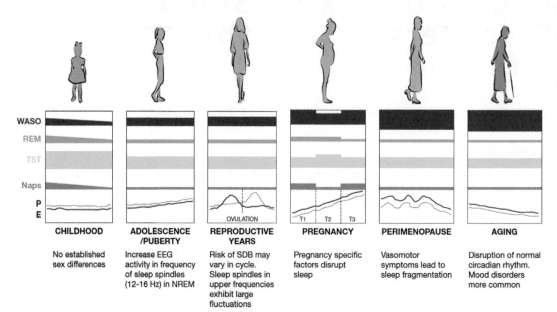

Fig. 1. Changes in sleep architecture through a woman's life. (*From* Pengo MF, Won CH, Bourjeily G. Sleep in Women Across the Life Span. *Chest.* 2018;154(1):196-206.)

similar in males and females, although some differences exist in sleep quality and quantity suggesting delayed central nervous system maturation in male infants.[4] Even though there may be further sex differences, this factor has not been studied fully owing to various confounding factors.[4] Prominent sex differences in sleep emerge once children reach puberty, when hormonal differences arise with the first menstrual cycle along with an increased prevalence of mood disorders.[7–9] For example, **Fig. 2** shows the development of the female predominance of insomnia as puberty progresses.

Hypersomnias

It has been reported that sleep problems and excessive daytime sleepiness (EDS) are more prevalent in the female adolescent and adult populations, but not in children.[9–11] The reported prevalence of EDS from various etiologies ranges from 10% to 20% in prepubertal children and is higher in adolescents (16%–47%). Sleep problems causing EDS in children and adolescents is estimated to be 25% to 40%.[12] A Korean study showed higher prevalence of EDS in girls (18.2% vs 14.9%) than boys along with significant differences in reported sleep duration. The girls also had statistically significant longer sleep latency and an increased frequency of nightmares and insomnia, whereas the boys had an increased prevalence of habitual snoring.[13] Another study showed that the female predominance of sleepiness starts after mid puberty; both puberty and

sex affect sleepiness via interaction with total time in bed and chronotype (females are more likely to have an evening chronotype).[14] For example, for females with a short time in bed, the prevalence of EDS was 3 times higher than males. In evening chronotypes, it was 6 times higher than males. Hence, the combined effect of mood disorders, insomnia, and an evening chronotype with pubertal maturation may contribute to increased EDS in female adolescents.[14]

A recent study of sleep disturbances in the Netherlands (aged >12 years) showed a prevalence of 27.3%, with 33.2% being females and 21.2% male.[15] A study in England showed that 49% of girls and 30% of boys reported experiencing sleeping difficulties; 36% of this age group reported not having enough sleep to be able to concentrate on school work.[16] Inadequate sleep hygiene, excessive social media use, later bedtime owing to more than 20 h/wk of work after school, and a greater need for sleep in these age groups could also contribute to hypersomnia.[17] The National Sleep Foundation's annual Sleep in America poll 2018 showed that only 10% of American adults prioritize sleep over other daily activities like fitness, nutrition, work, social life, and hobbies.[18]

Narcolepsy, a sleep disorder with clinical feature of EDS, cataplexy, hypnogogic and hypnopompic hallucinations, and/or sleep paralysis, and whose onset generally occurs in adolescence, has been shown to have higher prevalence in males than females (1.6–1.8 males per 1.0 female).[19,20] It is

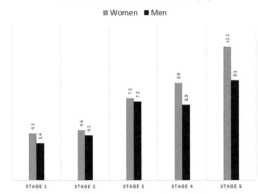

PREVALENCE OF INSOMNIA IN PUBERTAL CHILDREN BY TANNER STAGES (%)

■ Women ■ Men

Fig. 2. Pubertal maturation is associated with an increased prevalence of insomnia symptoms and emergence of female preponderance of insomnia severity during late puberty. (*Adapted from* Zhang J, Chan NY, Lam SP, et al. Emergence of Sex Differences in Insomnia Symptoms in Adolescents: A Large-Scale School-Based Study. *Sleep.* 2016;39(8):1563-1570.)

unknown if this is just a referral bias or a true sex difference, because in other studies it has been reported to have equal prevalence in males and females.[17]

Kleine–Levin syndrome is a rare disorder of recurrent severe hypersomnolence in association with cognitive, behavioral, dysautonomic, and psychiatric disturbances, which has a 4 times higher prevalence in men than women,[21] but longer disease duration in women.[22] Menstrual-related Kleine–Levin syndrome (18 women worldwide) is characterized by recurrent hypersomnia with or without other symptoms of Kleine–Levin syndrome associated with menstruation and/or the puerperium.[21] These symptoms last 3 to 15 days and recur fewer than 3 times a year with response to contraceptive doses of estrogen and progesterone in some cases, suggesting reproductive endocrine disturbances.[19]

A recent review showed varying estimates of hypersomnia in major depressive disorder across different ages and sex, with higher prevalence in females ranging anywhere from 8.9% in childhood (<13 years) to 75.8% in young adulthood.[23,24]

Sleep-Disordered Breathing

Obstructive sleep-disordered breathing (SDB) is characterized by a spectrum of severity with snoring being the characteristic feature reported in 35% of children as often or always present, and obstructive sleep apnea (OSA) at the severe end of the spectrum marked by intermittent hypoxia and sleep fragmentation reported in 1% to 6% of

children.[25] One study showed a greater prevalence of habitual snoring in boys compared with girls.[13] However, the prevalence and risk factors of SDB in children have not been well-studied and sex differences in children even less so. In contrast with adults, where the prevalence in SDB has been reported to be 24% to 84% in men and 9% to 77% in women,[26,27] only 1 study by Lumeng and colleagues showed significant differences in prevalence in before puberty, with higher rates in boys; other recent studies have shown no significant differences between girls and boys.[25,28–30] Brockman and colleagues showed the difference may be detectable in adolescents when obesity is coexistent, whereas Horne and colleagues showed no sex differences in the prevalence of SDB and its severity.[25,29] Like the inconsistent data of self-reported symptoms in adult men and women (likely owing to social and cultural factors), it is even more complex in children owing to the additional layer of parental or caregiver's perceptions in reporting. Particularly in girls, reporting bias could emerge from the social pressure to avoid stigmatization of an unfeminine condition, but this phenomenon has not been studied systematically.[29]

Obstructive SDB in young children is often caused by enlarged tonsils and adenoids; obesity also plays a role in adolescents.[29,31] Body mass index (BMI) is considered a strong modulating factor of OSA, even in adults.[32] In female adolescents, there is an association between OSA and obesity, increased androgen, and metabolic dysfunction.[29] Some studies in children and adolescents have shown no sex differences in the severity or consequences of SDB, whereas other studies show significant sex differences. One small study showed girls with OSA had greater upper airway space in imaging, along with less severe OSA and better sleep efficiency than boys.[30] Another study showed no sex differences in OSA severity among children, but that females less than 9 years old with moderate to severe sleep apnea had more internalizing problems (eg, mood disturbance, anxiety, depression, and social withdrawal) and a higher diastolic blood pressure than age-matched boys with a similar of severity OSA. Meanwhile, adolescent females with moderate to severe OSA had significantly worse scores for quality of life compared with males or younger children.[25]

In children with adenotonsillar hypertrophy, adenotonsillectomy is the mainstay of treatment and leads to improvement or complete resolution of symptoms.[33] There are no studies to indicate a differential treatment response between sexes for SDB.

Parasomnias

Parasomnias are abnormal events that occur in sleep causing major disruption in sleep and could be classified as occurring during REM sleep, non-REM (NREM) sleep, or independent of sleep stage. Persistence of parasomnias beyond puberty could be secondary to sleep disorders. NREM parasomnias include sleep terrors, confusional arousals, sleep walking, and sleep-related eating disorder. It has been shown that about 88% of children manifest at least 1 parasomnia in their lifetime.[34] Studies have reported no sex differences in parasomnias, except that boys with parasomnias had a significant increase in snoring and SDB, whereas girls with parasomnias had more complications while in utero or during delivery (suggesting immature or inappropriate neuronal circuit development).[35–37] An exception is sleep-related eating disorder, which is recurrent episodes of amnestic involuntary binge eating and drinking during period of partial arousals from NREM sleep with subsequent recall and problematic consequences.[19] The prevalence was noted to be 0.5% and is higher in patients with depression (3.4%) and in college students (4.6%). There is 60% to 83% female predominance of sleep-related eating disorder, which also corresponds with the female predominance in other eating disorders.[38]

There are no reported sex differences in children and teenagers with restless leg syndrome (RLS) in the US population, with a sex difference starting in adulthood with a higher prevalence in women.[39] However, a study conducted in Turkey showed higher prevalence in girls than boys that was prominent after 15 years of age.[40]

The most common REM parasomnia are nightmares characterized by extremely dysphoric dreams that lead to arousal in the latter one-half of the night with vivid recollection of the dream. It has been observed that there is an increase in nightmares in adolescent females and adult women with a strong sex difference in reporting around 10 to 15 years of age (with more females reporting).[35] This difference in reporting could be related to openness in discussing dreams and negative emotions in girls, but also should take into consideration the greater prevalence of depression, post-traumatic stress disorder, and childhood sexual abuse in females.[41]

Nocturnal enuresis—involuntary voiding at night—is the most common parasomnia occurring in both REM and NREM sleep and affects boys 2 to 3 times more often than girls.[35] Boys with nocturnal enuresis had higher chances of having SDB, whereas girls had greater chances of having other parasomnias as well.[42] Nocturnal decreases in antidiuretic hormone are thought to be the main reason for nocturnal enuresis in children. It is hypothesized that females may have an increased sensitivity to antidiuretic hormone.[43,44]

Circadian Disorders

Teenagers have a later bedtime owing to many social and cultural factors, despite the time constraints of school or work.[45] However, these factors alone are insufficient to explain delayed sleep onset in adolescents, which is typical of an evening chronotype.[45] Chronotype is the preferred time frame of daily activity with classification as an early (morning) or late (evening) chronotype. It depends on genetic and environmental factors, along with age.[46] Children are early chronotypes and progressively become later (delayed) in their adolescence, reaching maximum lateness around the age of 20 years, after which they become early (advancing) with age.[8] The significant shift in chronotype seen during adolescence in both boys and girls suggests a physiologic cause. Girls show delayed sleep onset 1 year earlier than boys and reach their maximum in lateness earlier (at 19.5 years of age). Boys reach theirs at around age 21 years and continue to remain a later chronotype most of their adulthood, with a greater magnitude of chronotype shift.[8,46] This sex difference in chronotype with age also points toward the involvement of hormonal factors.[8,47] A study showed that melatonin secretion was progressively shifted with puberty, likely owing to longer tau during adolescence or an increased sensitivity to evening light and decreased exposure to morning light.[48,49] All of these changes could explain the increased prevalence of delayed sleep phase syndrome (a disorder of symptomatic and maladaptive evening chronotype) in teenagers that peaks during adolescence (the prevalence ranges from 7% to 16% compared with 0.15% during adulthood).[50] Hence, with an evening type chronotype, adolescents are prone to have delayed bed and rise time. However, because they need to wake up early for work or school, evening chronotypes may develop delayed sleep phase syndrome and experience shortened nocturnal sleep with insufficient sleep hours, daytime sleepiness, and greater compensation of sleep over the weekend.[47] Because of these factors, a number of school districts have delayed school start time and promote middle and high school education about sleep and circadian principles along with sleep hygiene.[51]

PREGNANCY

Sleep disturbances are commonly reported during pregnancy, affecting more than one-half of all women and increasing as gestation progresses.[52] According to a poll by the National Sleep Foundation, 78% of women reported more disturbed sleep during pregnancy than at any other times of their lives. Relative to nonpregnant women, sleep during pregnancy is characterized by greater time awake after sleep onset, shorter sleep duration less rapid eye movement sleep, and more time in lighter sleep stages.[53]

The near-universal presence of sleep complaints during pregnancy may lead to a belief that these symptoms are normal or to be expected. Unfortunately, this perception may impede the accurate diagnosis of sleep disorders during this crucial time; 1 study found that fewer than 10% of pregnant patients were asked about symptoms of sleep apnea by their obstetric providers.[54] And, despite being a temporary state, poor sleep in pregnancy can lead to long-term health consequences, including an increased risk for hypertensive disorders of pregnancy and other adverse outcomes. Potential pathways linking sleep disturbances during pregnancy with adverse pregnancy outcomes are shown in **Fig. 3**.

Sleep Disruption and Insomnia

Factors contributing to sleep disruption in pregnancy include nausea, nocturia, fetal movements, oxytocin (which peaks at night may contribute to sleep fragmentation in late pregnancy), musculoskeletal discomfort, leg cramps, pregnancy-related anxiety and stress, and exacerbation of underlying medical conditions such as asthma, which often worsens at night. Studies suggest that not only the quality, but also the duration of sleep decreases throughout pregnancy, with more than one-third of women reporting 6 or fewer hours of sleep by the end of pregnancy.[55] An emerging literature suggests that short sleep duration and the presence of sleep disorders during pregnancy may increase the risk for adverse pregnancy outcomes, including higher rates of caesarean delivery and greater postpartum depression.[56] Poor sleep may disproportionately affect pregnant women of lower socioeconomic status and racial minorities, groups already at an increased risk for adverse pregnancy outcomes.[57,58]

Sleep disturbances during pregnancy have variable severity, and some women will meet the formal criteria for clinical insomnia, defined as difficulty falling or maintaining sleep at least 3 times per week for at least 3 months, and not attributable to another condition or substance.[59] Because of its association with adverse pregnancy outcomes, early screening for insomnia is important.[60,61]

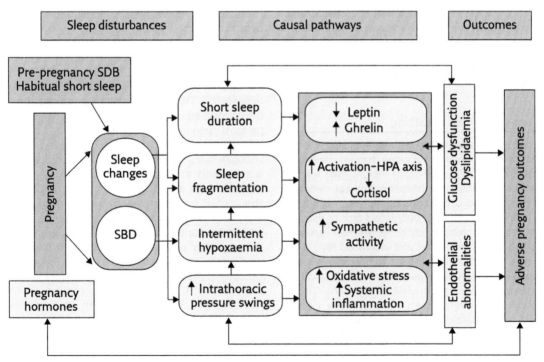

Fig. 3. Potential pathways linking sleep disturbances during pregnancy with adverse pregnancy outcomes. HPA, hypothalamic–pituitary–adrenal axis. (*Adapted from* Izci-Balserak B, Pien GW. The Relationship and Potential Mechanistic Pathways Between Sleep Disturbances and Maternal Hyperglycemia. *Current Diabetes Reports.* 2014;14(2).)

Several screening tools are available, including the Insomnia Symptom Questionnaire, which has been validated in pregnancy.[62]

Nonpharmacologic interventions are preferable during pregnancy. Cognitive behavioral therapy for insomnia is considered the first-line treatment for perinatal insomnia, and its efficacy in the pregnant population was supported by a recent randomized trial.[63] This multicomponent approach includes improving sleep hygiene, stimulus control, relaxation training, and sleep restriction therapy. Numerous studies in nonpregnant populations have shown cognitive behavioral therapy for insomnia to be at least as effective as pharmacologic therapy but more durable, and it spares potential fetal toxicity present with medications.

Although the safety of most sedative–hypnotic medications during pregnancy remains unclear, 1 in 25 pregnant women report using sleep medications at least 3 times weekly.[55] The decision about whether to continue or initiate pharmacologic therapy for insomnia requires a careful conversation between patient and provider that considers the severity of insomnia symptom and impact on quality of life, the potential for fetal harm, the availability of safer alternative therapy, and whether the risk of untreated disease may exceed that of the drug itself. The system of assigning medications a pregnancy category (ABCDX) was retired by the US Food and Drug Administration in 2015 because it was felt to be overly simplistic and often misinterpreted.[64] A discussion about safety and efficacy of specific pharmacologic agents in pregnancy is outside the scope of this article, but has been reviewed recently.[64]

Sleep-Disordered Breathing

Pregnancy is associated with several physiologic changes that may predispose toward development of SDB. These include weight gain with a central distribution; nasophargyngeal edema from increased circulating plasma volume, estrogen, and progesterone; decreased size of the upper airway; decreased functional residual capacity particularly while supine; and increased fetal oxygen consumption in the third trimester, resulting in a lower maternal oxygen reserve.[65] One-half of the reproductive age population begins their pregnancy either overweight or obese, even before they are exposed to the physiology of pregnancy.[66] Pregnant patients with OSA have a higher risk of pregnancy-specific complications, including gestational hypertension, gestational diabetes, and other medical and surgical complications, when compared with pregnant women without OSA (**Fig. 4**).[67]

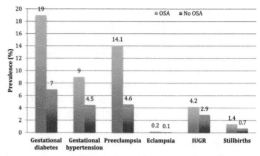

Fig. 4. OSA status and prevalence of pregnancy-specific complications. IUGR, intrauterine growth restriction. (*From* Bourjeily G, Danilack VA, Bublitz MH, et al. Obstructive sleep apnea in pregnancy is associated with adverse maternal outcomes: a national cohort. *Sleep Med.* 2017;38:50-57.)

The prevalence of sleep apnea in pregnancy depends on the particular demographic and at what time during pregnancy they are studied. The largest published cohort study of more than 3000 women observed an apnea-hypopnea index (AHI) of 5 or greater on ambulatory sleep testing in 4% and 8% of patients in early and mid pregnancy, respectively.[68] Another cohort of high-risk pregnancies found much higher prevalence estimates, with SDB present in nearly one-half of patients in the third trimester.[69]

Because pregnancy is a dynamic process, the best predictors of sleep apnea seem to vary by trimester. Prepregnancy BMI is the most powerful predictor of OSA in the first trimester, snoring best in the second trimester, and weight gain/BMI most significantly associated with OSA in the third trimester.[70] Traditional screening scales have been validated in the general population and often perform poorly in pregnant women.[71,72] For instance, the commonly used STOP-Bang Questionnaire has a sensitivity of only 53% in pregnant women and therefore cannot be relied on to exclude sleep apnea.[71] Furthermore, the optimal timing of screening is unknown. Screening in the first trimester is particularly insensitive, highlighting the importance of symptom reassessment as pregnancy progresses.[73] Data from the large multicenter prospective Nulliparous Pregnancy Outcomes: Monitoring Mothers-to-Be (nuMoM2b) study found that a logistic regression model including maternal age, frequent snoring, and BMI had good prediction of prevalent SDB.[74] Similarly, a 4-variable tool using self-reported frequent snoring, chronic hypertension, BMI, and age predicted sleep apnea in pregnancy with a sensitivity of 86% and specificity of 74%.[72]

The strongest associations between maternal sleep apnea and adverse outcomes have been demonstrated for the hypertensive disorders of pregnancy (gestational hypertension, pre-eclampsia and eclampsia) and for gestational diabetes. Pre-eclampsia, defined as new-onset hypertension and either proteinuria or end-organ damage with onset after 20 weeks gestation, is among the top causes of maternal deaths in the United States. Many of the pathophysiologic mechanisms that underlie OSA overlap with those involved in pre-eclampsia. These include a proinflammatory state, sympathetic nervous system activation, and endothelial dysfunction that may lead to vasoconstriction, hypertension, and proteinuria.[75] We now have robust evidence from several large studies demonstrating that sleep apnea during pregnancy is associated with a 2- to 3-fold increased risk of developing pre-eclampsia.[67,76–78] SDB during pregnancy is also associated with impaired glucose tolerance and gestational diabetes, independent of obesity.[68,79,80] Gestational diabetes confers risks for the mother and the fetus, including greater perinatal mortality, macrosomia, increased rates of caesarean section, and progression to type 2 diabetes in the postpartum period. Whether there exists a connection between sleep apnea in pregnancy and fetal outcomes is less well-established. Some studies have found that SDB is associated with intrauterine growth restriction and an increased risk of delivering small for gestational age infants, but larger studies are needed.[81,82]

Testing for sleep apnea in pregnancy may include polysomnography (PSG), the gold standard and most accurate method, or the more convenient but less sensitive ambulatory/home sleep testing. The decision about which study to order is often dictated by insurance. For pregnant women found not to have sleep apnea on testing performed early in pregnancy it is reasonable to considered repeat testing later in gestation, when the rates of sleep apnea are higher.

The management of SDB in pregnancy includes both behavioral strategies and positive airway pressure therapy; no specific practice guidelines exist. Behavioral interventions include behavioral measures such as limiting weight gain, avoidance of supine sleep, head-of-bed elevation, and avoidance of alcohol and sedatives that may contribute to airway relaxation and collapse. Definitive therapy involves application of positive airway pressure (eg, continuous positive airway pressure) therapy.[83] Alternative treatments for sleep apnea are typically impractical during pregnancy; for example, mandibular advancement devices, require time to fabricate and titrate. The few studies examining the impact of continuous positive airway pressure in pregnancy are limited by small sample sizes and short duration, but have generally demonstrated that continuous positive airway pressure is well-tolerated and beneficial.[84]

Restless Legs Syndrome

RLS is an unpleasant urge to move one's legs that worsens at night and while sedentary, and exhibits a clear predominance in women compared with men. RLS is very common in pregnancy, affecting up to 25% of pregnant women, a proportion significantly higher than the 2% to 15% prevalence in the general female population.[85] Two-thirds of pregnant women with RLS developed symptoms of the disorder newly during pregnancy, and the prevalence of RLS increases with advancing gestational age.[86] Gestational RLS has been linked to poor sleep quality, poor daytime function, daytime sleepiness, and a greater prevalence of pre-eclampsia, gestational hypertension, peripartum depression, daytime sleepiness, and decreased quality of life.[87,88]

RLS is a clinical diagnosis and the decision about whether to treat depends on symptom severity. A careful history is crucial to exclude disorders that may mimic RLS (**Box 1**). Treatment options are similar to those for nonpregnant women, including (1) the avoidance of inducers and aggravators such as prolonged immobility, caffeine, alcohol, smoking, certain medications (antihistamines, antiemetics), and sleep deprivation, (2) the assessment of a ferritin level and if less than 75 µg/L consideration of repletion with iron supplementation, and (3) pharmacologic agents after careful discussion of risks/benefits.[89] Whereas first-line pharmacologic therapy in nonpregnant women consists of gabapentinoids (gabapentin, pregabalin) and newer dopaminergic agents (ropinirole, pramipexole), carbidopa/levodopa is recommended as first-line during pregnancy, owing to greater safety data. Of note, dopaminergics may inhibit lactation and are therefore not recommending during breastfeeding. Most patients with new-onset RLS during pregnancy experience resolution of RLS symptoms within 1 week of delivery.[90]

LATE ADULTHOOD

Menopause affects women in the age range of 40 to 58 years, and at a median age of 51 years. The transition to menopause occurs when estrogen begins to decline with a concurrent increase in follicle-stimulating hormone. Sleep complaints are common in older women and affect approximately 40% to 60% of perimenopausal to postmenopausal women. Many recent studies demonstrate subjective sleep quality deterioration

<table>
<tr><td>

Box 1
Differential diagnosis of RLS during pregnancy

Common mimics

    Leg cramps

    Positional discomfort

    Venous stasis

    Leg edema

    Compression and stretch neuropathies

    Sore leg muscles

    Ligament sprain/tendon strain

    Positional ischemia (numbness)

    Dermatitis

    Bruises

Less common mimics

    Arthritis

    Other orthopedic disorders

    Peripheral neuropathy

    Radiculopathy

    Myelopathy

    Myopathy

    Fibromyalgia

    Complex region pain syndrome

    Drug-induced akathisia

    Sickle cell disease

Abbreviations: RLS, restless leg syndrome; WED, Willis-Ekbom disease.
From Picchietti DL, Hensley JG, Bainbridge JL, et al. Consensus clinical practice guidelines for the diagnosis and treatment of restless legs syndrome/Willis-Ekbom disease during pregnancy and lactation. *Sleep Med Rev.* 2015;22:64-77.

</td></tr>
</table>

starting in the perimenopausal period. Reported sleep changes relate to sleep fragmentation, increased awakenings, and nonrestorative or poor sleep quality (**Fig. 5**). Predictors of developing poor sleep during menopause include having premenopause depressive symptoms, crises, perceived poor health, daytime sleepiness, and central nervous system–active medications, according to a longitudinal study that followed premenopausal women for 5 years.[91] Menopause is also related to an increased risk of SDB for women. In fact, in postmenopausal women, sex differences in the occurrence and phenotype of OSA are less observed. These changes may be related to hormonal changes as well as the effects of aging.

Sleep Disruption and Insomnia

Chronic insomnia may develop in 31% to 42% of women during menopause.[92] There are many reasons for these changes in sleep during this period of her life: (1) nocturnal vasomotor symptoms, (2) direct hormonal effects on sleep, (3) direct age effects on sleep, (4) an increased risk for other sleep disorders such as OSA or RLS, (5) an increased risk for other medical disorders, (6) medications, and (7) an increased risk for depression and other psychiatric disorders. There are few studies measuring objective sleep findings during this period, and reporting variable outcomes. For example, PSG data in menopausal women show either no differences in sleep parameters, or worse sleep quality with decreased total sleep time, greater sleep fragmentation, and worse sleep efficiency compared with younger women.[93,94] In contrast, some longitudinal studies show better sleep architecture as women entered perimenopause, with longer total sleep time and slow wave sleep (SWS) compared with their premenopausal state.[95,96]

Sleep changes may reflect an aging process directly. Aging in women has been linked independently with fragmented sleep, insomnia, circadian derangements, and sleep architectural changes. Aged women show reduced sleep efficiency, increased wake after sleep onset, and decreased SWS and REM sleep.[97] A longitudinal cohort study following premenopausal women aged 46 years at baseline for approximately 6 years showed that both aging and hormonal changes impacted sleep architecture independently. Aging, independent of hormone status, was related to decreased total sleep time, increased awakenings, and worse sleep efficiency.

Night sweats and hot flashes occur in some women during menopause. Vasomotor symptoms are strongly associated with poor self-reported sleep quality. This finding is particularly true if vasomotor symptoms are perceived as severe and associated with night sweats.[98,99] Young women who had vasomotor symptoms induced with leuprolide (a gonadotropin-releasing hormone agonist) reported poorer sleep, more awakenings, and had worse scores on the Insomnia Severity Index and the Pittsburg Sleepiness Questionnaire Index.[100] The more severe the vasomotor symptoms, the more they were to develop chronic insomnia.[99,101–104] Objective sleep testing in women with vasomotor symptoms show more sleep fragmentation, poorer sleep efficiency, and increased wake after sleep onset. Similar findings of poor sleep are also shown on PSG or actigraphy when vasomotor activity is measured objectively

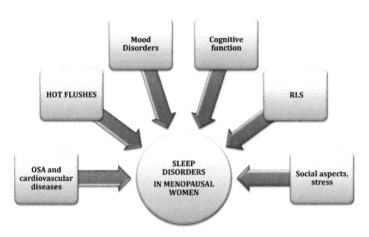

Fig. 5. Causes of sleep disturbance during menopause. (*From* Caretto M, Giannini A, Simoncini T. An integrated approach to diagnosing and managing sleep disorders in menopausal women. *Maturitas.* 2019;128:1-3.)

using skin conductance. The duration of a vasomotor event, but not the frequency of events, correlates with poorer sleep, including delayed REM sleep onset.[105] In addition, vasomotor activity in the first one-half of the night was more likely to relate to poor sleep, suggesting a possible sleep stage dependence of vasomotor activity on sleep quality.[106]

Hormonal changes, independent of vasomotor activity, may directly impact sleep. One study found that higher follicle-stimulating hormone levels were associated with more wakefulness on PSG in both premenopausal and perimenopausal women, even after adjusting for age, BMI, and vasomotor activity. In menopausal women from the Study of Women's Health Across the Nation (SWAN), a rapid increase in follicle-stimulating hormone (with low estrogen levels) had increased SWS as well as longer total sleep time. However, these women reported worse sleep quality on the Pittsburg Sleepiness Questionnaire Index.[107] It has been proposed that these findings actually reflected rebound SWS owing to generally poor sleep.

Hormonal therapy has been associated with serious risks such as breast cancer and heart disease; however, it remains an accepted treatment for sleep disturbances in some women.[108] Estrogen as monotherapy may effectively treat symptoms of vasomotor activity and improve sleep. In the Selective estrogens, Menopause and Response to Therapy (SMART) study, women with frequent vasomotor symptoms (ie, ≥7 severe symptoms/wk, or ≥50 events/wk) reported improved sleep quality with hormonal therapy, although it did not improve vasomotor symptoms.[109] Progesterone has a GABA-like effect and, although it has not shown to improve PSG features, subjective sleep quality is improved in older women. The withdrawal of hormone

therapies leads to rebound vasomotor symptoms and worse sleep disturbance.[108]

Whether hormonal or nonhormonal, treating vasomotor symptoms improves subjective sleep quality.[104,110,111] Nonhormonal therapies for vasomotor symptoms include selective serotonin reuptake inhibitors, serotonin-norepinephrine reuptake inhibitors, and GABA agonists. Older women with comorbid insomnia have been treated successfully with paroxetine, escitalopram, and venlafaxine. Gabapentin also treats hot flashes and sleep complaints.[108] Hypnotics such as zolpidem and eszopiclone may improve sleep onset and sleep maintenance in menopausal women. Eszopiclone in particular has been found to reduce the frequency of nocturnal but not daytime hot flashes.[112] Zolpidem has also been effective in concert with selective serotonin reuptake inhibitors at improving sleep disturbances.[113] Treatment with alternative therapies such as black cohosh, soy, and omega-3 have not been supported in randomized clinical trials. Exercise and cognitive behavioral therapy may also lead to improvements in vasomotor symptoms and sleep quality.[108]

Circadian Changes

Circadian disruption is a prominent feature of aging in both men and women and may be directly hormonally mediated. Postmenopausal women, as compared with premenopausal women, are more likely to be phase advanced by 1 hour and are more likely to be a "morning" chronotype.[114] Sleep onset is accompanied by a peak in melatonin secretion and a decrease in the core body temperature. Noradrenergic activation is decreased , and peripheral vasodilation with heat loss through the skin results. In postmenopausal women, however, this decrease in core body temperature, along with early morning cortisol levels, are blunted.

Nocturnal melatonin secretion generally decreases with age and decreases in relation to menopausal state.[115] It is speculated that melatonin could be playing a direct role in a woman's menopausal transition. The gonadotropin-releasing hormone–luteinizing hormone–ovarian axis is influenced by circadian rhythms; therefore, age-related circadian disruption may lead to amenorrhea. It has also been speculated that age-related alterations in melatonin secretion may lead to irregular pulsing of gonadotropin-releasing hormone and luteinizing hormone, causing vasomotor symptoms. The influence of melatonin in the menopausal transition is likely more complex, because exogenous melatonin does not relieve hot flashes or night sweats.[116] However, exogenous melatonin—whether through its circadian or hypnotic properties—improve mood and sleep symptoms in postmenopausal women.[117]

Sleep-Disordered Breathing

Hormonal differences may impact the occurrence and severity of sleep apnea. OSA is 3-fold more prevalent in postmenopausal compared with premenopausal women.[118] In the Wisconsin Sleep Cohort Study, the prevalence of OSA (defined by an AHI of ≥5) was 10.8%, 18.4%, and 29.1% in premenopausal, perimenopausal, and postmenopausal women, respectively.[96] Even after controlling for age, BMI, alcohol use, smoking, hypertension, exercise, cardiovascular disease, and health status, the risk for OSA remained 2.6 in postmenopausal compared with premenopausal women. They found a nonsignificant trend toward a decrease in the odds for OSA in hormone replacement therapy users. Bixler and colleagues also found a reduction in prevalence of OSA (defined by an AHI of ≥10) in postmenopausal women on hormone replacement therapy (1.1%), compared with those not on hormone replacement therapy (5.5%).[118]

In animal studies, progesterone shows hypnotic and anxiolytic properties, and estrogen increases the turnover of norepinephrine in brain regions expected to decrease REM sleep. Whether these sleep- related changes have protective effects on upper airway function and respiration during sleep is unclear. Medroxyprogesterone acts on central carbon dioxide receptors to stimulate ventilation during wakefulness. However, it has not been shown to affect ventilatory responses during sleep. The literature regarding the therapeutic utility of progesterone and/or estrogen replacement therapy for OSA in postmenopausal women is limited. Earlier studies showed medroxyprogesterone does not improve OSA in morbidly obese patients or eucapnic OSA.[119,120] A more recent study showed estrogen hormone therapy in postmenopausal women led to improvement in the AHI.[121]

Age impacts OSA prevalence and incidence in men and women differently. Tishler and colleagues[122] showed that the risk of OSA per 10-year age increase was 2.41 in women (95% confidence interval, 1.78–3.26) and 1.15 in men (95% confidence interval, 0.78–1.68). As a result, by age 60 years, the male predominance decreases and the prevalence rates among men and women become more similar. Older women are also more likely to have severe OSA compared with younger women, although older men continue to have greater incidences of severe OSA compared with age-matched women. In a middle-aged community sample, the incidence of moderate-to-severe OSA (an AHI of ≥15 events/h) over a 5-year period was 11.1% in men compared with 4.9% in women.[123]

BMI or weight also impart different risk for developing OSA among men and women. Men with a weight gain of more than 10 kg have a 5.2-fold increase in odds for an increase in AHI by more than 15 events per hour. In contrast, for a comparable weight gain, women have a 2.5-fold increase in odds for a similar increase in AHI.[124]

The symptoms of OSA also seem to change for women with age. In a study of 660 women (316 postmenopausal), premenopausal women were more likely to complain of fatigue, insomnia, cognitive dysfunction, irritability, sleepwalking, headaches, and muscle pain despite generally having a lower AHI.[125] Older women were more likely to present with traditionally male symptoms of snoring, gasping, and witnessed apneas. Premenopausal women with OSA were also more likely to have a lower BMI, more oral–facial clinical findings, and a greater occurrence of hypertension. Despite a lower AHI, younger women compared with older women required similar positive airway pressure settings for complete treatment of AHI and symptoms. Meanwhile, age seemed to impact men's symptoms much less. Therefore, the physiologic changes that occur with aging, including menopause, affect OSA progression differently in men and women.

Sleep Changes Related to Mood Disorders

Mood disorders are more prevalent in aging women compared with younger women or age-matched men. The occurrence of depression increases more than 2-fold during the menopausal transition.[126–128] Depression and anxiety can directly lead to poor sleep, while also aggravating vasomotor symptoms. In the SWAN study, comorbid anxiety led to more complaints of sleep and vasomotor symptoms in perimenopausal women.[129] Similarly, poor sleep may worsen mood disorders in women. A study following women aged 42 to 52 years for 3 years found subjective sleep reports, but not vasomotor symptoms, predicted negative mood the following day.[130]

Poor sleep rather than vasomotor symptoms may be a stronger correlate of depressed mood in older women. Many women have their first onset of depression during the menopausal transition when they are not experiencing vasomotor symptoms. Moreover, women with depressed mood and sleep disturbances do not have more vasomotor complaints than women without depressed mood. Finally, the pattern of sleep disruption related directly to depression versus vasomotor symptoms differ. Depressed midlife and elderly women more often will have longer sleep latency, shorter total sleep time, and disrupted REM sleep. In contrast, vasomotor-related sleep disturbances are more often characterized by frequent and prolonged awakenings.[100]

Other sleep disorders and medical disorders become more frequent with age that also impact sleep quality in older women. They include SDB, parasomnias, and movement disorders, among others, which altogether affect more than 53% of postmenopausal women.[131–133]

Restless Leg Syndrome

The prevalence of RLS has been estimated to be 5% to 7% in the general population, occurring more often in women and in the elderly population.[134] In the community-based Multi-ethnic Study of Atherosclerosis (MESA) cohort, a sample of ethnically diverse older individuals (mean age 68.4 ± 9.1 years), the occurrence of RLS was 16%.[135] Approximately 7% met criteria for electroclinical RLS, defined in this study as having both RLS by International Restless Legs Syndrome Study Group criteria and periodic limb movements on PSG (periodic limb movements index of >15/h). Electroclinical RLS was associated with advancing age. Periodic limb movements without RLS occurred in 21%. Periodic limb movements are also known to be associated with advanced age, but do not show a sex predilection.[136] Idiopathic RLS (RLS that is not associated with medical disease such as anemia or renal failure) is more common in women and is estimated to affect approximately 10% of the population older than 65 years of age. The symptoms are often progressive and tend to worsen with aging. The majority of persons with idiopathic RLS have a familial occurrence with an autosomal-dominant inheritance.

SUMMARY

Sex differences in sleep disorders generally occur after adolescence. Female sex is associated with higher rates of insomnia and RLS during reproductive hormonal shifts as seen with pregnancy and menopause. Meanwhile, SDB is more common in adult males. In women, SDB may develop or worsen during pregnancy and is associated with poor maternal and fetal outcomes. The menopausal transition is associated with significant objective and subjective sleep changes owing to hormonal changes, vasomotor symptoms, changes directly related to the aging process, an increase in comorbid medical and psychiatric conditions, and psychosocial changes that accompany this stage in a woman's life. These changes are important to study because poor sleep is associated with morbidities, including more incidences of chronic inflammation,[137] cardiovascular and metabolic disease,[138–143] and mood disorders. The timing of the onset of sex differences in sleep disorders very much suggest a sex hormone related process. Understanding the evolution of sleep across a woman's lifespan may lead to effective therapies that impact women's overall health and quality of life.

CLINICS CARE POINTS

- Nocturnal enuresis occurs more commonly in boys than girls. Otherwise, few sex differences in sleep disorders have been described during childhood.

- Sex differences in sleep disorders generally arise after adolescence, suggesting an impact of sex hormones on the development of sleep disorders.

- During adulthood, women are more likely to experience insomnia or RLS, while men are more likely to suffer from sleep disordered breathing.

- Pregnancy marks a unique period in a woman's life where the risk of sleep disruption, insomnia, RLS or sleep breathing disorders increases. The increased risk may be in part mediated by hormonal changes.

- The menopausal transition in women is accompanied by an increased risk for sleep disruption due to vasomotor symptoms, as well as insomnia. In later adulthood, women experience an increased risk for sleep disordered breathing.

DISCLOSURE

None of the authors have conflicts of interest to disclose.

REFERENCES

1. Theorell-Haglöw J, Miller CB, Bartlett DJ, et al. Gender differences in obstructive sleep apnoea, insomnia and restless legs syndrome in adults - what do we know? A clinical update. Sleep Med Rev 2018;38:28–38.

2. Auer M, Frauscher B, Hochleitner M, et al. Gender-specific differences in access to polysomnography and prevalence of sleep disorders. J Womens Health (Larchmt) 2018;27(4):525–30.

3. Pinto J, Van Zeller M, Amorim P, et al. Sleep quality in times of COVID-19 pandemic. Sleep Med 2020; 74:81–5.

4. Pengo MF, Won CH, Bourjeily G. Sleep in women across the life span. Chest 2018;154(1):196–206.

5. Bach V, Telliez F, Leke A, et al. Gender-related sleep differences in neonates in thermoneutral and cool environments. J Sleep Res 2000;9(3): 249–54.

6. Hoppenbrouwers T, Hodgman JE, Arakawa K, et al. Respiration during the first six months of life in normal infants. III. Computer identification of breathing pauses. Pediatr Res 1980;14(11): 1230–3.

7. Boukari R, Laouafa S, Ribon-Demars A, et al. Ovarian steroids act as respiratory stimulant and antioxidant against the causes and consequences of sleep-apnea in women. Respir Physiolo Neurobiol 2017;239:46–54.

8. Roenneberg T, Kuehnle T, Pramstaller PP, et al. A marker for the end of adolescence. Curr Biol 2004;14(24):R1038–9.

9. Kessler RC, Walters EE. Epidemiology of DSM-III-R major depression and minor depression among adolescents and young adults in the National Comorbidity Survey. Depress Anxiety 1998;7(1):3–14.

10. Lindberg E, Janson C, Gislason T, et al. Sleep disturbances in a young adult population: can gender differences be explained by differences in psychological status? Sleep 1997;20(6):381–7.

11. Yang C-K, Kim JK, Patel SR, et al. Age-related changes in sleep/wake patterns among Korean teenagers. Pediatrics 2005;115(Supplement 1): 250–6.

12. Owens JA, Babcock D, Weiss M. Evaluation and treatment of children and adolescents with excessive daytime sleepiness. Clin Pediatr 2020;59(4–5):340–51.

13. Joo S, Shin C, Kim J, et al. Prevalence and correlates of excessive daytime sleepiness in high school students in Korea. Psychiatry Clin Neurosci 2005;59(4):433–40.

14. Liu Y, Zhang J, Li SX, et al. Excessive daytime sleepiness among children and adolescents: prevalence, correlates, and pubertal effects. Sleep Med 2019;53:1–8.

15. Chattu VK, Manzar MD, Kumary S, et al. The global problem of insufficient sleep and its serious public health implications. Healthcare (Basel) 2018;7(1):1.

16. Bruce ES, Lunt L, McDonagh JE. Sleep in adolescents and young adults. Clin Med 2017;17(5): 424–8.

17. Kotagal S. Hypersomnia in children. Sleep Med Clin 2012;7(2):379–89.

18. National Sleep Foundation's 2018 Sleep in America® poll shows Americans failing to prioritize sleep. Available at: https://www.sleepfoundation.org/professionals/sleep-americar-polls/2018-sleep-prioritization-and-personal-effectiveness.

19. American Academy of Sleep Medicine. International classification of sleep disorders, 3rd ed. Darien (IL): American Academy of Sleep Medicine; 2014.

20. Kornum BR, Knudsen S, Ollila HM, et al. Narcolepsy. Nat Rev Dis Primers 2017;3(1):1–19.

21. Billiard M, Jaussent I, Dauvilliers Y, et al. Recurrent hypersomnia: a review of 339 cases. Sleep Med Rev 2011;15(4):247–57.

22. Arnulf I, Zeitzer JM, File J, et al. Kleine-Levin syndrome: a systematic review of 186 cases in the literature. Brain 2005;128(Pt 12):2763–76.

23. Dauvilliers Y, Lopez R, Ohayon M, et al. Hypersomnia and depressive symptoms: methodological and clinical aspects. BMC Med 2013;11(1):78.

24. Kaplan KA, Harvey AG. Hypersomnia across mood disorders: a review and synthesis. Sleep Med Rev 2009;13(4):275–85.

25. Horne RSC, Ong C, Weichard A, et al. Are there gender differences in the severity and consequences of sleep disordered in children? Sleep Med 2020;67:147–55.

26. Matsumoto T, Chin K. Prevalence of sleep disturbances: sleep disordered breathing, short sleep duration, and non-restorative sleep. Respir Investig 2019;57(3):227–37.

27. Heinzer R, Vat S, Marques-Vidal P, et al. Prevalence of sleep-disordered breathing in the general population: the HypnoLaus study. Lancet Respir Med 2015;3(4):310–8.

28. Lumeng JC, Chervin RD. Epidemiology of pediatric obstructive sleep apnea. Proc Am Thorac Soc 2008;5(2):242–52.

29. Brockmann PE, Koren D, Kheirandish-Gozal L, et al. Gender dimorphism in pediatric OSA: is it for real? Respir Physiolo Neurobiol 2017;245:83–8.

30. Inoshita A, Kasai T, Matsuoka R, et al. Age-stratified sex differences in polysomnographic findings and pharyngeal morphology among children with obstructive sleep apnea. J Thorac Dis 2018; 10(12):6702–10.

31. Kang K-T, Chou C-H, Weng W-C, et al. Associations between adenotonsillar hypertrophy, age, and obesity in children with obstructive sleep apnea. PLoS One 2013;8(10):e78666.

32. Dong J-Q, Chen X, Xiao Y, et al. Serum sex hormone levels in different severity of male adult obstructive sleep apnea-hypopnea syndrome in East Asians. J Huazhong Univ Sci Technology Med Sci 2015;35(4):553–7.

33. Todd CA, Bareiss AK, McCoul ED, et al. Adenotonsillectomy for obstructive sleep apnea and quality of life: systematic review and meta-analysis. Otolaryngol Head Neck Surg 2017;157(5):767–73.

34. Petit D, Touchette E, Tremblay RE, et al. Dyssomnias and parasomnias in early childhood. Pediatrics 2007;119(5):e1016–25.

35. Donskoy I. Gender differences in pediatric parasomnias. In: Attarian H, Viola-Saltzman M, editors. Sleep disorders in women: a guide to practical management. Cham: Springer International Publishing; 2020. p. 129–37.

36. Ozgun N, Sonmez FM, Topbas M, et al. Insomnia, parasomnia, and predisposing factors in Turkish school children. Pediatr Int 2016; 58(10):1014–22.

37. Nevsimalova S, Prihodova I, Kemlink D, et al. Childhood parasomnia – a disorder of sleep maturation? Eur J Paediatr Neurol 2013;17(6):615–9.

38. Irfan M, Schenck CH, Howell MJ. Non-rapid eye movement sleep and overlap parasomnias. Continuum (Minneap Minn) 2017;23(4, Sleep Neurology): 1035–50.

39. Picchietti D, Allen RP, Walters AS, et al. Restless legs syndrome: prevalence and impact in children and adolescents—The Peds REST Study. Pediatrics 2007;120(2):253–66.

40. Turkdogan D, Bekiroglu N, Zaimoglu S. A prevalence study of restless legs syndrome in Turkish children and adolescents. Sleep Med 2011;12(4):315–21.

41. Schredl M, Reinhard I. Gender differences in nightmare frequency: a meta-analysis. Sleep Med Rev 2011;15(2):115–21.

42. Ma J, Li S, Jiang F, et al. Relationship between sleep patterns, sleep problems, and childhood enuresis. Sleep Med 2018;50:14–20.

43. Mahler B, Kamperis K, Ankarberg-Lindgren C, et al. Puberty alters renal water handling. Am J Physiol Renal Physiol 2013;305(12):F1728–35.

44. Schroeder MK, Juul KV, Mahler B, et al. Desmopressin use in pediatric nocturnal enuresis patients: is there a sex difference in prescription patterns? Eur J Pediatr 2018;177(3):389–94.

45. Hagenauer MH, Perryman JI, Lee TM, et al. Adolescent changes in the homeostatic and circadian regulation of sleep. Dev Neurosci 2009;31(4):276–84.

46. Bailey M, Silver R. Sex differences in circadian timing systems: implications for disease. Front Neuroendocrinol 2014;35(1):111–39.

47. Gau S-F, Soong W-T. The transition of sleep-wake patterns in early adolescence. Sleep 2003;26(4): 449–54.

48. Carskadon MA, Acebo C, Richardson GS, et al. An approach to studying circadian rhythms of adolescent humans. J Biol Rhythms 1997;12(3):278–89.

49. Carskadon MA, Labyak SE, Acebo C, et al. Intrinsic circadian period of adolescent humans measured in conditions of forced desynchrony. Neurosci Lett 1999;260(2):129–32.

50. Jenni OG, Achermann P, Carskadon MA. Homeostatic sleep regulation in adolescents. Sleep 2005;28(11):1446–54.

51. Miano S. Circadian rhythm disorders in childhood. In: Nevšímalová S, Bruni O, editors. Sleep disorders in children. Cham: Springer International Publishing; 2017. p. 253–80.

52. Tomfohr LM, Buliga E, Letourneau NL, et al. Trajectories of sleep quality and associations with mood during the perinatal period. Sleep 2015;38(8): 1237–45.

53. Garbazza C, Hackethal S, Riccardi S, et al. Polysomnographic features of pregnancy: a systematic review. Sleep Med Rev 2020;50:101249.

54. Bourjeily G, Raker C, Paglia MJ, et al. Patient and provider perceptions of sleep disordered breathing assessment during prenatal care: a survey-based observational study. Ther Adv Respir Dis 2012; 6(4):211–9.

55. Mindell JA, Cook RA, Nikolovski J. Sleep patterns and sleep disturbances across pregnancy. Sleep Med 2015;16(4):483–8.

56. Sedov ID, Anderson NJ, Dhillon AK, et al. Insomnia symptoms during pregnancy: a meta-analysis. J Sleep Res 2021;30(1):e13207.

57. Silva-Perez LJ, Gonzalez-Cardenas N, Surani S, et al. Socioeconomic status in pregnant women and sleep quality during pregnancy. Cureus 2019;11(11):e6183.

58. Feinstein L, Mcwhorter KL, Gaston SA, et al. Racial/ethnic disparities in sleep duration and sleep disturbances among pregnant and non-pregnant women in the United States. J Sleep Res 2020; 29(5):e13000.

59. American Academy of Sleep Medicine. International Classification of Sleep Disorders – Third Edition (ICSD-3). Darien, IL: American Academy of Sleep Medicine; 2014.

60. Li R, Zhang J, Zhou R, et al. Sleep disturbances during pregnancy are associated with cesarean delivery and preterm birth. J Matern Fetal Neonatal Med 2017;30(6):733–8.

61. Dørheim SK, Bjorvatn B, Eberhard-Gran M. Insomnia and depressive symptoms in late pregnancy: a population-based study. Behav Sleep Med 2012;10(3):152–66.

62. Okun ML, Buysse DJ, Hall MH. Identifying insomnia in early pregnancy: validation of the insomnia symptoms questionnaire (ISQ) in pregnant women. J Clin Sleep Med 2015;11(06):645–54.

63. Manber R, Bei B, Simpson N, et al. Cognitive behavioral therapy for prenatal insomnia: a randomized controlled trial. Obstet Gynecol 2019;133(5):911–9.

64. Miller MA, Mehta N, Clark-Bilodeau C, et al. Sleep pharmacotherapy for common sleep disorders in pregnancy and lactation. Chest 2020;157(1):184–97.

65. Ayyar L, Shaib F, Guntupalli K. Sleep-disordered breathing in pregnancy. Sleep Med Clin 2018;13(3):349–57.

66. Martin JAHB, Osterman MJK, Driscoll AK. Births: final data for 2018. National vital statistics reports. Hyattsville, MD: National Center for Health Statistics; 2019.

67. Bourjeily G, Danilack VA, Bublitz MH, et al. Obstructive sleep apnea in pregnancy is associated with adverse maternal outcomes: a national cohort. Sleep Med 2017;38:50–7.

68. Facco FL, Parker CB, Reddy UM, et al. Association between sleep-disordered breathing and hypertensive disorders of pregnancy and gestational diabetes mellitus. Obstet Gynecol 2017;129(1):31–41.

69. Ouyang D, Zee P, Grobman W, et al. Sleep disordered breathing in a high-risk cohort prevalence and severity across pregnancy. Am J Perinatol 2014;31(10):899–904.

70. Tantrakul V, Sirijanchune P, Panburana P, et al. Screening of obstructive sleep apnea during pregnancy: differences in predictive values of questionnaires across trimesters. J Clin Sleep Med 2015;11(02):157–63.

71. Lockhart EM, Ben Abdallah A, Tuuli MG, et al. Obstructive sleep apnea in pregnancy: assessment of current screening tools. Obstet Gynecol 2015;126(1):93–102.

72. Facco FL, Ouyang DW, Zee PC, et al. Development of a pregnancy-specific screening tool for sleep apnea. J Clin Sleep Med 2012;08(04):389–94.

73. Pien GW, Pack AI, Jackson N, et al. Risk factors for sleep-disordered breathing in pregnancy. Thorax 2014;69(4):371–7.

74. Louis JM, Koch MA, Reddy UM, et al. Predictors of sleep-disordered breathing in pregnancy. Am J Obstet Gynecol 2018;218(5):521.e1–12.

75. Bourjeily G, Curran P, Butterfield K, et al. Placenta-secreted circulating markers in pregnant women with obstructive sleep apnea. J Perinat Med 2015;43(1):81–7.

76. Pamidi S, Pinto LM, Marc I, et al. Maternal sleep-disordered breathing and adverse pregnancy outcomes: a systematic review and metaanalysis. Am J Obstet Gynecol 2014;210(1):52.e1–14.

77. Chen Y-H, Kang J-H, Lin C-C, et al. Obstructive sleep apnea and the risk of adverse pregnancy outcomes. Am J Obstet Gynecol 2012;206(2):136.e1–5.

78. Bin YS, Cistulli PA, Ford JB. Population-based study of sleep apnea in pregnancy and maternal and infant outcomes. J Clin Sleep Med 2016;12(06):871–7.

79. Luque-Fernandez MA, Bain PA, Gelaye B, et al. Sleep-disordered breathing and gestational diabetes mellitus: a meta-analysis of 9,795 participants enrolled in epidemiological observational studies. Diabetes Care 2013;36(10):3353–60.

80. Pamidi S, Tasali E. Obstructive sleep apnea and type 2 diabetes: is there a link? Front Neurol 2012;3:126.

81. Fung AM, Wilson DL, Lappas M, et al. Effects of maternal obstructive sleep apnoea on fetal growth: a prospective cohort study. PLoS One 2013;8(7):e68057.

82. Pamidi S, Marc I, Simoneau G, et al. Maternal sleep-disordered breathing and the risk of delivering small for gestational age infants: a prospective cohort study. Thorax 2016;71(8):719–25.

83. Dominguez JE, Street L, Louis J. Management of obstructive sleep apnea in pregnancy. Obstet Gynecol Clin North Am 2018;45(2):233–47.

84. Pamidi S, Kimoff RJ. Maternal sleep-disordered breathing. Chest 2018;153(4):1052–66.

85. Darvishi N, Daneshkhah A, Khaledi-Paveh B, et al. The prevalence of Restless Legs Syndrome/Willis-Ekbom disease (RLS/WED) in the third trimester of pregnancy: a systematic review. BMC Neurol 2020;20(1):132.

86. Chen SJ, Shi L, Bao YP, et al. Prevalence of restless legs syndrome during pregnancy: a systematic review and meta-analysis. Sleep Med Rev 2018;40:43–54.

87. Steinweg K, Nippita T, Cistulli PA, et al. Maternal and neonatal outcomes associated with restless legs syndrome in pregnancy: a systematic review. Sleep Med Rev 2020;54:101359.

88. Dunietz GL, Lisabeth LD, Shedden K, et al. Restless legs syndrome and sleep-wake disturbances in pregnancy. J Clin Sleep Med 2017;13(07):863–70.

89. Picchietti DL, Hensley JG, Bainbridge JL, et al. Consensus clinical practice guidelines for the diagnosis and treatment of restless legs syndrome/Willis-Ekbom disease during pregnancy and lactation. Sleep Med Rev 2015;22:64–77.

90. Grover A, Clark-Bilodeau C, D'Ambrosio CM. Restless leg syndrome in pregnancy. Obstet Med 2015; 8(3):121–5.

91. Lampio L, Saaresranta T, Engblom J, et al. Predictors of sleep disturbance in menopausal transition. Maturitas 2016;94:137–42.

92. Ciano C, King TS, Wright RR, et al. Longitudinal study of insomnia symptoms among women during perimenopause. J Obstet Gynecol Neonatal Nurs 2017;46(6):804–13.

93. Xu M, Belanger L, Ivers H, et al. Comparison of subjective and objective sleep quality in menopausal and non-menopausal women with insomnia. Sleep Med 2011;12(1):65–9.

94. Freedman RR, Roehrs TA. Lack of sleep disturbance from menopausal hot flashes. Fertil Steril 2004;82(1):138–44.

95. Lampio L, Polo-Kantola P, Himanen SL, et al. Sleep during menopausal transition: a 6-year follow-up. Sleep 2017;40(7). https://doi.org/10.1093/sleep/zsx090.

96. Young T, Rabago D, Zgierska A, et al. Objective and subjective sleep quality in premenopausal, perimenopausal, and postmenopausal women in the Wisconsin Sleep Cohort Study. Sleep 2003; 26(6):667–72.

97. Ohayon MM, Carskadon MA, Guilleminault C, et al. Meta-analysis of quantitative sleep parameters from childhood to old age in healthy individuals: developing normative sleep values across the human lifespan. Sleep 2004;27(7):1255–73.

98. Joffe H, White DP, Crawford SL, et al. Adverse effects of induced hot flashes on objectively recorded and subjectively reported sleep: results of a gonadotropin-releasing hormone agonist experimental protocol. Menopause 2013;20(9):905–14.

99. Hartz A, Ross JJ, Noyes R, et al. Somatic symptoms and psychological characteristics associated with insomnia in postmenopausal women. Sleep Med 2013;14(1):71–8.

100. Joffe H, Crawford S, Economou N, et al. A gonadotropin-releasing hormone agonist model demonstrates that nocturnal hot flashes interrupt objective sleep. Sleep 2013;36(12):1977–85.

101. Xu Q, Lang CP. Examining the relationship between subjective sleep disturbance and menopause: a systematic review and meta-analysis. Menopause 2014;21(12):1301–18.

102. de Zambotti M, Colrain IM, Javitz HS, et al. Magnitude of the impact of hot flashes on sleep in perimenopausal women. Fertil Steril 2014;102(6): 1708–1715 e1701.

103. Ayers B, Hunter MS. Health-related quality of life of women with menopausal hot flushes and night sweats. Climacteric 2013;16(2):235–9.

104. Pinkerton JV, Abraham L, Bushmakin AG, et al. Relationship between changes in vasomotor symptoms and changes in menopause-specific quality of life and sleep parameters. Menopause 2016; 23(10):1060–6.

105. Savard MH, Savard J, Caplette-Gingras A, et al. Relationship between objectively recorded hot flashes and sleep disturbances among breast cancer patients: investigating hot flash characteristics other than frequency. Menopause 2013;20(10): 997–1005.

106. Freedman RR, Roehrs TA. Sleep disturbance in menopause. Menopause 2007;14(5):826–9.

107. Sowers MF, Zheng H, Kravitz HM, et al. Sex steroid hormone profiles are related to sleep measures from polysomnography and the Pittsburgh Sleep Quality Index. Sleep 2008;31(10):1339–49.

108. Eichling PS, Sahni J. Menopause related sleep disorders. J Clin Sleep Med 2005;1(3):291–300.

109. Stevenson JC, Chines A, Pan K, et al. A pooled analysis of the effects of conjugated estrogens/bazedoxifene on lipid parameters in postmenopausal women from the selective estrogens, menopause, and response to therapy (SMART) Trials. J Clin Endocrinol Metab 2015;100(6):2329–38.

110. Leeangkoonsathian E, Pantasri T, Chaovisitseree S, et al. The effect of different progestogens on sleep in postmenopausal women: a randomized trial. Gynecol Endocrinol 2017;33(12):933–6.

111. Cintron D, Lahr BD, Bailey KR, et al. Effects of oral versus transdermal menopausal hormone treatments on self-reported sleep domains and their association with vasomotor symptoms in recently menopausal women enrolled in the Kronos Early Estrogen Prevention Study (KEEPS). Menopause 2018;25(2):145–53.

112. Soares CN, Joffe H, Rubens R, et al. Eszopiclone in patients with insomnia during perimenopause and early postmenopause: a randomized controlled trial. Obstet Gynecol 2006;108(6):1402–10.

113. Dorsey CM, Lee KA, Scharf MB. Effect of zolpidem on sleep in women with perimenopausal and postmenopausal insomnia: a 4-week, randomized, multicenter, double-blind, placebo-controlled study. Clin Ther 2004;26(10):1578–86.

114. Gomez-Santos C, Saura CB, Lucas JA, et al. Menopause status is associated with circadian- and sleep-related alterations. Menopause 2016;23(6): 682–90.

115. Gursoy AY, Kiseli M, Caglar GS. Melatonin in aging women. Climacteric 2015;18(6):790–6.

116. Chen WY, Giobbie-Hurder A, Gantman K, et al. A randomized, placebo-controlled trial of melatonin on breast cancer survivors: impact on sleep,

mood, and hot flashes. Breast Cancer Res Treat 2014;145(2):381–8.

117. Kotlarczyk MP, Lassila HC, O'Neil CK, et al. Melatonin osteoporosis prevention study (MOPS): a randomized, double-blind, placebo-controlled study examining the effects of melatonin on bone health and quality of life in perimenopausal women. J Pineal Res 2012;52(4):414–26.

118. Bixler EO, Vgontzas AN, Lin HM, et al. Prevalence of sleep-disordered breathing in women: effects of gender. Am J Respir Crit Care Med 2001;163(3 Pt 1):608–13.

119. Cook WR, Benich JJ, Wooten SA. Indices of severity of obstructive sleep apnea syndrome do not change during medroxyprogesterone acetate therapy. Chest 1989;96(2):262–6.

120. Rajagopal KR, Abbrecht PH, Jabbari B. Effects of medroxyprogesterone acetate in obstructive sleep apnea. Chest 1986;90(6):815–21.

121. Manber R, Kuo TF, Cataldo N, et al. The effects of hormone replacement therapy on sleep-disordered breathing in postmenopausal women: a pilot study. Sleep 2003;26(2):163–8.

122. Tishler PV, Larkin EK, Schluchter MD, et al. Incidence of sleep-disordered breathing in an urban adult population: the relative importance of risk factors in the development of sleep-disordered breathing. JAMA 2003;289(17):2230–7.

123. Ware JC, McBrayer RH, Scott JA. Influence of sex and age on duration and frequency of sleep apnea events. Sleep 2000;23(2):165–70.

124. Newman AB, Foster G, Givelber R, et al. Progression and regression of sleep-disordered breathing with changes in weight: the Sleep Heart Health Study. Arch Intern Med 2005;165(20):2408–13.

125. Tantrakul V, Park CS, Guilleminault C. Sleep-disordered breathing in premenopausal women: differences between younger (less than 30 years old) and older women. Sleep Med 2012;13(6):656–62.

126. Freeman EW, Sammel MD, Boorman DW, et al. Longitudinal pattern of depressive symptoms around natural menopause. JAMA Psychiatry 2014;71(1):36–43.

127. Cohen LS, Soares CN, Vitonis AF, et al. Risk for new onset of depression during the menopausal transition: the Harvard study of moods and cycles. Arch Gen Psychiatry 2006;63(4):385–90.

128. Bromberger JT, Matthews KA, Schott LL, et al. Depressive symptoms during the menopausal transition: the study of women's health across the nation (SWAN). J Affect Disord 2007;103(1–3): 267–72.

129. Bromberger JT, Kravitz HM, Chang YF, et al. Major depression during and after the menopausal transition: study of women's health across the nation (SWAN). Psychol Med 2011;41(9):1879–88.

130. Burleson MH, Todd M, Trevathan WR. Daily vasomotor symptoms, sleep problems, and mood: using daily data to evaluate the domino hypothesis in middle-aged women. Menopause 2010;17(1): 87–95.

131. Mirer AG, Young T, Palta M, et al. Sleep-disordered breathing and the menopausal transition among participants in the Sleep in Midlife Women Study. Menopause 2017;24(2):157–62.

132. Galvan T, Camuso J, Sullivan K, et al. Association of estradiol with sleep apnea in depressed perimenopausal and postmenopausal women: a preliminary study. Menopause 2017;24(1):112–7.

133. Naufel MF, Frange C, Andersen ML, et al. Association between obesity and sleep disorders in postmenopausal women. Menopause 2018;25(2): 139–44.

134. Rye DB, Trotti LM. Restless legs syndrome and periodic leg movements of sleep. Neurol Clin 2012; 30(4):1137–66.

135. Doan TT, Koo BB, Ogilvie RP, et al. Restless legs syndrome and periodic limb movements during sleep in the Multi-Ethnic Study of Atherosclerosis. Sleep 2018;41(8):zsy106.

136. Ancoli-Israel S, Kripke DF, Klauber MR, et al. Periodic limb movements in sleep in community-dwelling elderly. Sleep 1991;14(6):496–500.

137. Huang WY, Huang CC, Chang CC, et al. Associations of self-reported sleep quality with circulating interferon gamma-inducible protein 10, interleukin 6, and high-sensitivity C-reactive protein in healthy menopausal women. PLoS One 2017;12(1): e0169216.

138. Zhou Y, Yang R, Li C, et al. Sleep disorder, an independent risk associated with arterial stiffness in menopause. Sci Rep 2017;7(1):1904.

139. Hita-Contreras F, Zagalaz-Anula N, Martinez-Amat A, et al. Sleep quality and its association with postural stability and fear of falling among Spanish postmenopausal women. Menopause 2017;25(1):62–9.

140. Chair SY, Wang Q, Cheng HY, et al. Relationship between sleep quality and cardiovascular disease risk in Chinese post-menopausal women. BMC Womens Health 2017;17(1):79.

141. Zhang J, Chan NY, Lam SP, et al. Emergence of sex differences in insomnia symptoms in adolescents: a large-scale school-based study. Sleep 2016;39(8):1563–70.

142. Izci-Balserak B, Pien GW. The relationship and potential mechanistic pathways between sleep disturbances and maternal hyperglycemia. Curr Diab Rep 2014;14(2):459.

143. Caretto M, Giannini A, Simoncini T. An integrated approach to diagnosing and managing sleep disorders in menopausal women. Maturitas 2019; 128:1–3.

Differences Between Men and Women with Chronic Obstructive Pulmonary Disease

Christine Jenkins, AM, MD, FRACP, FThorSoc[a,b,c],*

KEYWORDS

- Chronic obstructive lung disease • COPD • Sex and gender • Treatment outcomes

KEY POINTS

- COPD develops in response to a range of exposures and settings which may differ for men and women, resulting in different pathophysiologic and clinical features.
- Men and women also present at different stages of their disease with different symptom profiles and day to day impact.
- The results of large clinical trials of treatment for COPD have rarely been analysed for potential differences between men and women.
- It is crucial that we understand these differences in order to address them pro-actively, and to develop more effective, targeted approaches to the prevention and management of COPD in men and women.

Chronic obstructive pulmonary disease (COPD) is now the third most frequent cause of death in the world, behind ischemic heart disease and stroke. It will be a major ongoing public health problem for several decades to come because of its increasing international prevalence, aging populations, continued tobacco smoking, and indoor and outdoor and occupational pollution exposure, even though in some countries it is decreasing in prevalence and impact.[1,2] In others it may not decrease, despite reducing tobacco exposure, which is counterbalanced by increasing longevity[3] and reduced mortality from other chronic diseases, such as ischemic heart disease. It is becoming clear that COPD affects men and women differently,[4,5] develops in response to different exposures and doses,[6–9] may be characterized by different pathophysiologic features,[10] and presents differently clinically.[11–13] In an age of precision medicine, it is crucial that we understand these differences to address them

proactively, and to appreciate that more effective, targeted approaches to prevention and management of COPD in men and women will reduce its burden and impact on health, productivity, and mortality.

EPIDEMIOLOGY OF CHRONIC OBSTRUCTIVE PULMONARY DISEASE IN MEN AND WOMEN

Mortality and morbidity from chronic respiratory disease is falling slowly, but differently in men and women and in different parts of the world.[1,14] This change is due to varying exposures, sociodemographic factors, regional differences in access to care, and changes in life expectancy, particularly in high-income areas, where diagnostic improvements may also play a role. Over the period 1990 to 2017, the prevalence, mortality, and Disability Adjusted Life Years (DALY) rates per 100,000 people dropped by 14.3%, 42.6%, and 38.2%, respectively, but there are major regional

The author has nothing to disclose.

[a] Respiratory Group, The George Institute for Global Health, Sydney, Level 5, 1 King Street, Newtown, New South Wales 2042 Australia; [b] UNSW Medicine and Health, UNSW Sydney, NSW, Australia; [c] Concord Clinical School, University of Sydney, NSW, Australia

* PO Box M201, Missenden Road, New South Wales 2050, Australia.

E-mail address: christine.jenkins@sydney.edu.au

Clin Chest Med 42 (2021) 443–456
https://doi.org/10.1016/j.ccm.2021.06.001

differences in prevalence, morbidity, and mortality. Tobacco remains the most important contributor to risk of chronic airflow limitation,[9] but men and women have different rates of non–tobacco-associated airway disease, related especially to their occupational exposures, household air pollution, educational level, and poverty. Asia and Africa are the regions with the highest burden of chronic airways disease, which is only slightly different in men and women even though the causes differ significantly, men more often being tobacco smokers and women more often exposed to indoor air pollution.[9,15–17]

Prevalence of Chronic Obstructive Pulmonary Disease Differs in Men and Women

The prevalence of COPD in women is lower than in men in most studies, but higher than would be expected from tobacco smoke exposure alone.[6,9,18] In the international BOLD study, using a standardized protocol across 12 sites, the overall prevalence of GOLD stage II or higher COPD was 10.1% (SE 4.8), 11.8% (7.9) for men, and 8.5% (5.8) for women.[19] The prevalence increased with age, being 7.5% (95% confidence interval [CI] 5.7–9.4) among people aged $\geq$40 years and 29.2% (18.1–40.2) among people aged $\geq$75. In relation to tobacco smoke exposure, site-specific pack-year odds ratios varied significantly in women but not in men, suggesting there were several contributors to the risk of COPD in women, apart from tobacco exposure.

COPD prevalence has risen more rapidly in women than men in many high-income countries over the past 2 decades.[1,3] This may be a consequence of both the increased longevity and improved survival from cardiovascular disease, as well as the uptake of tobacco smoking by women, which began in the second half of the twentieth century. A significant proportion of men also gave up smoking, and gradually a similar prevalence of men and women smokers became the norm in high-income countries,[6,20,21] although there is considerable regional heterogeneity. In low-income to middle-income countries the prevalence of smoking among women is still relatively low compared with men, but women experience many other sources of smoke exposure, greatly increasing their risk of developing COPD. In the Global Burden of Disease analysis of temporal and geographic trends of mortality and disability from chronic respiratory disease 1990 to 2017, the leading risk factor for deaths and disability due to COPD was tobacco use, including smoking and second-hand smoke, which accounted for 1.41 (95% uncertainty

interval 1.27–1.54) million deaths from COPD and 33.01 (8.94–36.51) million DALYs in 2017.[6] The effect of smoking on deaths from COPD was greater in men than in women. Although the tobacco smoking rates over the period continued to decline in both sexes, a greater decline occurred in men, and thus disparity between the sexes in deaths due to COPD attributable to tobacco use narrowed over time.

In the same study, in regions with a high or middle sociodemographic index, tobacco was the most important risk factor for deaths from COPD, but the proportion of mortality attributable to tobacco decreased as the sociodemographic index declined and particulate matter pollution explained most of the deaths from COPD in regions with a low sociodemographic index. This is likely to mean increasing proportions of women compared with men account for deaths from COPD in low-income countries, secondary to household and outdoor air pollution, whereas in men tobacco remains the major risk factor for COPD.

This is evident in many studies undertaken in low-income countries. For example, in an Indian study tobacco smoking was the predominant smoke exposure in men, whereas smoke from biofuel burning was the predominant exposure in women. Compared with men, women were younger, reported more dyspnea, more severe bronchial obstruction, and more exacerbations. They smoked less and had airway-predominant disease compared with men, who had a higher prevalence of an emphysema-predominant phenotype.

Types of Environmental Exposure Differ Between Men and Women

Many similar studies have observed an increased risk of COPD with biomass smoke exposure, which is most marked in women. Exposure to coal and wood fuels for household cooking and heating increased the risk of incident COPD (adjusted hazard ratios [HRs] ranging from 1.06 to 1.21) in a prospective cohort of 475,827 adults in China (China Kadoorie Biobank), particularly in women and never-smokers, and with longer duration of exposure. The World Health Organization estimates that worldwide, more than 3 billion people are exposed to polluting energy sources from household cooking and heating, and that there are nearly 4 million deaths each year from exposure to household smoke emitted from solid fuels (https://www.who.int/airpollution/en/). In women who cook at home using polluting biomass fuel, it has been estimated that 13 years of exposure at 2 hours per day leads to lung function decline that is equivalent to 10 pack-years of cigarette smoking; however, it is also crucial to note that occupational exposure to fumes, dusts, and gases remain a major source of exposure for men.[1] The vast majority of deaths from chronic respiratory disease (among COPD, asthma, and pneumoconioses) were due to COPD arising from particulate dusts and gases and second-hand smoke.[16] The highest number of deaths and the highest rate of deaths from COPD due to occupational exposures occurred men who had 3 to 4 times the number and rate of deaths compared with women. However, the rate of DALYs increased considerably with age and was highest in the 75 to 84-year group for both men and women.[16]

Because environmental exposures leading to COPD other than active smoking may be more common in women, there is a greater proportion of never-smoking women with COPD than men in most studies. This is evident in the Rotterdam study in which participants were followed for 25 years for incidence and prevalence of COPD. The prevalence of COPD was 6.4% in never-smokers overall, but many more women with COPD were lifelong nonsmokers, the proportion being 27.2% compared with only 7.3% in men. Among the patients with incident COPD who never smoked, the proportion of passive smoking was 51%, and among these passive smokers, most were women (77%). High levels of nonsmoking COPD were also seen in the NHANES III study. Of the 24.9% of participants with mild-moderate COPD who had never smoked, most were women (82.5%). Similar high levels of COPD in nonsmoking adults have been found in studies in Norway (30.8%), Spain,[22] and Italy (33%).

Apart from exposure to indoor and outdoor air pollution, asthma is a significant factor contributing to the prevalence of COPD in nonsmokers. In never-smokers with COPD of all severities in the CanCOLD study, common independent associations were older age and a history of asthma. Among adults older than 40 years, the prevalence of spirometric features of COPD (forced expiratory volume in 1 second [FEV1]/forced vital capacity [FVC] <lower limits of normal) in never-smokers was 6.4%. In moderate-severe COPD, a history of hospitalization in childhood for respiratory illness was discriminative, whereas exposure to passive smoke and biomass fuel for heating was discriminative for women. In all, 47% of the Can-COLD population were never-smokers, and 10% of these had COPD, of whom nearly 70% were women. This could mean that women are either more susceptible or more exposed to nonsmoking risk factors associated with COPD. These

prevalence rates in never-smokers are consistent with reported proportions of 25% to 30% in the United States, Europe, and China.

Occupational Exposures Differ Between Men and Women

The role of the workplace in COPD causation is often underrecognized in women. In low-income and middle-income countries, cottage industries comprise a subgroup of informal, income-generating activities that are often conducted in the home or unregulated environments. Examples include brick making, fish smoking, tobacco curing, and leather working. In high-income countries, barriers to women being employed in traditional male-dominated occupations have progressively been broken down, and women increasingly work in industries such as construction, mining, engineering, manufacturing, road-building, farming, spray painting, and welding, with subsequent exposure to the associated hazards. These industries also continue to be major sources of dust, fume, and gas exposure for men, and many new industries such as the manufactured stone industry are recognized as causing dust diseases. Less often, however, are they recognized as important causes of COPD, sometimes additive with tobacco, but significant contributors to the development of chronic airflow limitation in nonsmokers also. Even so, particular exposures are mostly still typical of either men or women, examples being hairdressing exposures to fumes and dyes in women, and heavy industry gas and fumes exposure in men.

REASONS FOR DIFFERENT PREVALENCE OF CHRONIC OBSTRUCTIVE PULMONARY DISEASE IN MEN AND WOMEN
Different Impact of Cigarette Smoking in Men and Women

Women appear to be more susceptible to the effects of cigarette smoke than men, for a given number smoked per day, and total intake.[23–27] Evidence for this greater vulnerability is strongest in large population studies. In the UK Biobank study,[24] in the approximately 250,000 subjects with acceptable spirometry, the association of airflow obstruction with smoking status (current or previous smoking compared with lifetime nonsmoking) was stronger in women than in men. Among current smokers, the pattern was similar. For equal number of cigarettes per day and years of smoking, women showed greater risk of airflow obstruction than men. Not only were women at risk of airflow obstruction at lower doses of smoking than men (10 vs 19 pack-years), but as well, the risk of airflow obstruction for the same dose of smoking was greater among women than among men. The greatest risk of developing airflow obstruction was seen among those who started smoking at a young age, with the increase in risk at lower doses being steeper among women. For equal time since quitting, the reduction in risk among women seemed less marked than among men. This study highlights many aspects of the differences between men and women, of the impact of tobacco smoking and the contributions of years of smoking, starting age, pack-years, and duration.

In a study from Nanjing, China, exploring the relationship between cigarette smoking and COPD among urban and rural adults older than 35, the overall prevalence of diagnosed COPD was significantly higher among men than in women (7.2% vs 4.7%, $P<.0001$); however, the relationship between prevalence of COPD and total cigarette smoking was dose dependent by gradient in women, whereas only men with the highest cigarette smoking rates were more likely to have COPD.[28] Similarly, in an analysis[29] of the medical records of 844 patients with COPD in Finland, women reported significantly fewer pack-years than men. Compared with men, women had less advanced airway obstruction, but more severe gas transfer impairment. Parenchymal damage measured by diffusion capacity correlated more strongly with FEV1% predicted in women than men. This cohort showed several significant gender-dependent differences in their clinical presentation, including women having a lower body mass index, and more psychiatric conditions, especially depression, but men being more likely to have cardiovascular diseases, diabetes, and alcoholism.

Different Susceptibility to Smoke, Dusts, Fumes

There is also indirect evidence suggesting that for a given level of risk exposure, women are more susceptible to developing COPD or have more rapid disease progression than men. A study by Sørheim and colleagues[23] found that women were disproportionately represented in the subset of patients with COPD with severe disease despite minimal tobacco smoke exposure (defined as <20 pack-years). Women were also more likely to present with COPD before the age of 60. In a related observation in 2 Danish longitudinal population studies (combined N = 13,897) after adjusting for smoking, women had a greater risk of COPD-related hospitalization compared with men. It is not clear whether these differences in susceptibility are due to differences in genetic predisposition, physical differences (for example airway and lung size), hormonal influences, or second-hand risk exposure. A recent study by Hardin and colleagues suggests that there may be variations between different subgroups of female patients that influence susceptibility to parenchymal destruction; however, more research is needed to fully elucidate these and other findings.

Potential Differences in Mechanisms for Development of Chronic Obstructive Pulmonary Disease

Although the reasons for these differences have not been clearly elucidated, the explanations are likely to be multifactorial. There are many possible mechanisms, including different molecular and metabolic responses to cigarette and biomass smoke, different airway geometry, patterns of inhalation, intensity and diversity of exposure, and cellular vulnerability.[27–31] In a study examining the pattern of smoke inhalation in 28 actively smoking men and women, it was shown that while smoking, women preferentially recruited the rib cage with lesser contribution of the abdomen, whereas men preferentially recruit the abdominal compartment. These differing patterns of chest expansion may result in different exposure of small airways and lung parenchyma to inhaled smoke.[30]

At a cellular level, there are many potential metabolic and hormonal pathways that are significantly different in men and women that could potentially influence susceptibility to the effects of cigarette smoke.[31] In proteomic analyses of broncoalveolar lavage (BAL), significant gender differences were seen in the cell proteome in female but not male patients with COPD.[32] In a related study,[33] the investigators confirmed these findings showing that cells from female smokers with normal lung function and early-stage COPD showed more pronounced alterations compared with male smokers in whom alterations were minor. These changes involved dysregulation of phagocytosis and increase in oxidative stress, which correlated well with specific clinical features, including measures of emphysema, FEV1 and FEV1/FVC.

In another BAL study, T-cell chemokine receptor expression was examined demonstrating disparate profiles of T-cell recruitment to the lower airways of women and men. Among female smokers with COPD, T-cell immune responses were linked to BAL macrophage numbers and goblet cell density, and T-helper:T-cytotoxic cell response was associated with emphysema on high-resolution computed tomography. The highly gender-dependent T-cell profile in COPD suggested different links between cellular events and clinical manifestations in women compared with men, which are potential explanations for different impacts of smoking. These differences in activation of inflammatory pathways and cellular mechanisms may help explain the difference in smoke susceptibility, clinical manifestations, and course of COPD in female patients compared with male patients.

Reasons for smoking may differ between genders. Female empowerment through tobacco smoking was a concept widely and deftly promoted by tobacco companies for a number of decades, as was smoking as a means to control body weight. Both are direct appeals to women and likely to be more persuasive reasons to smoke for women than men. In addition, once a smoking habit is established, several lines of evidence suggest that cessation efforts are less successful in women than men; various contributory factors for this have been suggested that require further study. For example, a large, national community study in Canada indicated that women with COPD who smoke have higher rates of nicotine addiction than their male counterparts.

PATTERNS OF PRESENTATION AND SYMPTOM DEVELOPMENT BETWEEN MEN AND WOMEN

It is now well recognized that there are differences in the frequency of particular COPD phenotypes affecting men and women.[34,35] These phenotypes may underpin differing presentations and symptom profiles of men and women. Women appear more likely to exhibit small airway disease (bronchiolitis), whereas men are more prone to develop an emphysematous phenotype.[36–39] Women who develop COPD from biomass exposure are more likely to develop a chronic bronchitic, mucus hypersecretion phenotype, with a slower rate of decline in lung function. Nevertheless, in relation to tobacco smoking also, women are more likely to present with airway-predominant features,[8,40] especially chronic bronchitis and wheeze.[41] Women have more severe symptoms when they do have an emphysema phenotype,[39] but in most studies still have a better life expectancy.[42]

Although it is well accepted that men and women respond differently to the presence of symptoms, it is perhaps not recognized that physiologic features, rather than behavioral features alone, contribute significantly to these different patterns of presentation.[41,43,44] Although in most studies, women are more likely to respond to symptoms by seeking health care advice,[45,46]

this is not the case in all parts of the world, and is strongly influenced by culture, socioeconomic factors, rurality, and access to care.[47–50]

Delayed and Misdiagnosis

Several studies have shown that women are also more likely to be given an asthma diagnosis, even when they have a significant smoking history. This is especially the case in countries in which smoking prevalence is traditionally much higher in men, resulting in a higher rate of misdiagnosis in women with COPD compared with men, potentially leading to suboptimal treatment.[51–54] In one Canadian study, when spirometry was added, a COPD diagnosis became more probable.[52] Another recent Canadian study[29] identified many missed opportunities for care when symptomatic patients presented frequently before diagnosis, to pharmacy, primary care, and specialists. In the 2 years before diagnosis, 72.1% of patients with COPD had a respiratory-related primary care visit that did not result in a COPD diagnosis. Although no gender analysis is reported in that study, similar if not more concerning data from the United Kingdom showed that opportunities for diagnosis were missed in 85% of patients in the 5 years immediately preceding diagnosis of COPD.[55] In this dataset, from 16 years before diagnosis of COPD, and each year until diagnosis, female patients had consistently more missed opportunities in terms of lower respiratory consultations and lower respiratory prescribing consultations than did male patients. The investigators noted that men were more likely to have a chest radiography requested in the year before diagnosis than were women, yet women were more likely to be admitted to hospital in the 2 years before diagnosis than were men. In addition, in relation to diagnostic spirometry, patients with available FEV1 data were more likely to be men, have their smoking status available, and be current or ex-smokers. This suggests that a stereotyped notion of a patients with COPD guides some initial investigations, and that women may be less likely to be seen as being at risk of having COPD, contributing to later diagnosis and treatment.[56]

Although the gender bias in diagnosis is reduced by the use of spirometry, spirometry in general remains underused for the diagnosis and monitoring of COPD, particularly in women,[52] although in a Swedish online survey using case histories, all clinicians identified spirometry as a key diagnostic test and no gender bias was evident.[57] However, in practice it is in primary care where most patients first present and receive their initial diagnosis of COPD.[58–60] Spirometry performance in that setting is low in most countries, giving a higher probability that neither men nor women will receive a COPD diagnosis and optimum treatment when that is the true nature of their disease.[61,62]

Different Symptom Patterns

Prominent airway symptoms, along with a higher prevalence of airway hyperresponsiveness in women may partly account for this tendency to more readily diagnose asthma than COPD in women.[63] Although this tendency is not evident in some studies,[14] a number of investigators have shown that women are more likely to experience delay in the diagnosis of COPD even though they may present earlier.[54,61] This may be a consequence of being more likely to receive an asthma diagnosis than men, even with a similar smoking history,[64] due to coexisting obesity[65] or a spectrum of different comorbidities.[66,67] As different treatment strategies are applied to asthma and COPD, and inhaled corticosteroids (ICS)–long-acting beta agonists (LABA) should not be the correct initial treatment for both, it is important that when possible the 2 diseases are correctly identified and managed.[65]

Men and women appear to experience different spectrums and severity of symptoms for a given severity of spirometric abnormality. In a Spanish study, women were younger, smoked less, had better Pao_2 and lower $Paco_2$, but more exacerbations in the last year and fewer comorbidities; however, they performed poorer in walking distance, had worse St George's Respiratory Questionnaire (SGRQ) total, symptoms, and activity scores, and had a higher degree of dyspnea than men.[68] Comorbidities have been shown to be different in a range of studies, with a greater predominance of anxiety, depression, osteoporosis, and sleep disturbance but a lower prevalence of cardiovascular diagnoses[46,54,69] in women.

Several studies show that for a similar degree of airway obstruction, women have worse scores on health status questionnaires than men, including for SGRQ domains.[70] Women may also experience greater psychosocial impairment related to COPD than men[71] and have greater levels of anxiety and depression.[12,29,67,72–74] This aligns with studies demonstrating lower scores in the mental component of the Short Form-12 health status questionnaire compared with men.[69] Younger women in particular may have a higher symptom burden with worse dyspnea, airflow limitation, greater risk for exacerbations, and more likely categorization in GOLD groups B and D compared to men with COPD[75]

DIFFERENT APPROACHES TO CARE OCCUR FOR MEN AND WOMEN

Men and women also receive different treatments, both pharmacologic and nonpharmacologic for their COPD, although it is highly variable around the world, men receiving more interventions and earlier treatment and diagnosis in some settings,[11] and women in others.[76]

Tobacco Uptake and Cessation in Men and Women

The potential major benefits from smoking reduction that have occurred in many countries may differ for men and women also. Such differences were seen in the Tromso Study, where COPD morbidity decreased between 2001 and 2017, associated with daily smoking reduction from 29.9% to 14.1% among women and from 31.4% to 12.8% among men ($P<.0001$). The age-standardized prevalence of COPD dropped from 7.6% to 5.6% among women ($P = .2$) and from 7.3% to 5.6% among men ($P = .003$). This significant drop among men was associated with a decreased hospitalization rate and reduced dispensing of oral corticosteroids or/and antibiotics for COPD exacerbations. These data highlight the opportunity to target smoking cessation and to maintain public health initiatives to reduce the uptake of smoking among young people. These data, along with those from the UK Biobank study, highlight the vulnerability of women in particular to the damaging effects of tobacco smoke at an early age should be included in health messaging regarding the harms of tobacco.

In support of this relationship between increased tobacco smoking and adverse health effects becoming more evident in women, the high prevalence of smoking among French women since the 1970s is evident from a review of National Health surveys, smoking prevalence, and health outcomes.[77] The incidence of COPD increased by 100% among women between 2002 and 2015; for other tobacco-related diseases, such as myocardial infarction before the age of 65, the incidence increased by 50% between 2002 and 2015 in women versus 16% in men. In this study, the estimated number of women who died as a result of smoking more than doubled between 2000 and 2014 (7% vs 3% of all deaths).

There is mixed evidence on the comparative success rates of men and women in smoking cessation. Some evidence suggests that women may be less successful with long-term smoking cessation than men,[4,78] especially with nicotine replacement therapy, although some pharmacologic interventions appear to be equally effective in men and women.[79] In most studies, women with COPD have a higher prevalence of anxiety and depression than men as comorbidities associated with their COPD,[67,80,81] and this may complicate their attempts to stop smoking, and add to their tendency to relapse. These mental health issues may require specific therapy, both pharmacologic and behavioral to maximize the possibility of success with specific tobacco cessation approaches.

In a recent analysis of helpline callers with COPD,[82] 81.4% were current smokers. This did not show a gender bias but highlights the need for tobacco cessation support, including both behavioral support and pharmacotherapy. On the other hand, specific needs in addressing tobacco dependency for men and women have been highlighted by previous authors along with the necessity for a gendered approach[83] to better understand the factors underlying tobacco dependency and to help all people with tailored cessation strategies. This is especially important, as active promotion of tobacco is occurring in low-income countries and most of what we have learned about cessation derives from populations of smokers in high-income countries.

Multiple studies from different regions of the world have suggested that women experience higher levels of health care need, particularly hospital presentation and admission, than men with COPD. Two longitudinal Danish studies,[6] the Copenhagen City Heart Study and the Glostrup Population Study combined, found that after adjusting for smoking, women had a 1.5 times greater probability of COPD-related hospitalizations than men, which could not be accounted for by higher rates of hospitalization in women in general. Women were also more likely to present with COPD before the age of 60 years and are disproportionately represented in the subset of patients with COPD with severe disease despite significantly lower tobacco smoke exposure.[7]

Acute Exacerbations of Chronic Obstructive Pulmonary Disease

Several studies report a higher rate of exacerbations in women versus men with COPD,[41] although generally women have better short-term and long-term survival after severe exacerbations requiring hospitalization.[42,84] This is despite the fact that mortality rates in many high-income countries are increasing for women and declining for men,[85,86] and in some, women's COPD-mortality rates are now higher overall.[87] Exacerbation rates and symptom burden have been higher in women

recruited into several large COPD clinical trials as well as in large population cohorts.[41] In the ECLIPSE cohort, the rate of exacerbations was significantly higher in women than men at each GOLD stage.[88] In a post hoc analysis of the POET-COPD trial, the risk of first exacerbation was higher for women compared with men (HR 1.31; 95% CI 1.19–1.43).[89] In the TORCH study, the time to first exacerbation was shorter and the rate of exacerbations was 25% higher in women than in men ($P<0.001$; 95% CI 16–34), although the number of hospital admissions caused by exacerbations was similar.[90] Although several studies show that women are more likely to be admitted to hospital for an exacerbation,[91] they appear less likely to die in hospital.[92] In a population of more than 40,000 participants in the Quebec Insurance databases, men had a significantly increased risk of death (adjusted HR 1.45; 95% CI 1.42–1.49) and rehospitalization for COPD (adjusted HR 1.12; 95% CI 1.09–1.15).[93]

Differences in admission rates and in-hospital management may be both culture-sensitive and country-sensitive. In an Italian retrospective cohort study based on administrative data, hospital admissions among residents aged ≥65 years showed higher rates of readmission for men with COPD than women. The investigators referred to a study suggesting that direct costs for management are higher in male than in female patients,[94] although perhaps more importantly as a general observation, men use primary care health services less frequently than women, are less likely to adopt preventive initiatives, and are less health literate.[95] In a UK study of hospitalized patients for general medical conditions, risk factors for men but not women for readmission within 30 days included having no primary care physician visit within 30 days. As well in a self-reported survey, fewer men than women understood and attended their follow-up appointments after acute hospitalization.[96]

By contrast, in a nationwide Chinese study published more than 10 years ago, profound differences in women and men were noted in relation to COPD diagnosis, care, and health knowledge.[11] Fewer women reported having a severe exacerbation resulting in hospitalization in the previous year and more women reported that they never heard of COPD before. Fewer had pulmonary function tests done initially or annually, reported not having had pulmonary rehabilitation and not knowing that COPD should be given combined therapy and long-term treatment. Although some of these differences were relatively small between men and women, and may not apply so starkly now, they suggest consistency in gender bias. Many differences have been reported globally, which points to specific factors that are best understood at a local level to be properly addressed.[13,14,57,97–100]

Treatment for Stable Chronic Obstructive Pulmonary Disease

Smoking cessation is the most important initial step in COPD management. The Lung Health Study suggests that women may benefit more from smoking cessation than men, even though other studies suggest they may have more difficulty giving it up.[101,102] There are no studies designed to examine sex-related differences in the effects of nicotine replacement therapy, and smoking cessation medications (such as bupropion and varenicline) appear to be equally effective in men and women.[4,53,78,79] As women may have greater levels of anxiety and greater smoking dependence than men, they may benefit also from a tailored behavioral approach.[78] Pulmonary rehabilitation is also a key nonpharmacologic intervention for patients with COPD, but very few studies report any differences between men and women and most enroll more men than women, although most who do suggest there are no consistent differences,[103,104] and a systematic review concluded that there was insufficient evidence to support or refute gender-associated differences in pulmonary rehabilitation outcomes.[105]

Among other nonpharmacologic therapies, in a recent report of a German COPD cohort,[106] self-report of having received a recommendation for nondrug treatments did not differ according to sex. However, women showed significantly higher utilization rates than men for all interventions except influenza vaccination. Utilization of nonpharmacological interventions was lower in men and current smokers. By contrast, in a recently reported UK primary care cohort of more than 80,000 participants in a national COPD audit,[107] patients who were older, female, more deprived, or had a comorbidity of diabetes, asthma, or painful condition had significantly lower odds of referral to pulmonary rehabilitation.

In pharmacologic trials, only recently have gendered analyses been undertaken and they remain very uncommon in the statistical analysis plan as prespecified analyses. Studies may be underpowered for analyses based on sex, particularly when women are underrepresented, but this is the case for many prespecified subanalyses even when the primary outcome is highly significant. Some studies, however, have published results that inform us regarding potential sex-related benefits or harms from interventions in randomized clinical trials, going as far back as the EUROSCOP study,[108] in which the improvement in phlegm on budesonide was limited to men. Longitudinally, men showed a greater response based on their symptom reporting to cigarette exposure (worsening) and treatment (improvement). Women initially reported greater remission of symptoms in the first year of follow-up but over the 3-year period, the symptom prevalence differences between men and women disappeared.

In the TORCH study,[90] in which just over 75% of the patients were male, baseline characteristics differed between men and women; women were on average younger, and had higher FEV1 and worse St. George's Respiratory Questionnaire and Medical Research Council (MRC) dyspnea scores. After adjusting for differences in baseline factors, the risk of dying was 16% higher in men than in women, although not statistically significant. As already mentioned, the mean exacerbation rate was 25% higher in women than in men, and women reported worse dyspnea and health status scores than men.

More recently, a post hoc analysis by gender was undertaken in the FLAME study, comparing response to indacaterol/glycopyrronium to salmeterol/fluticasone in patients with exacerbating COPD. The dual bronchodilator demonstrated similar trends for exacerbation prevention and lung function improvement in men and women with moderate-to-very severe COPD and a history of exacerbations compared with salmeterol fluticasone. Of great interest were the similar observations in FLAME as TORCH regarding the differences between men and women, which add great value in understanding the potential for different outcomes, clinical features, and treatment effects. Similarly, 76% of the total population were men. At baseline, women were significantly younger, and had longer duration of COPD compared with men. A higher proportion of women than men were current smokers, and women were found to have a lower cumulative smoking habit. A greater number of men had more severe COPD and airflow limitation than women at baseline; however, a higher proportion of women had a history of $\geq$2 exacerbations in the previous year. The modified MRC score at baseline was similar between men and women, but COPD assessment test score was higher in women, although women had better lung function. The investigators commented that minor differences seen between men and women need to be prospectively studied given the small numbers in the analyses.

Adherence

In general, women are thought to be less adherent to medication than their male counterparts; however, the data are inconclusive in COPD. This may be because adherence to inhaled therapies may be deliberate or inadvertent, the commonest reason for unintentional lack of adherence being poor inhaler technique, but complexity of regimens, polypharmacy, and a range of different inhaler types adds to the risk of poor adherence in COPD.[109] Knowledge and skills can be improved. In the Lung Health Study, women were more likely to report good adherence, but no more likely than men to be adherent, as objectively recorded by canister weights.[110]

Some limited data suggest that women with COPD are less likely to be controlled and content with their COPD treatment than men.[4] As already indicated, generally women have a higher symptom burden, particularly dyspnea, but overall worse quality-of-life scores, suggesting they may have greater need for their daily medications. In some studies, women with COPD are more adherent with long-term medications than men[97,111] and in others less so.[112]

It is well known that patients may progressively reduce their prescribed medications over time, tending to resume them for worsening symptoms and exacerbations. In a Canadian study,[113] there was an increased risk of both long-acting muscarinic antagonist and LABA/ICS medications being discontinued in patients who had COPD for more than 2 years, but discontinuation did not differ between men and women, although men were less likely to deliberately cease their medications in the previously cited study.[109] Whether men or women are more or less adherent, outside of clinical trials, adherence is uniformly low over time and associated with worse clinical outcomes.[114,115] Regular review of inhaler technique and adherence is a key clinical intervention that can significantly improve outcomes.[116]

Considering the increasing and expansive literature on COPD management, there have been far too many missed opportunities to better understand the different outcomes of treatment in men and women with COPD. As a consequence, there is scant information from clinical trials to support physicians with tailored, gender-focused pharmacologic treatment of COPD[117] and current guidelines tend to minimize or ignore this potential effect because major randomized trials have not addressed it.[118–120] The lack of gender-specific recommendations could be because there is no difference in the effectiveness or efficacy of treatments; however, this is not known. Analyses suggest that clinical trials populations differ from real-world patients, particularly in gender distribution.

As the rate of smoking in women has increased and will inevitably be reflected in increased COPD morbidity and mortality in future decades,[17,77,121] and as indoor and outdoor air pollution continue to contribute so significantly to obstructive lung disease, there is an urgent need for future trials to redress this information deficit. Further, as many women and children in low-income countries will be exposed to biomass fuels for heating and cooking for decades to come,[122,123] specific studies examining the effects of treatment in those with a biomass-chronic bronchitis phenotype of COPD are urgently needed. Randomized controlled trials should adopt strategies to recruit women who have been until very recently, grossly underrepresented in randomized trials, and to prespecify subanalyses based on gender to assess responses to treatment and their determinants. Systematic reviews and meta-analyses, as well as less robust but potentially informative post hoc analyses should be undertaken to explore gender-related treatment effects and to plan future studies. These analyses would be hypothesis generating and would help identify differential effects of treatment and target therapy to reduce the impact of COPD in both men and women.

SUMMARY

There are many differences between men and women in risk factor vulnerability and impact, symptom development, presentation, clinical manifestations, and outcomes of COPD. These differences have been very inadequately explored, which is of particular concern in view of the delay in diagnosis and treatment that occurs for both men and women, as well as the need to use all therapies in a targeted and tailored way for best clinical gain and least harm. Taking a gendered approach to study design and treatment assessment, which includes prespecifying analyses that enable a better understanding of differences between men and women with COPD, would make a major contribution to achieving better outcomes.

CLINICS CARE POINTS

- Sex and gender related differences in COPD aetiology and pathophysiology manifest as different clinical phenotypes, with differing symptoms, time of presentation and prognosis in the trajectory of COPD.

- These different clinical profiles have important consequences for diagnosis and management but there is a scarcity of research into targeting treatment to address these differences to achieve best possible outcomes for men and women with COPD.

- COPD is a heterogeneous disease and develops differently in men and women, depending on susceptibility, the underlying contributors and continuing exposures. The impact and burden of symptoms of COPD are also different for men and women in their daily lives. Taking a detailed history which explores and acknowledges these differences will help clinicians develop a tailored treatment plan for each patient.

- Research is urgently needed to further refine our understanding of sex and gender related responses to treatment and the importance of this in determining optimal management for men and women with COPD.

REFERENCES

1. Prevalence and attributable health burden of chronic respiratory diseases, 1990-2017: a systematic analysis for the Global Burden of Disease Study 2017. Lancet Respir Med 2020;8(6):585–96.
2. Backman H, Vanfleteren L, Lindberg A, et al. Decreased COPD prevalence in Sweden after decades of decrease in smoking. Respir Res 2020; 21(1):283.
3. Wen H, Xie C, Wang L, et al. Difference in long-term trends in COPD mortality between China and the U.S., 1992-2017: an age-period-cohort analysis. Int J Environ Res Public Health 2019;16(9):30.
4. Aryal S, Diaz-Guzman E, Mannino DM. Influence of sex on chronic obstructive pulmonary disease risk and treatment outcomes. Int J Chron Obstruct Pulmon Dis 2014;9:1145–54.
5. Jordan RE, Miller MR, Lam K, et al. Sex, susceptibility to smoking and chronic obstructive pulmonary disease: the effect of different diagnostic criteria. Analysis of the Health Survey for England. Thorax 2012;67(7):600–5.
6. Li X, Cao X, Guo M, et al. Trends and risk factors of mortality and disability adjusted life years for chronic respiratory diseases from 1990 to 2017: systematic analysis for the Global Burden of Disease Study 2017. BMJ 2020;368:m234.
7. Moll M, Regan EA, Hokanson JE, et al. The association of multiparity with lung function and chronic obstructive pulmonary disease-related phenotypes. Chronic Obstructive Pulm Dis 2020;7(2): 86–98.
8. Po JY, FitzGerald JM, Carlsten C. Respiratory disease associated with solid biomass fuel exposure in rural women and children: systematic review and meta-analysis. Thorax 2011;66(3):232–9.
9. Burney P, Patel J, Minelli C, et al. Prevalence and population attributable risk for chronic airflow obstruction in a large multinational study. Am J Respir Crit Care Med 2020;10:10.
10. Young KA, Regan EA, Han MK, et al. Subtypes of COPD have unique distributions and differential risk of mortality. Chronic Obstructive Pulm Dis 2019;6(5):400–13.
11. Jia G, Lu M, Wu R, et al. Gender difference on the knowledge, attitude, and practice of COPD diagnosis and treatment: a national, multicenter, cross-sectional survey in China. Int J Chron Obstruct Pulmon Dis 2018;13:3269–80.
12. Roche N, Deslee G, Caillaud D, et al. Impact of gender on COPD expression in a real-life cohort. Respir Res 2014;15:20.
13. Amegadzie JE, Gamble JM, Farrell J, et al. Gender differences in inhaled pharmacotherapy utilization in patients with obstructive airway diseases (OADs): a population-based study. Int J Chron Obstruct Pulmon Dis 2020;15:2355–66.
14. Lamprecht B, Soriano JB, Studnicka M, et al. Determinants of underdiagnosis of COPD in national and international surveys. Chest 2015;148(4):971–85.
15. Babatola SS. Global burden of diseases attributable to air pollution. J Public Health Africa 2018; 9(3):813.
16. Occupational Chronic Respiratory Risk Factors Collaborators. Global and regional burden of chronic respiratory disease in 2016 arising from non-infectious airborne occupational exposures: a systematic analysis for the Global Burden of Disease Study 2016. Occup Environ Med 2020; 77(3):142–50.
17. Burney P, Jithoo A, Kato B, et al. Chronic obstructive pulmonary disease mortality and prevalence: the associations with smoking and poverty–a BOLD analysis. Thorax 2014;69(5):465–73.
18. Abramson MJ, Wigmann C, Altug H, et al. Ambient air pollution is associated with airway inflammation in older women: a nested cross-sectional analysis. BMJ Open Respir Res 2020;7(1):e000549.
19. Buist AS, McBurnie MA, Vollmer WM, et al. International variation in the prevalence of COPD (The BOLD Study): a population-based prevalence study. Lancet 2007;370(9589):741–50.
20. Ng R, Sutradhar R, Yao Z, et al. Smoking, drinking, diet and physical activity-modifiable lifestyle risk factors and their associations with age to first chronic disease. Int J Epidemiol 2020;49(1): 113–30.
21. Melbye H, Helgeland J, Karlstad O, et al. Is the disease burden from COPD in Norway falling off? A study of time trends in three different data sources. Int J Chron Obstruct Pulmon Dis 2020;15:323–34.

22. Trigueros JA, Riesco JA, Alcazar-Navarrete B, et al. Clinical features of women with COPD: sex differences in a cross-sectional study in Spain ("The ESPIRAL-ES study"). Int J Chron Obstruct Pulmon Dis 2019;14:2469–78.

23. Sørheim I-C, Johannessen A, Gulsvik A, et al. Gender differences in COPD: are women more susceptible to smoking effects than men? Thorax 2010;65(6):480–5.

24. Amaral AFS, Strachan DP, Burney PGJ, et al. Female smokers are at greater risk of airflow obstruction than male smokers. UK Biobank. Am J Respir Crit Care Med 2017;195(9):1226–35.

25. Sansores RH, Ramirez-Venegas A. COPD in women: susceptibility or vulnerability? Eur Respir J 2016;47(1):19–22.

26. Wang B, Xiao D, Wang C. Smoking and chronic obstructive pulmonary disease in Chinese population: a meta-analysis. Clin Respir J 2015;9(2):165–75.

27. Downs SH, Brandli O, Zellweger JP, et al. Accelerated decline in lung function in smoking women with airway obstruction: SAPALDIA 2 cohort study. Respir Res 2005;6:45.

28. Xu F, Yin X, Zhang M, et al. Prevalence of physician-diagnosed COPD and its association with smoking among urban and rural residents in regional mainland China. Chest 2005;128(4):2818–23.

29. Laitinen THU, Kupiainen H, Tammilehto L, et al. Real-world clinical data identifies gender-related profiles in chronic obstructive pulmonary disease. J Chronic Obstructive Pulm Dis 2009;6:6.

30. Polverino M, Capuozzo A, Cicchitto G, et al. Smoking pattern in men and women: a possible contributor to gender differences in smoke-related lung diseases. Am J Respir Crit Care Med 2020;202(7):1048–51.

31. Han MK. Chronic obstructive pulmonary disease in women: a biologically focused review with a systematic search strategy. Int J Chron Obstruct Pulmon Dis 2020;15:711–21.

32. Kohler M, Sandberg A, Kjellqvist S, et al. Gender differences in the bronchoalveolar lavage cell proteome of patients with chronic obstructive pulmonary disease. J Allergy Clin Immunol 2013;131(3):743–51.

33. Yang M, Kohler M, Heyder T, et al. Proteomic profiling of lung immune cells reveals dysregulation of phagocytotic pathways in female-dominated molecular COPD phenotype. Respir Res 2018;19(1):39.

34. Salvi SS, Brashier BB, Londhe J, et al. Phenotypic comparison between smoking and non-smoking chronic obstructive pulmonary disease. Respir Res 2020;21(1):50.

35. Grabicki M, Kuznar-Kaminska B, Rubinsztajn R, et al. COPD course and comorbidities: are there gender differences? Adv Exp Med Biol 2019;1113:43–51.

36. Hardin M, Foreman M, Dransfield MT, et al. Sex-specific features of emphysema among current and former smokers with COPD. Eur Respir J 2016;47(1):104–12.

37. Camp PG, Coxson HO, Levy RD, et al. Sex differences in emphysema and airway disease in smokers. Chest 2009;136(6):1480–8.

38. Han MK, Kazerooni EA, Lynch DA, et al. Chronic obstructive pulmonary disease exacerbations in the COPDGene study: associated radiologic phenotypes. Radiology 2011;261(1):274–82.

39. Martinez FJ, Curtis JL, Sciurba F, et al. Sex differences in severe pulmonary emphysema. Am J Respir Crit Care Med 2007;176(3):243–52.

40. Regalado J, Perez-Padilla R, Sansores R, et al. The effect of biomass burning on respiratory symptoms and lung function in rural Mexican women. Am J Respir Crit Care Med 2006;174(8):901–5.

41. Sundh J, Johansson G, Larsson K, et al. The phenotype of concurrent chronic bronchitis and frequent exacerbations in patients with severe COPD attending Swedish secondary care units. Int J Chron Obstruct Pulmon Dis 2015;10:2327–34.

42. de Torres JP, Cote CG, Lopez MV, et al. Sex differences in mortality in patients with COPD. Eur Respir J 2009;33(3):528–35.

43. Xiao T, Qiu H, Chen Y, et al. Prevalence of anxiety and depression symptoms and their associated factors in mild COPD patients from community settings, Shanghai, China: a cross-sectional study. BMC Psychiatry 2018;18(1):89.

44. Kim V, Davey A, Comellas AP, et al. Clinical and computed tomographic predictors of chronic bronchitis in COPD: a cross sectional analysis of the COPDGene study. Respir Res 2014;15:52.

45. Barsky AJ, Borus JF. Somatic symptom reporting in women and men. J Gen Intern Med 2001;16:266–75.

46. Watson L, Vestbo J, Postma DS, et al. Gender differences in the management and experience of chronic obstructive pulmonary disease. Respir Med 2004;98(12):1207–13.

47. Hwang YI, Park YB, Yoon HK, et al. Male current smokers have low awareness and optimistic bias about COPD: field survey results about COPD in Korea. Int J Chron Obstruct Pulmon Dis 2019;14:271–7.

48. Choi JY, Kim SY, Lee JH, et al. Clinical characteristics of chronic obstructive pulmonary disease in female patients: findings from a KOCOSS cohort. Int J Chron Obstruct Pulmon Dis 2020;15:2217–24.

49. Abramson MJ, Kaushik S, Benke GP, et al. Symptoms and lung function decline in a middle-aged

cohort of males and females in Australia. Int J Chron Obstruct Pulmon Dis 2016;11:1097–103.

50. Cai L, Wang XM, Fan LM, et al. Socioeconomic variations in chronic obstructive pulmonary disease prevalence, diagnosis, and treatment in rural Southwest China. BMC Public Health 2020;20(1):536.

51. Ancochea J, Miravitlles M, García-Río F, et al. Underdiagnosis of chronic obstructive pulmonary disease in women: quantification of the problem, determinants and proposed actions. Arch Bronconeumol 2013;49(6):223–9.

52. Chapman KR, Tashkin DP, Pye DJ. Gender bias in the diagnosis of COPD. Chest 2001;119(6):1691–5.

53. Han MK, Postma D, Mannino DM, et al. Gender and chronic obstructive pulmonary disease: why it matters. Am J Respir Crit Care Med 2007;176(12):1179–84.

54. Martinez CH, Raparla S, Plauschinat CA, et al. Gender differences in symptoms and care delivery for chronic obstructive pulmonary disease. J Womens Health (Larchmt) 2012;21(12):1267–74.

55. Jones RCM, Price D, Ryan D, et al. Opportunities to diagnose chronic obstructive pulmonary disease in routine care in the UK: a retrospective study of a clinical cohort. Lancet Respir Med 2014;2(4):267–76.

56. Ohar J, Fromer L, Donohue JF. Reconsidering sex-based stereotypes of COPD. Prim Care Respir J 2011;20(4):370–8.

57. Akbarshahi H, Ahmadi Z, Currow DC, et al. No gender-related bias in COPD diagnosis and treatment in Sweden: a randomised, controlled, case-based trial. ERJ Open Res 2020;6(4):00342–2020.

58. Miravitlles M, Andreu I, Romero Y, et al. Difficulties in differential diagnosis of COPD and asthma in primary care. Br J Gen Pract 2012;62(595):e68–75.

59. Llordes M, Jaen A, Almagro P, et al. Prevalence, risk factors and diagnostic accuracy of COPD among smokers in primary care. COPD 2015;12(4):404–12.

60. Barrecheguren M, Monteagudo M, Ferrer J, et al. Treatment patterns in COPD patients newly diagnosed in primary care. A population-based study. Respir Med 2016;111:47–53.

61. Roberts NJ, Patel IS, Partridge MR. The diagnosis of COPD in primary care; gender differences and the role of spirometry. Respir Med 2016;111:60–3.

62. Walker PP, Mitchell P, Diamantea F, et al. Effect of primary-care spirometry on the diagnosis and management of COPD. Eur Respir J 2006;28(5):945–52.

63. Anthonisen NR. Lessons from the lung health study. Proc Am Thorac Soc 2004;1(2):143–5.

64. Martinez CH, Raparla S, Plauschinat CA, et al. Gender differences in symptoms and care delivery for COPD. J Womens Health 2012;21(12):1267–74.

65. Walters JA, Walters EH, Nelson M, et al. Factors associated with misdiagnosis of COPD in primary care. Prim Care Respir J 2011;20(4):396–402.

66. Sillen MJ, Franssen FM, Delbressine JM, et al. Heterogeneity in clinical characteristics and co-morbidities in dyspneic individuals with COPD GOLD D: findings of the DICES trial. Respir Med 2013;107(8):1186–94.

67. Raherison C, Tillie-Leblond I, Prudhomme A, et al. Clinical characteristics and quality of life in women with COPD: an observational study. BMC Womens Health 2014;14(1):31.

68. de Torres J, Casanova C, Herna'ndez C, et al. Gender and COPD in patients attending a pulmonary clinic. Chest 2005;128:2012–6.

69. Carrasco-Garrido P, de Miguel-Diez J, Rejas-Gutierrez J, et al. Characteristics of chronic obstructive pulmonary disease in Spain from a gender perspective. BMC Pulm Med 2009;9:2.

70. Ferrari R, Tanni SE, Lucheta PA, et al. Gender differences in predictors of health status in patients with COPD. J Bras Pneumol 2010;36(1):37–43.

71. Low G, Gutman G. Examining the role of gender in health-related quality of life: perceptions of older adults with chronic obstructive pulmonary disease. J Gerontol Nurs 2006;32(11):42–9.

72. Naberan K, Azpeitia A, Cantoni J, et al. Impairment of quality of life in women with chronic obstructive pulmonary disease. Respir Med 2012;106(3):367–73.

73. Dowson C, Laing R, Barraclough R, et al. The use of the Hospital Anxiety and Depression Scale (HADS) in patients with chronic obstructive pulmonary disease: a pilot study. N Z Med J 2001;114(1141):447–9.

74. Gudmundsson G, Gislason T, Janson C, et al. Depression, anxiety and health status after hospitalisation for COPD: a multicentre study in the Nordic countries. Respir Med 2006;100(1):87–93.

75. DeMeo DL, Ramagopalan S, Kavati A, et al. Women manifest more severe COPD symptoms across the life course. Int J Chron Obstruct Pulmon Dis 2018;13:3021–9.

76. Aberg J, Hasselgren M, Montgomery S, et al. Sex-related differences in management of Swedish patients with a clinical diagnosis of chronic obstructive pulmonary disease. Int J Chron Obstruct Pulmon Dis 2019;14:961–9.

77. Olie V, Pasquereau A, Assogba FAG, et al. Changes in tobacco-related morbidity and mortality in French women: worrying trends. Eur J Public Health 2020;30(2):380–5.

78. Rahmanian SD, Diaz PT, Wewers ME. Tobacco use and cessation among women: research and treatment-related issues. J Womens Health 2011;20(3):349–57.

79. Gonzales D, Rennard SI, Nides M, et al. Vareni-cline, an alpha4beta2 nicotinic acetylcholine receptor partial agonist, vs sustained-release bupropion and placebo for smoking cessation: a randomized controlled trial. JAMA 2006;296(1):47–55.

80. Yohannes AM, Mullerova H, Hanania NA, et al. Long-term course of depression trajectories in patients with COPD: a 3-year follow-up analysis of the evaluation of COPD longitudinally to identify predictive surrogate endpoints cohort. Chest 2016;149(4):916–26.

81. Sawalha S, Hedman L, Backman H, et al. The impact of comorbidities on mortality among men and women with COPD: report from the OLIN COPD study. Ther Adv Respir Dis 2019;13. 1753466619860058.

82. Mathew AR, Guzman M, Bridges C, et al. Assessment of self-management treatment needs among COPD helpline callers. COPD 2019;16(1):82–8.

83. Amos A, Greaves L, Nichter M, et al. Women and tobacco: a call for including gender in tobacco control research, policy and practice. Tob Control 2012;21(2):236–43.

84. Doucet M, Rochette L, Hamel D. Incidence, prevalence, and mortality trends in chronic obstructive pulmonary disease over 2001 to 2011: a public health point of view of the burden. Can Respir J 2016;2016:7518287.

85. Mannino D, Brown C, Giovino G. Obstructive lung disease deaths in the United States from 1979 through 1993: an analysis using multiple-cause mortality data. Am J Respir Crit Care Med 1997;156:814–8.

86. Gershon A, Hwee J, Victor JC, et al. Mortality trends in women and men with COPD in Ontario, Canada, 1996-2012. Thorax 2015;70(2):121–6.

87. Ringbaek T, Seersholm N, Viskum K. Standardised mortality rates in females and males with COPD and asthma. Eur Respir J 2005;25(5):891–5.

88. Agusti A, Calverley PM, Celli B, et al. Characterisation of COPD heterogeneity in the ECLIPSE cohort. Respir Res 2010;11:122.

89. Beeh KM, Glaab T, Stowasser S, et al. Characterisation of exacerbation risk and exacerbator phenotypes in the POET-COPD trial. Respir Res 2013;14(1):116.

90. Celli B, Vestbo J, Jenkins CR, et al. Sex differences in mortality and clinical expressions of patients with chronic obstructive pulmonary disease the TORCH experience. Am J Respir Crit Care Med 2011;183(3):317–22.

91. Prescott E, Bjerg AM, Andersen PK, et al. Gender difference in smoking effects on lung function and risk of hospitalization for COPD: results from a Danish longitudinal population stud. Eur Respir J 1997;10:822–7.

92. Ekstrom MP, Jogreus C, Strom KE. Comorbidity and sex-related differences in mortality in oxygen-dependent chronic obstructive pulmonary disease. PLoS One 2012;7(4):e35806.

93. Gonzalez AV, Suissa S, Ernst P. Gender differences in survival following hospitalisation for COPD. Thorax 2011;66(1):38–42.

94. Dal Negro R, Rossi A, Cerveri I. The burden of COPD in Italy: results from the Confronting COPD survey. Respir Med 2003;97(Suppl C):S43–50.

95. Galdas PM, Cheater F, Marshall P. Men and health help-seeking behaviour: literature review. J Adv Nurs 2005;49(6):616–23.

96. Woz S, Mitchell S, Hesko C, et al. Gender as risk factor for 30 days post-discharge hospital utilisation: a secondary data analysis. BMJ Open 2012;2:e000428.

97. Nishi SPE, Maslonka M, Zhang W, et al. Pattern and adherence to maintenance medication use in medicare beneficiaries with chronic obstructive pulmonary disease: 2008-2013. Chronic Obstr Pulm Dis 2018;5(1):16–26.

98. Fernandez-Garcia S, Represas-Represas C, Ruano-Ravina A, et al. Social profile of patients admitted for COPD exacerbations. A gender analysis. Arch Bronconeumol 2020;56(2):84–9.

99. Goncalves-Macedo L, Lacerda EM, Markman-Filho B, et al. Trends in morbidity and mortality from COPD in Brazil, 2000 to 2016. J Bras Pneumol 2019;45(6):e20180402.

100. Papaioannou AI, Bania E, Alexopoulos EC, et al. Sex discrepancies in COPD patients and burden of the disease in females: a nationwide study in Greece (Greek Obstructive Lung Disease Epidemiology and health ecoNomics: GOLDEN study). Int J Chron Obstruct Pulmon Dis 2014;9:203–13.

101. Connett JE, Murray RP, Buist AS, et al. Changes in smoking status affect women more than men: results of the Lung Health Study. Am J Epidemiol 2003;157(11):973–9.

102. Vozoris NT, Stanbrook MB. Smoking prevalence, behaviours, and cessation among individuals with COPD or asthma. Respir Med 2011;105(3):477–84.

103. Haave E, Skumlien S, Hyland ME. Gender considerations in pulmonary rehabilitation. J Cardiopulm Rehabil Prev 2008;28(3):215–9.

104. Grosbois JM, Gephine S, Diot AS, et al. Gender does not impact the short- or long-term outcomes of home-based pulmonary rehabilitation in patients with COPD. ERJ Open Res 2020;6(4):00032–2020.

105. Robles PG, Brooks D, Goldstein R, et al. Gender-associated differences in pulmonary rehabilitation outcomes in people with chronic obstructive pulmonary disease: a systematic review. J Cardiopulm Rehabil Prev 2014;34(2):87–97.

106. Lutter JI, Lukas M, Schwarzkopf L, et al. Utilization and determinants of use of non-pharmacological interventions in COPD: results of the COSYCONET cohort. Respir Med 2020;171:106087.

107. Stone PW, Hickman K, Steiner MC, et al. Predictors of referral to pulmonary rehabilitation from UK primary care. Int J Chron Obstruct Pulmon Dis 2020; 15:2941–52.

108. Watson L, Schouten JP, Lofdahl CG, et al. Predictors of COPD symptoms: does the sex of the patient matter? Eur Respir J 2006;28(2):311–8.

109. Laforest L, Denis F, Van Ganse E, et al. Correlates of adherence to respiratory drugs in COPD patients. Prim Care Respir J 2010;19(2):148–54.

110. Simmons MS, Nides MA, Rand CS, et al. Unpredictability of deception in compliance with physician-prescribed bronchodilator inhaler use in a clinical trial. Chest 2000;118(2):290–5.

111. Darba J, Ramirez G, Sicras A, et al. The importance of inhaler devices: the choice of inhaler device may lead to suboptimal adherence in COPD patients. Int J Chron Obstruct Pulmon Dis 2015; 10:2335–45.

112. Kilic H, Kokturk N, Sari G, et al. Do females behave differently in COPD exacerbation? Int J Chron Obstruct Pulmon Dis 2015;10:823–30.

113. Gershon AS, McGihon RE, Thiruchelvam D, et al. Medication discontinuation in adults with COPD discharged from the hospital: a population-based cohort study. Chest 2020;159(3):975–84.

114. Montes de Oca M, Menezes A, Wehrmeister FC, et al. Adherence to inhaled therapies of COPD patients from seven Latin American countries: the LASSYC study. PLoS One 2017;12(11):e0186777.

115. Vestbo J, Anderson JA, Calverley PMA, et al. Adherence to inhaled therapy, mortality and hospital admission in COPD. Thorax 2009;64(11): 939–43.

116. Bhattarai B, Walpola R, Mey A, et al. Barriers and strategies for improving medication adherence among people living with COPD: a systematic review. Respir Care 2020;65(11):1738–50.

117. Becklake MR, Kauffmann F. Gender differences in airway behaviour over the human life span. Thorax 1999;54(12):1119–38.

118. Bateman ED, Ferguson GT, Barnes N, et al. Dual bronchodilation with QVA149 versus single bronchodilator therapy: the SHINE study. Eur Respir J 2013;42(6):1484–94.

119. Decramer M, Anzueto A, Kerwin E, et al. Efficacy and safety of umeclidinium plus vilanterol versus tiotropium, vilanterol, or umeclidinium monotherapies over 24 weeks in patients with chronic obstructive pulmonary disease: results from two multicentre, blinded, randomised controlled trials. Lancet Respir Med 2014;2(6):472–86.

120. Global Initiative for Chronic Obstructive Lung Disease (GOLD). Global strategy for the diagnosis, management, and prevention of chronic obstructive pulmonary disease 2015. Available at: wwwgoldcopdorg/uploads/users/files/GOLD_Report_2015pdf http://www.goldcopd.org/uploads/users/files/GOLD_Report_2015.pdf. Accessed November 17, 2015.

121. Burgel PR, Laurendeau C, Raherison C, et al. An attempt at modeling COPD epidemiological trends in France. Respir Res 2018;19(1):130.

122. Hernandez-Garduno E, Ocana-Servin HL. Temporal trends in chronic obstructive pulmonary disease mortality in Mexico, 1999-2014. Int J Tuberc Lung Dis 2017;21(3):357–62.

123. India State-Level Disease Burden Initiative CRDC. The burden of chronic respiratory diseases and their heterogeneity across the states of India: the Global Burden of Disease Study 1990-2016. Lancet Glob Health 2018;6(12):e1363–74.

Sex Differences and the Role of Sex Hormones in Pulmonary Hypertension

Hannah Takahashi Oakland, MD, Phillip Joseph, MD*

KEYWORDS

• Sex differences • Hormones • Estrogen • Adipose • Pulmonary hypertension

KEY POINTS

- Enumerate the major contributions of the sex hormones to pulmonary hypertension pathophysiology.
- Describe how sex influences the prevalence and survival of patients with pulmonary hypertension.
- Introduce future directions related to sex differences in pulmonary hypertension.

INTRODUCTION

The global burden of pulmonary hypertension (PH) numbers in the millions of cases, and there is a high degree of associated morbidity and mortality. The 6th World Symposium on Pulmonary Hypertension defines PH as a mean pulmonary artery pressure (mPAP) greater than 20 mm Hg, with pulmonary arterial hypertension (PAH) further characterized by the hemodynamic parameters of pulmonary vascular resistance (PVR) greater than 3 Wood units (WU) and pulmonary arterial wedge pressure (PAWP) less than or equal to 15 mm Hg.[1] Mechanistic explanations for PH include vasoconstriction, metabolic flux, inflammation, and imbalance between cellular proliferation and apoptosis, leading to pulmonary vascular (PV) remodeling and eventual right heart failure. Contributing to the pathophysiology of PH are the sex hormones, specifically estrogen, its metabolites, and their influence in multiple signaling pathways. This has led to a phenomenon known as the female paradox, that is, the increased prevalence of PH among women despite a seemingly paradoxical, protective effect.

A wealth of literature exists that address the pathophysiologic mechanisms underpinning sex differences in PH, although a fuller understanding continues to be pursued. The regulatory effects of estrogen in this context are far-reaching and influence numerous components of the pathways that lead to disease pathogenesis of the pulmonary vasculature. Discoveries of sex-related differences have led to clinical trials of potential therapeutics that involve both men and women, including aromatase and dehydroepiandrosterone (DHEA). In this article, the authors aim to describe sex differences in PH presentation, disease course, and outcomes, detail the role of the sex hormones in PH pathophysiology, and introduce related future directions.

PREVALENCE AND SURVIVAL

Sex has long been associated with prevalence of PH. Dresdale and colleagues'[2] 1951 report of known cases of idiopathic PAH (IPAH) documented that 60% of the reviewed cases were female. This estimate was corroborated in the first national prospective cohort study undertaken by the National Institutes of Health in 1981, the results of which showed a 1.7:1 female-to-male prevalence.[3] This study further noted that female patients tended to have more severe symptoms at presentation, 75% of whom were diagnosed with New York Heart Association functional class III or class IV symptoms as opposed to 64% of male patients ($P = .08$).

Pulmonary, Critical Care, and Sleep Medicine, Yale New Haven Hospital/Yale School of Medicine, 20 York Street, New Haven, CT 06519, USA
* Corresponding author.
E-mail address: phillip.joseph@yale.edu

Clin Chest Med 42 (2021) 457–465
https://doi.org/10.1016/j.ccm.2021.04.006
0272-5231/21/© 2021 Elsevier Inc. All rights reserved.

A review of modern registries of PH show that the overall proportion of PAH patients who are female ranges from 65% to 80%.[4] One of the largest registries created, REVEAL, had one of the highest female preponderances of female sex at 78%, with the highest female-to-male ratios in Hispanic (4.7:1) and black (5.5:1) patients.[5]

The increased prevalence of PAH in women is thought to be related to hormonal differences between the sexes. This is supported by registry data showing an increased female-to-male ratio of 2.3:1 in patients less than 65 years in age compared with 1.2:1 for those greater than 65 years.[6] Despite the increased prevalence, multiple registries have demonstrated improved survival in women with PAH in both prevalent and incident cases, supporting the concept of the female paradox.[7,8] For example, in a multicenter cohort study from the French Network on Pulmonary Hypertension of 354 prospectively enrolled patients with idiopathic, familial, or anorexigen-associated PAH, female patients made up 63% of incident and prevalent cases yet had a 62.5% improved chance of survival. On multivariable analysis, only greater baseline 6-minute walk distance (6MWD) and cardiac output (CO) also were associated with risk reduction.[9]

Furthermore, in another large series of 15,646 US military veterans (3% of whom were women) who had right heart catheterization–diagnosed PH (defined as mPAP $\geq$25 mm Hg), women had a higher average PVR (3.1 WU vs 2.5 WU, respectively; $P = .005$) at diagnosis. Despite this, women with PH had an 18% greater survival compared with men ($P = .020$) and women with precapillary PH, additionally defined as having a PVR greater than or equal to 3 WU and PAWP less than or equal to 15 mm Hg, were 29% more likely to survive than their male counterparts.[10] A caveat to using hemodynamic criteria for prognostication, however, is that CO is lower in healthy women compared with men in both the resting and exercise states; this discrepancy affects the calculation of PVR by Ohm's law.[11] Hemodynamic cutoffs for defining PH have not accounted for these sex differences.

In addition to hormonal mechanisms, discussed previously, the unequal burden of comorbidities between the sexes is an important contributor to this disparity and, in some studies, is thought to fully explain it. In the study of US veterans, described previously, men were more likely to use tobacco and have chronic obstructive pulmonary disease (COPD), heart failure, coronary artery disease, atrial fibrillation, and chronic kidney disease, whereas women were more likely to have connective tissue disease and depression.[10]

In an investigation into the Swedish Pulmonary Arterial Hypertension Register of 271 patients with IPAH, women were half as likely to have 2 or more comorbidities and a third as likely to have ischemic heart disease.[12] A more modern cohort with older patients (median age 68) and only 56% women, this study observed that among this group of Swedish patients, women were diagnosed at a younger age. Additionally, they had higher PVR at diagnosis and more often were started with combination PAH-targeted therapies than men. Men had decreased survival rates (hazard ratio [HR] 1.49; CI, 1.02–2.18; $P = .038$) but, when adjusted for age, this difference was no longer statistically significant (HR 1.30; CI, 0.89–1.90; $P = .178$), suggesting that in this cohort, adjustment for the older age and higher comorbidity burden of male patients explained the difference in outcome (**Fig. 1**).

Further supporting this concept is the divergence of survival between sexes as age progresses. This was shown in an analysis of the REVEAL registry, which at the time included 2318 women and 651 men.[13] In this series of US patients, differences in cardiovascular disease prevalence were less pronounced and mortality rates were similar among women and men under the age of 60. Survival curves diverged with aging, however, as men over age 60 experienced worse prognoses (HR 1.72; CI, 1.32–2.25; $P < .001$) (**Fig. 2**). Consequently, male patients over the age of 60 receive additional points in the REVEAL 2.0 Registry Risk Score for Pulmonary Arterial Hypertension, which predicts mortality among PAH patients.[7,14]

HEMODYNAMIC CHARACTERISTICS

RV function is well-established as a strong prognostic indicator in PH. Sex differences in RV function long have been noted. In 1973, invasive hemodynamics were obtained in pigs who were exposed to 4 weeks of a simulated high-altitude environment of 5490 meters in the form of a hypobaric chamber with a pressure of inspired oxygen of 70 mm Hg.[15] The pigs developed marked PH and mPAP almost quadrupled. Although both sexes developed right ventricular hypertrophy (RVH), male pigs developed significantly more.

Sex differences in RV function also have been observed in modern studies of humans. In a study of 40 patients with treatment-naïve IPAH, men had lower RVEF and stroke volume (SV), despite having similar mPAP and PAWP.[16] The higher SV in women persisted even when corrected for age, sex, and body surface area. These investigators found that RV mass, when adjusted for predicted

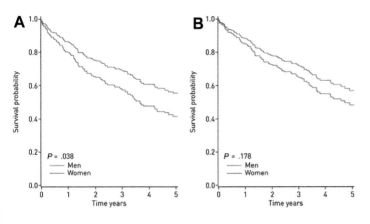

Fig. 1. Survival of patients (n = 271) stratified by sex. (*A*) Unadjusted; (*B*) adjusted for age. (*From* Kjellström B, Nisell M, Kylhammar D, et al. Sex-specific differences and survival in patients with idiopathic pulmonary arterial hypertension 2008-2016. *ERJ Open Res.* 2019;5(3).)

values for age and sex, was similar between the sexes.

RV function also has been investigated in PH due to left heart disease. In a study of 96 patients with heart failure with preserved ejection fraction (HFpEF) who had an average mPAP of 36 mm Hg, male sex was associated with a substantially increased risk of RV dysfunction (OR 6.1; 95% CI, 2.5–16; $P < 001$).[17] This persisted even after the investigators adjusted for coronary artery disease. In this study, the investigators also showed that RV dysfunction was the strongest single predictor of mortality in HFpEF patients (HR 2.4; 95% CI, 1.6–2.6; $P < .0001$).

There is evidence that part of the difference in mortality between men and women with PH can be explained by the response of the RV to treatment. In a retrospective study of 101 patients with PAH, female patients and male patients had a similar average baseline PVR and right ventricular ejection fraction (RVEF) as measured by cardiac magnetic resonance imaging (cMRI).[18] After treatment, however, RVEF improved by 3.6% in women but declined by 1% in men. Furthermore, the male RVs remained more dilated and hypertrophied. After treatment, male sex was associated with a worse functional class and 6MWD even when adjusted for initial hemodynamic values. The established difference in ejection fraction accounted for 39% of improvement in survival.

Limited data exist on the sex-specific selection of the 3 major treatment pathways of PAH or of combination therapy. A meta-analysis of trials of endothelin receptor antagonists showed increased 6MWD in women compared with men,[19] potentially explained by higher circulating endothelin levels in men.[20]

THE ESTROGEN PARADOX

Estrogen and progesterone are the steroids that comprise female sex hormones. There exist 3

endogenous isoforms: estrone (E1), estradiol (E2), and estriol (E3) (**Fig. 3**). Estradiol predominates in premenopausal women and serum concentrations range between 100 pg/mL and 600 pg/mL, depending on the phase of the menstrual cycle. The levels of estradiol fall to 5 pg/mL to 20 pg/mL after menopause, similar to or lower than men of the same age,[21] and estrone becomes the most active isoform seen in postmenopausal women. Steroid hormones are synthesized primarily in the adrenal glands and gonads but also can be created by placental, hepatic, cutaneous, and adipose tissues.

On first inspection, seemingly contradictory evidence regarding the role of estrogen in the pathophysiology of PH emerges. As reviewed later,

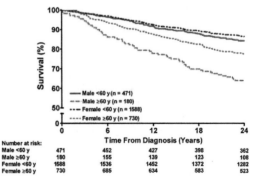

Fig. 2. Two-year survival from time of enrollment in the REVEAL registry, ages less than 60 years versus ages greater than or equal to 60 years groups, by sex. Age less than 60 years: men, 84.3% ± 1.7%, and women, 86.4% ± 0.9%; $P = .24$. Age greater than or equal to 60 years: men, 64.0% ± 3.6%, and women, 77.5% ± 1.6%; $P<.001$. (*From* Shapiro S, Traiger GL, Turner M, McGoon MD, Wason P, Barst RJ. Sex differences in the diagnosis, treatment, and outcome of patients with pulmonary arterial hypertension enrolled in the registry to evaluate early and long-term pulmonary arterial hypertension disease management. *Chest.* 2012;141(2):363-373.)

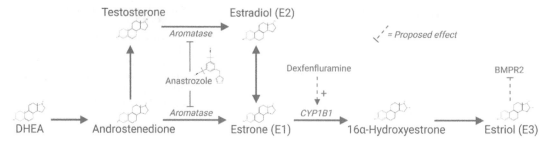

Fig. 3. The estrogen and testosterone metabolism pathway with proposed external effects, as discussed in this article. (Created with BioRender.com.)

inhibition of estrogen synthesis with anastrozole has been shown to treat and prevent PH through several mechanisms. Over-expression of the serotonin receptor—via a pathway influenced by estrogen—induces PH in female mice that can be reversed by ovariectomy.[22] Additionally, inhibition of estrogen receptor-α in a female, hypoxic, PH mouse model attenuates elevations in right ventricular systolic pressure (RVSP) and PV remodeling.[23]

In spite of extensive literature implicating estrogen as pathophysiologic, there is some evidence supporting its protective qualities. For example, administration of 17β-estradiol in studies of male mice showed improvement in hypoxic PH endpoints, including RVSP, CO, hypoxic PV remodeling, and hypoxia-induced right ventricular (RV) remodeling.[24] In another study of a male PH rat model, estrogen restored RV function and structure.[25] Additionally, there is suggestion that estrogen may have some RV inotropic properties and may protect against PV remodeling, as shown in a hypoxemia-induced PAH mouse model.[26] The contradictory effects of estrogen contributing to PV remodeling and attenuating RV failure may play a role in the mechanism of the female paradox. The use of male-only or female-only murine models in many studies further complicates the calculus, because unaccounted for sex-related differences in these unbalanced cohorts may play a role.

AROMATASE

A member of the cytochrome P450 (CYP) superfamily, the enzyme aromatase is responsible for critical steps in the synthesis of estrogens. Its primary role is to catalyze the conversion of androstenedione to estrogen and testosterone to estradiol (see **Fig. 3**). Aromatase levels are higher in the pulmonary arterial smooth muscle cells (PASMCs) of both healthy and hypoxic rodent and female humans as opposed to male humans. Additionally, levels are significantly higher in hypoxic mice as opposed to normoxic mice of both sexes.[23]

Anastrozole is a potent and selective aromatase inhibitor that is used primarily in the treatment of breast cancer but is also used to treat other gynecologic cancers and to reduce the risk of breast cancer in postmenopausal women. In an important investigation into its experimental effects on PH, anastrozole was found to significantly improve hypoxia-induced increases in RVSP, right ventricular hypertrophy (RVH), and PV remodeling in female PH-modeled mice. The same was not found in male mice in the same experiment. The absence of improvement in these parameters in the male mice correlated with a lack of reduction in serum estrogen and estradiol levels in male rodent models as opposed to female rodents, in which levels decreased significantly.[23] These findings were further corroborated by a study in which bone morphogenic protein receptor 2 (BMPR2) mutant mice were treated with anastrozole and fulvestrant, an estrogen receptor antagonist. These medications were able both to prevent expected increases in RVSP and to improve RVSP in mice with established PH.[27]

These findings have led to trials of anastrozole for therapeutic use in humans with PH. In a small, randomized, double-blind, placebo-controlled trial of 18 patients with PAH, anastrozole reduced 17β-estradiol levels and improved 6MWD compared with placebo. It did not, however, affect tricuspid annular plane systolic excursion, functional class, or health-related quality-of-life scores.[28] The Pulmonary Hypertension and Anastrozole Trial (PHANTOM [NCT03229499]), a larger, randomized, blinded, phase 2 clinical trial of group 1 PH patients currently is enrolling.[29]

CYTOCHROME P450 1B1

CYP1B1 creates hydroxylated forms of estrogen, which are thought to be pathogenic in some patients with PH, in particular 16α-hydroxyestrone. Estrogen metabolism occurs mostly via hydroxylation by CYP enzymes and conjugation in the liver, where reactive oxygen intermediates are primed for elimination from the body. A notable exception is CYP1B1, which is found primarily outside the liver and has high concentrations in the PV wall in both humans with PAH and murine models of PAH.[30] It has been shown, for example, that RVSP and RVH are ameliorated in CYP1B1 (−/−) PAH murine models. Similarly, a strong CYP1B1 inhibitor attenuated PASMCs proliferation in human and murine models.[30] 16α-Hydroxyestrone has been shown to induce reactive oxygen species generation, which leads to PV remodeling and proliferation of PASMCs. In this study, estrogen's effects were inhibited by CYP1B1 blockade.[31]

In a related mechanism, increased activity in serotonin signaling results in estrogen-dependent PH; serotonin and estrogen metabolic pathways are intricately linked.[22] Mouse models that overexpress the serotonin receptor have high levels of expression of CYP1B1 and develop PH. Administration of a CYP1B1 inhibitor to these mice attenuated elevations in RVSP and even improved survival in another mouse model.[32] Dexfenfluramine (Dfen) is an anorexic drug known to cause PAH via a serotonergic pathway.[33] Dfen administration similarly has been shown to cause an increase in CYP1B1 levels and cause PAH (see **Fig. 3**). Conversely, administration of Dfen to CYP1B1 (−/−) mice did not result in PAH, strongly suggesting that the cytochrome is integral to the pathogenesis of the disease.[34]

There has been novel investigation into genetic variation in the expression of sex hormone pathways with RV function. By correlating levels of expression of relevant single-nucleotide polymorphisms (SNPs) to cMRI findings, researchers have associated the CYP1B1 SNP rs162561 with increased RVEF in African American women. Additionally, haplotype analysis of this SNP along with two others with which it is in tight linkage disequilibrium showed significant association of RVEF in both African American and white women.[35] One of the additional SNPs has been associated with higher PAH penetrance in BMPR2 carriers, which highlights the complex interplay of multiple levels of phenotypic determination, as discussed later.[36]

BONE MORPHOGENETIC PROTEIN RECEPTOR 2

BMPR2 is a member of the transforming growth factor β (TGF-β) superfamily. It currently is estimated that 70% to 80% of families with PAH and 10% to 20% of IPAH cases are caused by BMPR mutations.[37] Familial primary PH is an autosomal dominant disease resulting from 300 distinct BMPR2 mutations that result in haploinsufficiency.[38] There is considerable heterogeneity

in this familial form of PH, which on aggregate presents at a younger age and is associated with a worse clinical course and higher risk of death or transplantation.[39] The male penetrance is lower than the female penetrance, estimated at 14% and 42%, respectively, driving investigation into the cause of this disparity.[40]

In healthy, non-PH patients, messenger RNA and protein expression of BMPR2 is lower in female patients than in male patients. In vitro assessment of these patients' PASMCs showed that estrogen attenuated the expression of downstream mediators of BMPR2 signaling.[41] In an important mouse model study on the role of estrogen in the regulation of BMPR2, the baseline levels of lung transcription of the protein were lower in female mice. Further supporting the idea that estrogen negatively regulates BMPR2, administration of anastrozole resulted in up-regulation of BMPR2 in female mice but had no effect on male mice.[23] An estrogen-binding site has been identified on the BMPR2 promoter, which is conserved across humans and several other animals which, when bound, down-regulates BMPR2 gene expression (see **Fig. 3**).[42]

The pathophysiology of BMPR2 mutations may extend beyond the PV and into RV. In a study of 28 patients with a known BMPR2 mutation and 67 patients with idiopathic or familial BMPR2 without a mutation, RVEF was lower in patients with a BMPR2 mutation despite the groups having similar mPAP and PVR. In a subset of these patients, RV tissue and left ventricle tissue were obtained and compared with controls, which showed that BMPR2 signaling was similar between mutation carriers and noncarriers.[43]

ADIPOSE AND SEX HORMONES

Obesity is an important and common comorbidity of PH, affecting 33.3% of patients in the REVEAL registry, as published in 2010.[44] Adipose tissue is responsible for a significant proportion of the interconversion of sex hormones; it is responsible almost exclusively for the production of circulating estrogen in postmenopausal women[45] and up to half in premenopausal women.[46] Furthermore, the gene encoding CYP1B1 was 1 of the 2 genes expressed most commonly in a compilation of genome-wide sequencing studies of obesity.[47]

In the commonly used leptin-deficient obese mouse (ob/ob) model, an increase in RVSP and PV remodeling is seen in both male mice and female mice. Administration of anastrozole reverses increases in RVSP in both sexes as well as RVH and PV remodeling in female ob/ob mice. In accordance with the human genomic findings, discussed previously, CYP1B1 is up-regulated in white adipose tissue of obese mice and administration of a CYP1B1 inhibitor attenuates the elevated RVSP and PV remodeling seen in the ob/ob model.[48] These findings, when taken together, strongly suggest that part of the pathogenesis of obesity in PH is mediated via sex hormones.

TESTOSTERONE AND DEHYDROEPIANDROSTERONE

Both the male sex hormone testosterone and its precursor DHEA have been shown to be potent vasodilators in the pulmonary arteries (PAs).[49,50] In rat models, DHEA has been shown to prevent hypoxic PH and to reverse established hypoxic PH.[51] It also has shown beneficial effects on the RV, restoring cardiac index (CI) and inhibiting RV capillary rarefaction, apoptosis, fibrosis, and oxidative stress in a rat PH model.[52] In a case-control study comparing plasma levels of sex hormones associated with PAH in male patients, hormones were implicated as follows:

- Testosterone levels were similar between the groups.
- Higher levels of DHEA-sulfate levels were associated with a reduced risk of PAH, lower right atrial pressure, and lower PVR.
- Higher estradiol levels were associated with a higher risk of PAH and reduced 6MWD.[53]

Additionally, 2 SNPs in the androgen receptor gene have been associated with increased risk of RVH and RV end-diastolic volume as measured by cMRI in multivariate analysis.[35]

These data, among other studies, have led to the proposed use of DHEA supplementation in the treatment of PH. A pilot study of 8 patients with PH associated with chronic obstructive pulmonary disease (COPD) showed that oral DHEA given for 3 months improved 6MWD, mPAP, PVR, and carbon monoxide diffusing capacity (DLCO) of the lung.[54] A phase 2 crossover, randomized, placebo-controlled clinical trial, DHEA in Pulmonary Hypertension (EDIPHY [NCT03648385]), is recruiting. The primary outcome is change in RV longitudinal strain as measured by cMRI; secondary outcomes include RVEF, N-terminal–prohormone of brain natriuretic peptide, sex hormone levels, 6MWD, functional class, and quality of life scores.[55]

PULMONARY HYPERTENSION IN PREGNANCY

Although a full discussion of the pathophysiology, diagnosis, and management of PH in pregnancy lies beyond the scope of this article, it remains important to note that pregnancy carries high morbidity and mortality in PH. Management remains challenging. CO is expected to rise by approximately 50% in pregnancy, and changes in the sex hormones estrogen and progesterone cause a rapid decrease in systemic vascular resistance, leading to relative hypotension. Significant hemodynamic changes occur at 20 weeks to 24 weeks of gestation (peak in plasma volume) as well as at 32 weeks to 34 weeks (peak in CO), changes that often cannot be tolerated by patients with PH. Maternal mortality remains at approximately 25% in the modern era in most series.[56,57] In 1 large review of a modern European cohort, mortality was much lower, 5%, but more than one-quarter of patients still developed heart failure during pregnancy, and half required hospitalization.[58] The 1-month postpartum period retains the highest mortality, usually from RV failure or shock.[56]

These concerning observations have led to the general recommendation that women with PH should avoid pregnancy, and termination should be considered.[59] The evidence does suggest that outcomes have significantly improved in the past few decades, and standard of care should involve referral to expert centers with multidisciplinary teams composed of specialists in PV disease, maternal-fetal medicine, anesthesia, and neonatology.[60]

FUTURE DIRECTIONS

Sex differences are being elucidated through increasingly sophisticated characterizations of RV performance. In a study of 57 patients with PAH and chronic thromboembolic PH (CTEPH), single-beat and multibeat pressure-volume analysis was used to determine RV-PA coupling in patients with PAH.[61] RV contractility was significantly higher in female patients compared with their male counterparts despite having a similar degree of afterload. This led to a higher RV-PA coupling ratio (0.92 in female patients vs 0.59 in male patients; $P = .03$); the cutoff for a failing RV has been proposed at 0.805 and normal is approximately 1.5.[62] This indicates that female RVs were better able to match the afterload imposed by their disease. Consistent with most prior studies, RV mass index as given by cMRI was lower in the female patients as opposed to the male patients (34 vs 46, respectively; $P = .01$). Furthermore, female patients additionally showed better early diastolic relaxation. Further characterization of how sex may affect RV performance will be critical, given the importance of RV failure in the natural history of PH.

Additionally, the remarkable work, described previously, which has shed light on the pathophysiologic mechanisms of hormonal dysregulation in PH, has led to clinical trials of drugs that manipulate these pathways. As discussed previously, the following clinical trials currently are under way in the United States:

- PHANTOM currently is clarifying the possible therapeutic effects of estrogen blockade.[29]
- The EDIPHY trial seeks to clarify if the vasodilator and testosterone precursor DHEA has clinical benefit in the treatment of PH.[55]

Finally, as has been pointed out by leading experts in the field,[63] measurement of estrogen and estrogen metabolite levels during clinical care and in research settings has the potential to advance both treatment and knowledge of the sex-based pathophysiology of PH.

SUMMARY

Sex hormones contribute to the pathophysiology of PH. Estrogen and its metabolites have both harmful and protective effects on the PV and RV, leading to the female paradox. Additionally, sex hormones have interplay with other signaling pathways that contribute to PH pathophysiology, which include BMPR2, serotonin, and adipose tissue. Due to differences between the sexes, these hormones have led to increased prevalence and survival among women. Future studies seek to expand on the current understanding of this pathophysiology and develop new therapeutic targets.

CLINICS CARE POINTS

- Sex differences in PH may be caused by differential regulation of estrogen and its metabolites between the sexes.
- While estrogen may contribute to the increased prevalence of PH in female patients, it may also have a protective effect among female patients, thus leading to the "female paradox."
- Studies targeting pathways in estrogen and testosterone metabolism are ongoing and may offer future therapeutics for PH.

DISCLOSURE

The authors have nothing to disclose.

REFERENCES

1. Simonneau G, Montani D, Celermajer DS, et al. Haemodynamic definitions and updated clinical classification of pulmonary hypertension. Eur Respir J 2019;53(1).
2. Dresdale DT, Schultz M, Michtom RJ. Primary pulmonary hypertension. I. Clinical and hemodynamic study. Am J Med 1951;11(6):686–705.
3. Rich S, Dantzker DR, Ayres SM, et al. Primary pulmonary hypertension. A national prospective study. Ann Intern Med 1987;107(2):216–23.
4. McGoon MD, Benza RL, Escribano-Subias P, et al. Pulmonary arterial hypertension: epidemiology and registries. J Am Coll Cardiol 2013;62(25 Suppl): D51–9.
5. Frost AE, Badesch DB, Barst RJ, et al. The changing picture of patients with pulmonary arterial hypertension in the United States: how REVEAL differs from historic and non-US Contemporary Registries. Chest 2011;139(1):128–37.
6. Hoeper MM, Huscher D, Ghofrani HA, et al. Elderly patients diagnosed with idiopathic pulmonary arterial hypertension: results from the COMPERA registry. Int J Cardiol 2013;168(2):871–80.
7. Benza RL, Miller DP, Gomberg-Maitland M, et al. Predicting survival in pulmonary arterial hypertension: insights from the registry to evaluate early and long-term pulmonary arterial hypertension disease management (REVEAL). Circulation 2010; 122(2):164–72.
8. Humbert M, Sitbon O, Chaouat A, et al. Pulmonary arterial hypertension in France: results from a national registry. Am J Respir Crit Care Med 2006; 173(9):1023–30.
9. Humbert M, Sitbon O, Chaouat A, et al. Survival in patients with idiopathic, familial, and anorexigen-associated pulmonary arterial hypertension in the modern management era. Circulation 2010;122(2): 156–63.
10. Ventetuolo CE, Hess E, Austin ED, et al. Sex-based differences in veterans with pulmonary hypertension: results from the veterans affairs-clinical assessment reporting and tracking database. PLoS One 2017;12(11):e0187734.
11. Wheatley CM, Snyder EM, Johnson BD, et al. Sex differences in cardiovascular function during submaximal exercise in humans. Springerplus 2014;3: 445.
12. Kjellström B, Nisell M, Kylhammar D, et al. Sex-specific differences and survival in patients with idiopathic pulmonary arterial hypertension 2008-2016. ERJ Open Res 2019;5(3).

13. Shapiro S, Traiger GL, Turner M, et al. Sex differences in the diagnosis, treatment, and outcome of patients with pulmonary arterial hypertension enrolled in the registry to evaluate early and long-term pulmonary arterial hypertension disease management. Chest 2012;141(2):363–73.

14. Benza RL, Gomberg-Maitland M, Elliott CG, et al. Predicting survival in patients with pulmonary arterial hypertension: the REVEAL risk score calculator 2.0 and comparison with ESC/ERS-Based risk assessment strategies. Chest 2019;156(2):323–37.

15. McMurtry IF, Frith CH, Will DH. Cardiopulmonary responses of male and female swine to simulated high altitude. J Appl Phys 1973;35(4):459–62.

16. Swift AJ, Capener D, Hammerton C, et al. Right ventricular sex differences in patients with idiopathic pulmonary arterial hypertension characterised by magnetic resonance imaging: pair-matched case controlled study. PLoS One 2015;10(5):e0127415.

17. Melenovsky V, Hwang SJ, Lin G, et al. Right heart dysfunction in heart failure with preserved ejection fraction. Eur Heart J 2014;35(48):3452–62.

18. Jacobs W, van de Veerdonk MC, Trip P, et al. The right ventricle explains sex differences in survival in idiopathic pulmonary arterial hypertension. Chest 2014;145(6):1230–6.

19. Gabler NB, French B, Strom BL, et al. Race and sex differences in response to endothelin receptor antagonists for pulmonary arterial hypertension. Chest 2012;141(1):20–6.

20. Polderman KH, Stehouwer CD, van Kamp GJ, et al. Influence of sex hormones on plasma endothelin levels. Ann Intern Med 1993;118(6):429–32.

21. Mendelsohn ME, Karas RH. The protective effects of estrogen on the cardiovascular system. N Engl J Med 1999;340(23):1801–11.

22. White K, Dempsie Y, Nilsen M, et al. The serotonin transporter, gender, and 17β oestradiol in the development of pulmonary arterial hypertension. Cardiovasc Res 2011;90(2):373–82.

23. Mair KM, Wright AF, Duggan N, et al. Sex-dependent influence of endogenous estrogen in pulmonary hypertension. Am J Respir Crit Care Med 2014;190(4):456–67.

24. Lahm T, Albrecht M, Fisher AJ, et al. 17β-Estradiol attenuates hypoxic pulmonary hypertension via estrogen receptor-mediated effects. Am J Respir Crit Care Med 2012;185(9):965–80.

25. Umar S, Iorga A, Matori H, et al. Estrogen rescues preexisting severe pulmonary hypertension in rats. Am J Respir Crit Care Med 2011;184(6):715–23.

26. Liu A, Schreier D, Tian L, et al. Direct and indirect protection of right ventricular function by estrogen in an experimental model of pulmonary arterial hypertension. Am J Physiol Heart Circ Physiol 2014; 307(3):H273–83.

27. Chen X, Austin ED, Talati M, et al. Oestrogen inhibition reverses pulmonary arterial hypertension and associated metabolic defects. Eur Respir J 2017;50(2).

28. Kawut SM, Archer-Chicko CL, DeMichele A, et al. Anastrozole in pulmonary arterial hypertension. A randomized, double-blind, placebo-controlled trial. Am J Respir Crit Care Med 2017;195(3):360–8.

29. U.S., NLoM. Pulmonary hypertension and anastrazole trial (PHANTOM). Identifier NCT03229499. (December 7, 2017). Available: https://clinicaltrials.gov/ct2/show/NCT03229499. Accessed December, 2020.

30. White K, Johansen AK, Nilsen M, et al. Activity of the estrogen-metabolizing enzyme cytochrome P450 1B1 influences the development of pulmonary arterial hypertension. Circulation 2012;126(9):1087–98.

31. Hood KY, Montezano AC, Harvey AP, et al. Nicotinamide adenine dinucleotide phosphate oxidase-mediated redox signaling and vascular remodeling by 16α-hydroxyestrone in human pulmonary artery cells: implications in pulmonary arterial hypertension. Hypertension 2016;68(3):796–808.

32. Johansen AK, Dean A, Morecroft I, et al. The serotonin transporter promotes a pathological estrogen metabolic pathway in pulmonary hypertension via cytochrome P450 1B1. Pulm Circ 2016;6(1):82–92.

33. Rothman RB, Ayestas MA, Dersch CM, et al. Aminorex, fenfluramine, and chlorphentermine are serotonin transporter substrates. Implications for primary pulmonary hypertension. Circulation 1999;100(8):869–75.

34. Dempsie Y, MacRitchie NA, White K, et al. Dexfenfluramine and the oestrogen-metabolizing enzyme CYP1B1 in the development of pulmonary arterial hypertension. Cardiovasc Res 2013;99(1):24–34.

35. Ventetuolo CE, Mitra N, Wan F, et al. Oestradiol metabolism and androgen receptor genotypes are associated with right ventricular function. Eur Respir J 2016;47(2):553–63.

36. Austin ED, Cogan JD, West JD, et al. Alterations in oestrogen metabolism: implications for higher penetrance of familial pulmonary arterial hypertension in females. Eur Respir J 2009;34(5):1093–9.

37. Morrell NW, Aldred MA, Chung WK, et al. Genetics and genomics of pulmonary arterial hypertension. Eur Respir J 2019;53(1).

38. Machado RD, Pauciulo MW, Thomson JR, et al. BMPR2 haploinsufficiency as the inherited molecular mechanism for primary pulmonary hypertension. Am J Hum Genet 2001;68(1):92–102.

39. Evans JD, Girerd B, Montani D, et al. BMPR2 mutations and survival in pulmonary arterial hypertension: an individual participant data meta-analysis. Lancet Respir Med 2016;4(2):129–37.

40. Larkin EK, Newman JH, Austin ED, et al. Longitudinal analysis casts doubt on the presence of genetic

anticipation in heritable pulmonary arterial hypertension. Am J Respir Crit Care Med 2012;186(9):892–6.

41. Mair KM, Yang XD, Long L, et al. Sex affects bone morphogenetic protein type II receptor signaling in pulmonary artery smooth muscle cells. Am J Respir Crit Care Med 2015;191(6):693–703.

42. Austin ED, Hamid R, Hemnes AR, et al. BMPR2 expression is suppressed by signaling through the estrogen receptor. Biol Sex Differ 2012;3(1):6.

43. van der Bruggen CE, Happé CM, Dorfmüller P, et al. Bone morphogenetic protein receptor type 2 mutation in pulmonary arterial hypertension: a view on the right ventricle. Circulation 2016;133(18): 1747–60.

44. Badesch DB, Raskob GE, Elliott CG, et al. Pulmonary arterial hypertension: baseline characteristics from the REVEAL Registry. Chest 2010;137(2): 376–87.

45. Grodin JM, Siiteri PK, MacDonald PC. Source of estrogen production in postmenopausal women. J Clin Endocrinol Metab 1973;36(2):207–14.

46. Meseguer A, Puche C, Cabero A. Sex steroid biosynthesis in white adipose tissue. Horm Metab Res 2002;34(11–12):731–6.

47. English SB, Butte AJ. Evaluation and integration of 49 genome-wide experiments and the prediction of previously unknown obesity-related genes. Bioinformatics 2007;23(21):2910–7.

48. Mair KM, Harvey KY, Henry AD, et al. Obesity alters oestrogen metabolism and contributes to pulmonary arterial hypertension. Eur Respir J 2019;53(6).

49. Rowell KO, Hall J, Pugh PJ, et al. Testosterone acts as an efficacious vasodilator in isolated human pulmonary arteries and veins: evidence for a biphasic effect at physiological and supra-physiological concentrations. J Endocrinol Invest 2009;32(9):718–23.

50. Farrukh IS, Peng W, Orlinska U, et al. Effect of dehydroepiandrosterone on hypoxic pulmonary vasoconstriction: a Ca(2+)-activated K(+)-channel opener. Am J Physiol 1998;274(2):L186–95.

51. Oka M, Karoor V, Homma N, et al. Dehydroepiandrosterone upregulates soluble guanylate cyclase and inhibits hypoxic pulmonary hypertension. Cardiovasc Res 2007;74(3):377–87.

52. Alzoubi A, Toba M, Abe K, et al. Dehydroepiandrosterone restores right ventricular structure and function in rats with severe pulmonary arterial hypertension. Am J Physiol Heart Circ Physiol 2013;304(12):H1708–18.

53. Ventetuolo CE, Baird GL, Barr RG, et al. Higher estradiol and lower dehydroepiandrosterone-sulfate levels are associated with pulmonary arterial hypertension in men. Am J Respir Crit Care Med 2016; 193(10):1168–75.

54. Dumas de La Roque E, Savineau JP, Metivier AC, et al. Dehydroepiandrosterone (DHEA) improves pulmonary hypertension in chronic obstructive pulmonary disease (COPD): a pilot study. Ann Endocrinol (Paris) 2012;73(1):20–5.

55. U.S.) NLoM. Effects of DHEA in Pulmonary Hypertension (EDIPHY). Identifier NCT03648385. (January 9, 2019). Available: https://clinicaltrials.gov/ct2/show/NCT03648385. Accessed December, 2020.

56. Bedard E, Dimopoulos K, Gatzoulis MA. Has there been any progress made on pregnancy outcomes among women with pulmonary arterial hypertension? Eur Heart J 2009;30(3):256–65.

57. Thomas E, Yang J, Xu J, et al. Pulmonary hypertension and pregnancy outcomes: insights from the national inpatient sample. J Am Heart Assoc 2017; 6(10).

58. Sliwa K, van Hagen IM, Budts W, et al. Pulmonary hypertension and pregnancy outcomes: data from the registry of pregnancy and cardiac disease (ROPAC) of the European Society of Cardiology. Eur J Heart Fail 2016;18(9):1119–28.

59. Hemnes AR, Kiely DG, Cockrill BA, et al. Statement on pregnancy in pulmonary hypertension from the pulmonary vascular research Institute. Pulm Circ 2015;5(3):435–65.

60. Kiely DG, Condliffe R, Webster V, et al. Improved survival in pregnancy and pulmonary hypertension using a multiprofessional approach. BJOG 2010; 117(5):565–74.

61. Tello K, Richter MJ, Yogeswaran A, et al. Sex differences in right ventricular-pulmonary arterial coupling in pulmonary arterial hypertension. Am J Respir Crit Care Med 2020;202(7):1042–6.

62. Tello K, Dalmer A, Axmann J, et al. Reserve of right ventricular-arterial coupling in the setting of chronic overload. Circ Heart Fail 2019;12(1):e005512.

63. Morris H, Denver N, Gaw R, et al. Sex differences in pulmonary hypertension. Clin Chest Med 2021; 42(1):217–28.

Women and Lung Cancer

Lynn T. Tanoue, MD, MBA

KEYWORDS

- Lung cancer in women • Sex differences in lung cancer • Lung cancer in nonsmokers
- Epidermal growth factor receptor • Hormonal factors in lung cancer
- Lung cancer survival in women

KEY POINTS

- Lung cancer is the leading cause of cancer death in women in industrialized countries, and is a growing cause of cancer death around the world.
- Smoking is the most important risk factor for lung cancer in women.
- Lung cancer is more common in never-smoking women than men.
- Sex-related differences occur in hormonal, environmental, and molecular factors.
- Lung cancer outcomes are better in women compared with men.

INTRODUCTION

Lung cancer is the leading cause of cancer mortality globally, with an estimated 1.8 million deaths occurring worldwide this year. Historically, lung cancer incidence and mortality rates have been higher in men than in women. The landmark 1964 US Surgeon General report on the health consequences of smoking concluded definitively that, "Cigarette smoking is causally related to lung cancer in men," but with a weaker comment that "The data for women … point in the same direction."[1] A short 16 years later, the 1980 US Surgeon General report dedicated to women and smoking declared that, "signs of an epidemic of smoking-related disease among women are now appearing,"[2] and by 1987 lung cancer surpassed and continues to exceed breast cancer as the leading cause of cancer death in American women. Although lung cancer mortality rates are now declining in the United States in both men and women, lung cancer in this country still causes more deaths annually than breast, colon, and prostate cancers combined.[3] Moreover, trends in the opposite direction with lung cancer incidence and mortality rates on the rise are the unfortunate reality across the globe, particularly in countries with lower human development indices (HDIs).

Fifty years ago, lung cancer was largely considered a disease of men. We know that this distinction largely reflected the reality that cigarette smoking was a societal norm for men long before it was acceptable in women, a trend that unfortunately is being recapitulated now across the globe. Lung cancer levies a catastrophic toll of disease and downstream health and economic consequences on both sexes. We should not assume that the disease is the same in men and women. A growing body of evidence supports sex-based differences in risk factors, both modifiable and nonmodifiable, as well as biologic factors influencing carcinogenesis, which merit investigation and better understanding to achieve best outcomes for women with lung cancer.

EPIDEMIOLOGY

In 1964, at the time of the first Surgeon General's report on the health consequences of smoking, lung cancer was an uncommon cause of cancer in women. In stark sequence, by 1987, lung cancer had surpassed breast cancer as the leading cause of cancer death in women in the United States. This rapid shift is a testament to how powerfully modifiable risk factors such as cigarette smoking can influence health. Globally, breast cancer remains the most common cause of cancer

Dr L.T. Tanoue has no commercial or financial conflicts of interest with this article.
Yale School of Medicine, Boardman Building 110, 333 Cedar Street, New Haven, CT 06510, USA
E-mail address: lynn.tanoue@yale.edu

Clin Chest Med 42 (2021) 467–482
https://doi.org/10.1016/j.ccm.2021.04.007

incidence and mortality in women, but with trends unfortunately following what has been observed in the United States. **Fig. 1** shows a map of the world identifying the leading cause of cancer death in women by country in 2020 as reported by the International Agency for Research on Cancer (IARC), which monitors trends in cancer burden over time for the World Health Organization (WHO).[4,5] IARC data demonstrate that, among the 5 most common causes of cancer in women globally in 2020, the incidence of breast cancer is triple that of lung cancer.[6] However, the outcomes with lung cancer are far worse, with the number of deaths and cumulative risk of mortality attributable to lung cancer very close to those observed for breast cancer (**Table 1**).[6] Lung cancer is now the most common cause of cancer death in women in 28 industrialized countries with high HDI, including the United States, Canada, Australia, China, much of Western Europe, and Scandinavia. Martin-Sanchez and colleagues[7] recently reported on age-standardized mortality rates (ASMR) for lung and breast cancer in women from 2015 to 2030 in 52 countries (33 high-income and 19 low-income or middle-income) selected based on population of at least 1 million and WHO mortality data available for at least 4 years from 2008 to 2014. As would be anticipated from the IARC data, the first countries where lung cancer mortality exceeded breast cancer mortality were mostly high-income countries. This shift toward more mortality burden from lung cancer was conjectured as attributable to widespread efforts at breast cancer screening and early detection as well as improvements in treatment, coincident with a more established tobacco

epidemic in women. Overall, the median ASMR in all 52 countries by 2030 was projected to decline for breast cancer from 16.1 to 14.7 per 100,000, with an anticipated increase for lung cancer from 11.2 to 16.0 per 100,000.

In high HDI countries such as the United States, lung cancer incidence and mortality are declining in both men and women. The graphs shown in **Fig. 2** demonstrate mortality rates since 1930 for lung cancer (in red) and other cancers in men and women in the United States since 1930.[3] The steep increases in lung cancer mortality in men up from 1930 to 1990 and in women from 1960 to 2005 are largely attributable to cigarette smoking. Similarly, much, though not all, of the declines in lung cancer mortality thereafter are related to public health efforts targeted at tobacco control. A deeper examination of these data demonstrates that the decrease in both lung cancer incidence and mortality in women has been at a lesser rate than in men, the notable consequence of which is that the historic male preponderance in lung cancer has shifted. Jemal and colleagues[8] performed an analysis of age-specific lung cancer incidence from 1970 to 2016 in the North American Association of Central Cancer Registries, with specific reference to race or ethnic group, age at diagnosis, and birth year cohort, and correlated those data with prevalence of cigarette smoking in the same time period recorded by the National Health Survey. They observed that female-to-male incidence rate ratios among Hispanic and non-Hispanic white individuals born after the mid-1960s in the age groups of 30 to 34, 35 to 39, 40 to 44, and 45 to 59 years exceeded 1.0, indicating that lung cancer incidence rates in these

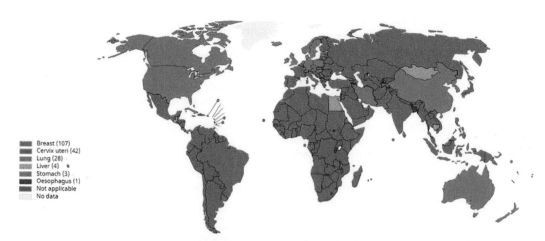

Breast (107)
Cervix uteri (42)
Lung (28)
Liver (4)
Stomach (3)
Oesophagus (1)
Not applicable
No data

Fig. 1. Leading cause of cancer mortality in women age ≥30 years, by country, 2020. (*From* International Agency for Research on Cancer, World Health Organization. Cancer Today. Estimated age-standardized incidence rates (World) in 2020, all cancers, females, ages 30+. 2020; https://gco.iarc.fr/today/online-analysis-map accessed 12/31/2020.)

Table 1
Estimated statistics for the 5 most common causes of cancer in women aged 30 to 84, worldwide in 2020

Cancer	Number of Incident Cases	Age-Standardized Incidence per 100,000	Number of Deaths	Cumulative Risk of Mortality
Breast	2.138,134	105.1	619,339	1.48
Lung	698,664	31.4	539,062	1.34
Cervix uteri	571,050	28.8	325,727	0.81
Colon	471,585	20.8	215.367	0.45
Corpus uteri	401,411	19.5	87,085	0.22

Data from International Agency for Research on Cancer, World Health Organization. Cancer Today. Estimated number of new cases in 2020, worldwide, both sexes, all ages. 2020; https://gco.iarc.fr/today/online-analysis-table accessed 1/2/2021.

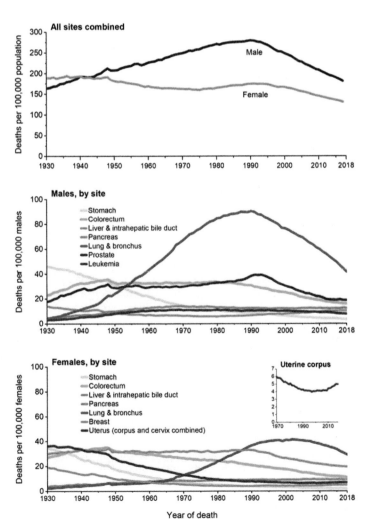

Fig. 2. Trends in cancer mortality rates by sex overall and for selected cancers, United States, 1930 to 2018. Rates are age-adjusted to the 2000 US standard population. Due to improvements in International Classification of Diseases coding over time, numerator data for cancers of the lung and bronchus, colon and rectum, liver, and uterus differ from those for the contemporary time period. For example, rates for lung and bronchus include pleura, trachea, mediastinum, and other respiratory organs. (*From* Siegel RL, Miller KD, Fuchs HE et al. Cancer Statistics, 2021;71:7-33.)

groups were higher in women than in men. This shift could not be explained by sex differences in smoking behaviors. The average number of cigarettes smoked per day was lower among women, and further, women tended not to consume other tobacco products, such as cigars or chewing tobacco, and were more likely to smoke menthol cigarettes, which are not associated with a higher risk of lung cancer.[9–11] This study highlights 2 areas of concern in the discussion of sex differences in lung cancer, particularly in the younger population. The first is a hypothesis that has received much attention, although no firm proof, that women are more susceptible to the carcinogenic effects of tobacco. The second is that sex-specific factors other than smoking behaviors are likely important determinants of lung cancer development and outcomes in both women and men.

LUNG CANCER SCREENING

Lung cancer screening with low-dose chest computed tomography (LDCT) scan was first recommended by the US Preventive Services Task Force (USPSTF) in 2013 for persons in the United States aged 55 to 80, who have smoked at least 30 pack-years and are currently smoking or quit smoking within the past 15 years.[12] This recommendation was largely based on the results of the National Lung Screening Trial (NLST), a randomized study including more than 50,000 participants, which demonstrated a lung cancer mortality benefit of 20% with screening with LDCT versus chest radiograph annually.[13] In addition, modeling studies performed by the National Cancer Institute Cancer Intervention Surveillance and Modeling Network (CISNET) using data from NLST and the Prostate, Lung, Colorectal and Ovarian Cancer Screening Trial identified this strategy as most advantageously balancing benefits and potential harms of screening.[14] Another large randomized study in Europe, the Dutch-Belgian Lung Cancer Screening (NELSON) trial, compared screening with volume-based LDCT compared with no screening, and demonstrated a 24% reduction in lung cancer mortality over 10 years of follow-up.[15] Based on a systematic evidence synthesis including NELSON and other studies published since NLST, as well as a new CISNET modeling study, USPSTF updated and expanded its recommendations for screening in 2021.[16–18] Lung cancer screening is now recommended for individuals ages 50 to 80, who have smoked at least 20 pack-years and are currently smoking or quit smoking within the past 15 years.[16]

Women were underrepresented in both NLST and NELSON, representing 41% of participants in NLST and only 16% of participants in NELSON. In NLST, the rate ratio for lung cancer mortality was lower (ie, greater percentage reduction in mortality with LDCT screening) in women than men, although the interaction of sex and trial arm was not statistically significant.[19] In the NELSON trial, the imbalance of gender representation resulted in a primary analysis in men (13,195 subjects) demonstrating a 24% reduction in lung cancer mortality after 10 years of follow-up. A subgroup analysis in the much smaller group of women (2594 subjects) showed significant reductions in lung cancer mortality at 7 (64%), 8 (69%), and 9 (48%) years of follow-up, although that benefit was not sustained at 10 years. The results of NLST and NELSON, as well as those of the recently reported German Lung Cancer Screening Intervention (LUSI) trial suggest that screening for lung cancer with LDCT results in a larger reduction in lung cancer mortality among women than men.[20]

LUNG CANCER RISK
Cigarette Smoking

Cigarette smoking is the leading cause of preventable disease and death in the United States and increasingly around the globe. Tobacco use is implicated causally in cardiovascular disease, stroke, chronic obstructive pulmonary disease, and multiple cancers. Approximately 80% to 90% of lung cancers in women are attributable to smoking.[21,22]

The history of smoking in women is a lesson in the power of targeted marketing, one that should not be ignored in the context of the current globalization of tobacco. At the turn of the twentieth century, societal norms prevented women from smoking, but the tobacco industry quickly and successfully identified women as a potential lucrative market segment. In 1928, George Washington Hill, president of the American Tobacco company, was described as stating, "It will be like opening a new gold mine in our front yard."[23] In the 1920s and 1930s in the United States, targeted marketing focused on normalization of social attitudes toward women smoking, intentionally elevating smoking by linking cigarettes to ideals of independence and emancipation, including the infamous identification of cigarettes as "torches of freedom."[24] Advertising embraced cigarettes as symbols of fashion, purposefully linking cigarettes with movie stars and glamour. A new American ideal of female thinness as a requisite for beauty was capitalized on by the Lucky Strike campaign launched in 1925, encouraging women to "reach for a Lucky instead of a sweet."[25] These campaigns were enormously successful in opening a new, highly profitable market segment of female smokers, with the result that 34% of American women were smoking at the time of the 1964 Surgeon General report.[2] The industry continues to pursue this targeted approach, focusing on emerging markets to entice women around the world to smoke. To the detriment of women's health, similar strategies continue to intentionally encourage cigarette smoking among women in countries around the world where smoking is not yet widely adopted, who represent an untapped and potentially lucrative market.

The most recent Centers for Disease Control and Prevention (CDC) summary on tobacco use among adults in the United States based on the National Health Interview Survey reported that in 2019, approximately 1 of every 5 adult Americans (20.8%) used tobacco products, 80.5% of which were combustible tobacco products, most commonly cigarettes.[26] Despite the success of health initiatives informing the public of the health hazards of smoking, 14% (34.1 million) of adults in the United States smoke cigarettes. Other forms of combustible tobacco are also highly prevalent, with e-cigarettes used by 4.5% (10.9 million), cigars by 3.6% (8.7 million), and smokeless tobacco by 2.4% (5.9 million). As has been historically the case, the prevalence of any tobacco use was higher among men (26.2%) than women (15.7%), and among the population <65 compared with ≥65 years of age. Higher prevalence of tobacco use was also associated with factors correlating with socioeconomic or environmental stress, including GED as the level of highest education, marital status divorced/separated/widowed or single, annual household income <$35,000, lesbian/gay/bisexual identification, uninsured or insured by Medicaid or other public insurance, and self-reporting of disability or anxiety.

Whether women are more susceptible to the effects of tobacco carcinogens is an area of considerable controversy. Case control studies in the 1990s suggested that, given the same exposure to cigarettes, women had a 1.5 to 2.0 times higher risk for developing all major histologic types of lung cancer.[27–29] Other studies suggested that lung cancer in women occurred at younger age relative to smoking initiation, and with less exposure to cigarettes when compared with men.[30,31] A more recent analysis of the UK Health Improvement Network database reported that women who smoked more than 20 cigarettes per day had a higher likelihood of developing lung cancer than men with similar smoking exposure, with odds ratios (OR) of 19.2 (95% confidence interval [CI] 17.1–21.3) versus 13.0 (95% CI 11.7–14.5).[32]

Several prospective studies have not borne these findings out. In an analysis of the Nurses' Health Study in women and the Health Professionals Follow-up Study in men, Bain and colleagues[33] demonstrated that, after adjusting for age, number of cigarettes smoked per day, age at start of smoking, and time since quitting, incidence rates and hazard ratios of lung cancer were no different in women and men. Similarly, in a prospective study performed in Denmark, rate ratios of lung cancer did not differ between women and men after adjustment for pack-years and age.[34] The most recent Surgeon General report on the health consequences of smoking points out that studies addressing sex-associated differences in lung cancer risk such as those noted previously were performed 2 to 3 decades ago, in older cohorts smoking cigarettes with less lung cancer risk than currently on the market.[35] Although the hypothesis that women are more susceptible to development of smoking-related lung cancer remains unproven, an increasing body of evidence suggests that other sex-related genetic and biologic factors may play important roles in determining the ultimate carcinogenic effects of tobacco smoke exposure.

Lung Cancer in Never-Smokers

There is a growing appreciation that a substantial portion of lung cancers occur in never-smokers, and that the preponderance of this subgroup of lung cancer occurs in women. In the United States, approximately 15% to 20% of lung cancers in women occur in never-smokers, compared with 7% to 9% in men, and with never-smokers accounting for approximately 10% to 15% of all non–small-cell lung cancers (NSCLC) in both sexes combined.[8,36] Globally, it is estimated that 15% of men and 53% of women with lung cancer are never-smokers, accounting for 25% of all lung cancers worldwide.[37,38] Substantial geographic variation is observed between countries around the world. In South Asia, the proportion of female never-smokers with lung cancer is reported as high as 83%, whereas industrialized countries in Europe report patterns more similar to that observed in the United States.[37,39–41] Studies in Asian countries have reported an earlier age at diagnosis for never-smokers, although this has not been observed in the United States or Europe.[42,43] A number of studies have reported an association with better clinical outcome for never-smokers, independent of stage, treatment, or comorbidities.[42,44,45]

It is not completely clear whether the incidence of never-smoking lung cancer cases is increasing or whether their proportion is simply rising because of falling incidence of smoking-related lung cancers. Arguments have been made for both sides of this controversy. The observation that lung cancer was so uncommon at the turn of the twentieth century by itself argues that the incidence of lung cancers in never-smokers must have risen. In a study performed in 3 large institutions in the United States, including 10,593 NSCLC cases, the proportion of never-smoker patients with NSCLC increased from 8.0% in 1990 to 1995, to 14.9% in 2011 to 2013, a difference that persisted after controlling for sex, stage at diagnosis, and race/ethnicity.[36] Never-smokers were more likely to be female (17.5%) as opposed to male (6.9%). Similarly, a retrospective study of 2170 patients who underwent surgery for lung cancer at the center with highest surgical activity for lung cancer in the United Kingdom showed an increase in annual frequency of lung cancer in never-smokers from 13% to 28% over the period 2008 to 2014, with 67% of never-smoking lung cancer cases occurring in women.[46] Regardless of whether incidence is truly rising, the absolute number of lung cancer cases in never-smokers is substantial, estimated at more than 300,000 cases per year globally, and making lung cancer in never-smokers as a distinct entity the seventh leading cause of cancer death in the world.[37]

A consistent observation in never-smokers with lung cancer is that the most common histologic subtype is adenocarcinoma, which cannot be explained by a general trend toward an increase in lung adenocarcinomas over time.[37,47] Moreover, although genomic mutations that may predispose to carcinogenesis predictably occur more frequently in smokers exposed to tobacco carcinogens, never-smokers have a higher prevalence of driver mutations, the first examples of which were described in the epidermal growth factor receptor (EGFR) gene.[41] Activating mutations in EGFR, typically an exon 19 deletion or exon 21 mutation, are identified in 40% to 60% of lung adenocarcinomas in never-smokers, compared with approximately 15% in a general population of lung adenocarcinomas in the United States, and are more common in women and persons of Asian ethnicity.[48–52]

Preliminary data from the Taiwan Lung Cancer Screening for Never-Smoker Trial (TALENT) suggest that a positive family history of lung cancer is a significant contributor to lung cancer risk in never-smokers.[53] In Taiwan, 53% of lung cancer deaths occur in never-smokers. TALENT included 12,011 never-smoking individuals aged 55 to 75 years with a high-risk feature (family history of lung cancer, history of chronic lung disease, cooking without ventilation, and cooking with high intensity of frying); 73.8% of the study population were women. The prevalence of lung cancer over 6 years of follow-up was 2.6%, higher than lung cancer detection rates in NLST or NELSON. Strikingly, patients with a family history of lung cancer had a lung cancer detection rate of 3.2%. Even higher risk was observed if the affected family member was a first-degree compared with more distant relation, as well as with the number of family members with lung cancer.

Biologic Factors

Although cigarettes remain the primary cause of lung cancer in both women and men, a growing body of evidence supports the hypothesis that multiple biologic factors contribute to susceptibility differences in women and men relative to the development of lung cancer. Jemal and colleagues[8] noted that sex differences in smoking behaviors do not fully explain the higher incidence rates of lung cancer observed among non-Hispanic white and Hispanic women born since the mid-1960s. Moreover, the important observation that lung cancer in never-smokers is more frequent in women by itself suggests that there are sex-related differences in carcinogenesis influenced by hormonal, genetic, and environmental factors (**Table 2**).

Histology of lung cancer in women
The distribution of histology among lung cancers in women and men have consistently differed. Over time, adenocarcinoma has become the most common histologic type in both women and men, but male smokers are still more likely to develop squamous cell carcinoma than female smokers.[54–56] Rates of small cell carcinoma have remained similar in men and women.[27,56] The preponderance of adenocarcinoma in women as well as the rising proportion of adenocarcinoma in men has been hypothesized as related to changes in tar concentration of cigarettes as well as behaviors of cigarette inhalation between sexes and over time, although these are unproven.[57] Interest in understanding why lung cancer histology distribution is different in women and men has increasingly focused on sex-associated variations in genetic factors and molecular variations associated with or caused by smoking and other carcinogenic exposures.

Molecular factors
DNA adducts are covalent modifications of DNA resulting from exposure to carcinogens. With reference to smoking, reactive metabolites of tobacco smoke carcinogens, typically polycyclic aromatic hydrocarbons, are known to bind to DNA and form adducts. These molecular alterations

Table 2
Brief summary of sex-related differences in lung cancer

Susceptibility to carcinogenic effects of cigarette smoking	• Controversial. Definite causality of cigarettes in women who smoke, but no consistent evidence supporting increased susceptibility based on female sex
Lung cancer in never-smokers	• 15%–20% of women compared with 7%–9% of men with lung cancer in the United States are never-smokers • Globally, 53% of women and 15% of men with lung cancer are never-smokers
Histology	• Higher likelihood of adenocarcinoma histology in women compared with men
Molecular and genetic factors	• Higher DNA adduct accumulation in women • Higher likelihood of activating mutations in *EGFR* in women
Hormonal factors	• Controversial; no consistent evidence supporting effect of estrogen or other reproductive hormones on lung cancer development or outcomes
Environmental factors	• Domestic radon exposure implicated in 26% of lung cancers in never-smokers in United States • Women in less industrialized countries have higher exposure to carcinogens and particulates from combustion of biomass fuels
Ionizing radiation	• Relative risk of lung cancer is increased in women who receive adjuvant radiation therapy for breast cancer and who smoke
Screening	• Results from several studies (National Lung Screening Trial, Dutch-Belgian Lung Cancer Screening Trial, German Lung Cancer Screening Intervention) suggest larger reduction in lung cancer mortality in women than men related to screening
Outcomes	• Women have better 5-year lung cancer survival, regardless of age, stage, treatment

may serve as biomarkers of carcinogenic exposure, and there has been great interest in their potential application as predictors of cancer risk.[58,59] If not repaired by normal mechanisms, DNA adducts may result in enduring mutations, with the potential to alter transcription of tumor suppressor genes or oncogenes.[59] Higher levels of DNA adducts are associated with more intense cigarette use.[60] Women smokers appear to accumulate DNA adducts with less tobacco exposure than men, suggesting either increased susceptibility to development of adducts or decreased DNA repair capability or both.[61,62] This has been proposed as a potential biologic explanation supporting the hypothesis that women have increased susceptibility to the carcinogenic effects of cigarette smoking.

Some somatic gene mutations have strong associations with lung cancer. The most common of these are activating mutations in the Kirsten rat sarcoma viral oncogene (KRAS) and EGFR. The higher frequency of EGFR mutations in women and never-smokers has already been discussed previously. In contrast, mutations in KRAS occur more commonly in adenocarcinomas in smokers, are highly associated with DNA adduct formation, and do not demonstrate differences in prevalence between sexes.[63–65] ALK rearrangements are more commonly identified in never-smokers, but, like KRAS, these and other mutations and gene alterations, including ROS-1 translocations and mutations in HER2 and BRAF, do not appear to have any sex-related differences in prevalence.[66,67]

Hormonal factors

The hypothesis, albeit unproven, that women have increased susceptibility to carcinogenic effects of cigarette smoking, the higher prevalence of lung cancer in never-smoking women, and the observed differences between men and women in histology, molecular factors such as EGFR mutations, and outcomes have led to questions as to the potential role of female reproductive hormones, particularly estrogen, in lung cancer. Of the 2 types of classical estrogen receptors, ERα (or ESR1) is normally distributed in breast, ovary, and endometrium, whereas ERβ (or ESR2) is normally distributed in a wide array of organs. In the lung, ERβ is highly expressed in pneumocytes and bronchial epithelial cells and appears to be integral to maintenance of extracellular matrix.[68]

The estrogen signaling pathway is clearly critical in the pathogenesis of breast cancer and has been extensively investigated in that context, with consequential impact on treatment. Several observations have raised speculation that estrogens may also play an important role in lung carcinogenesis.[68] First, estrogen receptors have been found in lung cancer cell lines and lung cancer tissues from both women and men, predominantly ERβ in adenocarcinoma.[69–71] Aromatase, the rate-limiting enzyme in estrogen synthesis, has also been demonstrated in both lung cancer cell lines and human specimens, suggesting that release of estrogen can occur in the tumor microenvironment.[72,73] Second, older women (age >60 years) have been observed to have better survival outcome than men or their younger female counterparts, leading to speculation that postmenopausal status may be protective.[74] Third, lung cancer is more frequent in never-smoking women than never-smoking men, with younger, premenopausal women comprising a significant subgroup of these patients.[36,37,41,46]

Whether exogenous hormone replacement therapy (HRT) has an effect on lung cancer is an area of controversy. A number of studies have suggested an association between HRT and increased lung cancer risk[52,75–80] The Women's Health Initiative trial, a double-blind, placebo-controlled, randomized trial that included 16,608 women aged 50 to 79 years and compared estrogen plus progestin versus placebo, was stopped early because of an increased risk of malignancy in the intervention group.[77,78] In the estrogen-progestin arm, there was a significantly higher number of deaths from NSCLC (0.11% vs 0.06%; HR 1.71; 95% CI 1.16–2.52). However, the trial did not show any significant increase in incidence of lung cancer, and other prospective studies examining the impact of menopause and HRT have not demonstrated any sex-related difference in lung cancer rates.[81–84] Further, some studies have reported a protective effect of HRT against lung cancer.[85,86] The multiple conflicting studies clearly indicate that much more research is needed to understand the influence of reproductive hormones, endogenous or exogenous, on lung cancer risk and outcomes.

Occupational and environmental exposures

Many occupational and environmental carcinogens are known to be associated with increased lung cancer risk. Men have had a much higher likelihood of exposure to carcinogens in the workplace including, for example, asbestos in construction or insulation work, and radon gas in mining. Women have historically had more exposure to carcinogens in the domestic environment, including radon or byproducts of burning of biomass fuels in the home. Differences between women and men appear to relate predominantly to the likelihood of exposure and its intensity, with less known about whether sex-related differences in susceptibility to the effects of specific exposures exist.

Radon Radon is a decay product of uranium-238 and radium-226 that is widely distributed in rock, soil, and groundwater. It is associated with increased lung cancer risk and has an interactive effect with cigarette smoking. In its 1999 publication on the Biological Effects of Ionizing Radiation (BEIR VI) and the health effects of exposure to indoor radon, the National Research Council indicated that radon was the second most important cause of lung cancer in the United States.[87] In a report on assessment of risks from domestic radon in the United States, the Environmental Protection Agency estimated that radon was implicated in 26% of lung cancers in never-smokers and in 13.4% of lung cancers overall, with cigarette exposure being a co-carcinogen in many but not all cases.[88]

Biomass fuels Around the world and particularly in less industrialized countries, women are more likely to be exposed to smoke and byproducts of the indoor burning of coal or biomass fuels (wood, charcoal, plant materials, or dung) for heating and cooking. Emissions from combustion of these fuels generate high concentrations of polycyclic aromatic hydrocarbons that are similar to those in tobacco smoke.[89] Moreover, burning of these fuels creates particulates of small diameter (<2.5 μm) that have been implicated in the deposition of adherent carcinogens in the lung.[37] Emissions of chemical byproducts and particulates will be compounded in dwellings that are poorly ventilated. In a retrospective cohort study of more than 30,000 individuals in Xuanwei, China, lifelong use of bituminous ("smoky") compared with anthracite ("smokeless") coal for heating was associated with a significantly increased risk of lung cancer death in men (HR 36; 95% CI 20–65) and an even higher risk of lung cancer death in women (HR 99; 95% CI 37–266).[90] Domestic exposure to wood smoke has similarly been associated with lung cancer. Kurmi and colleagues[89] performed a meta-analysis evaluating the association of solid fuel use and lung cancer. Their analysis included 28 studies performed in 15 countries, with 12,419 pooled lung cancer cases and 34,609 pooled controls. An overall higher likelihood of lung cancer was observed in users of wood fuel for cooking and heating (OR 1.50; 95% CI 1.17–1.94). Combining all solid fuel exposures, the risk of lung cancer was significantly increased in women (OR 1.81; 95% CI 1.54–2.12) but not in men (OR 1.16; 95% CI 0.79–1.69). These findings merit particular attention in understanding the high frequency of never-smoking status in women with lung cancer in East and South Asia and less developed areas of the world.

Radiation therapy Therapeutic radiation is known to increase the risk of secondary malignancies, including lung cancer. This was firmly established in the follow-up of patients surviving Hodgkin lymphoma who received radiation therapy to the chest. In a systematic review of studies reporting long-term complications in more than 32,000 patients treated for Hodgkin lymphoma, the relative risk (RR) of developing any solid tumor by 25 years after lymphoma diagnosis was doubled (RR = 2.0), with lung cancer having the highest risk (RR = 2.9).[91] Development of lung cancer was associated with increasing radiation dose, increasing age at lymphoma diagnosis, duration of time after lymphoma treatment, and cigarette smoking, with a synergistic interaction observed between radiation and smoking. Most, but not all, secondary lung cancers occurred within or on the edge of the treatment field.[92–94] It should be noted that many of the patients included in this 2005 review had been treated with mantle radiation, and that the type of radiation given as well as the extent of treated fields have evolved since then. Further, no difference in risk by sex was observed. Nonetheless, the observations in these patients provides an important background for consideration of the potential harms of both therapeutic and diagnostic radiation used presently.

Radiation therapy is an important component of the treatment approach to breast cancer. Adjuvant radiation is often recommended after lumpectomy or mastectomy to reduce the risk of locoregional recurrence and improve survival. The decision to include radiation as part of treatment will be informed by tumor characteristics, including stage, size, number of sites, status of lymphatic or vascular invasion, completeness of surgical resection, and involvement of lymph nodes or skin, as well as by patient-specific factors including patient preference. A meta-analysis of lung and heart complications associated with breast cancer regimens in studies published from 2010 to 2015 and including 40,781 women demonstrated that, ≥10 years after treatment, lung cancer incidence was increased with RR 2.10 (95% CI 1.48–2.98).[95] As was observed in the Hodgkin lymphoma population, this effect was particularly pronounced in patients with breast cancer who were long-term continuing smokers (absolute risk 4%) compared with non-smokers (absolute risk 0.3%). Modern radiation techniques such as intensity modulated radiation therapy may limit radiation dose to nonbreast tissue, but long-term impact on the incidence of secondary lung malignancy will not be known for decades. For all women with breast cancer being considered for adjuvant radiation therapy, smoking status should be established, tobacco cessation interventions offered when appropriate, and a discussion held to consider the benefit to survival versus risk of secondary lung malignancy.

A discussion of lung cancer risk from radiation necessitates consideration of the risks of radiation exposure incurred with lung cancer screening with LDCT scanning (LDCT). The current recommendations for screening in the United States include annual LDCT imaging. By definition, radiation dose with LDCT is low, but serial screening inevitably will result in cumulative exposure. At a very high level, women are generally felt to have more health risk related to ionizing radiation than men.[96] There is some organ-specificity to this, with higher risk in women related to irradiation of the breast and thyroid and higher risk in men related to irradiation of the liver and colon. In particular, breast tissue is known to be one of the most radiation-sensitive tissues in humans, particularly in younger women.[96–98] Assuming a screening protocol such as was used in the NLST, one study incorporating risk modeling from the 2006 National Academies of Science Biologic Effects of Ionizing Radiation report (BIER VII)[99] estimated a lifetime attributable risk of radiation-related lung cancer mortality from lung cancer screening at approximately 0.07% in men and 0.14% in women,[100] whereas another study projected that 1 cancer death would be anticipated for every 2500 persons screened.[101] In the Continuous Observation of Smoking Subjects (COSMOS) lung cancer screening study performed in Italy, at 10 years of follow-up, the actual median cumulative effective radiation dose, inclusive of all LDCT and PET CT scans done in the context of screening, was 9.3 mSv for men and 13.0 mSv for women.[20] As reference, the typical radiation dose for a standard chest CT scan is in the range of 7 to 8 mSv, and the average annual radiation dose from background sources (eg, radon in rock/soil/water/building materials, radioactive isotopes in the food chain, cosmic radiation) in the United States is estimated at 3.6 mSv.[102–105] The COSMOS study concluded that 1 radiation-induced lung cancer would be expected for every 173 lung cancers detected, and 1 radiation-induced major cancer other than lung cancer would be expected for every 108 lung cancers detected through screening.[20] The lifetime attributable risk for developing cancer was greater for women than for men, with RR up to 4 times greater for lung cancer and up to 3 times greater for major cancers. The COSMOS investigators felt

that the higher risk of screening-induced cancer in women in their study was due to the increased sensitivity of women to radiation overall as well as specifically to their increased risk of breast cancer.[99]

The capability and utilization of imaging modalities has increased dramatically with technology innovation. In 2006, the per capita radiation dose from diagnostic medical exposure had increased almost 600% compared with 1982, largely related to CT and nuclear imaging, with an average annual radiation rising to equal natural background radiation.[104,106] In other words, the average American is now exposed to twice the amount of annual radiation as was the case in the 1980s, largely due to health care–related radiation.[104] Responsible use of medical imaging, including for lung cancer screening, is an expectation for high quality practice, and particularly for female patients.

OUTCOMES

Studies performed in large population databases have demonstrated that, at every stage of disease, the prognosis of women with lung cancer is better than that of men. The Cancer Registry of Norway (CRN), the repository for mandatory cancer reporting in Norway, collected 40,118 cases of lung cancer over the period 1988 to 2007.[107] Of these, 14,139 (35%) were women and 25,979 (65%) were men. In the first 5 years of study (1988–1992), 71% of lung cancer cases occurred in men and 29% in women (total 8245 cases). In the last 5 years of study (2003–2007), there were more lung cancer cases (total 12,096 cases) with 60% occurring in men and 40% in women. Over the entire study duration, average age-adjusted annual incidence increased more in women than in men (4.9% vs 1.4%). Examination of 1- and 5-year survival over 5-year periods of the entire study duration demonstrated improvement in survival with each consecutive period, and with both 1- and 5-year survival consistently higher in women than in men. Multivariate analysis demonstrated that the observed superior survival of women compared with men was independent of age, stage, histology, or period of diagnosis (Table 3).

The observations of the CRN study are mirrored in populations in other parts of the world. Multivariate analysis of the Osaka Cancer Registry in Japan, including 79,330 cases of lung cancer grouped in 5-year intervals from 1975 to 2007, demonstrated that women had better 5-year survival than men.[108] After adjusting for age, stage, histologic type, and treatment, the hazard ratio for death in men compared with women was 1.19 (95% CI 1.16–1.21). In the United States, an

Table 3
Cancer Registry of Norway, lung cancer cases 1988 to 2007

	Women (n = 13,983) HR 95% CI	Men (n = 25,721) HR 95% CI	P Value
Histology (adjusted for stage, age and diagnostic period)			
Adenocarcinoma	1.000	1.244 (1.191–1.298)	<.001
NOS	1.000	1.141 (1.078–1.207)	<.001
Squamous cell carcinoma	1.000	1.048 (0.994–1.105)	.084
Small cell carcinoma	1.000	1.052 (1.001–1.105)	.045
Large cell carcinoma	1.000	1.147 (1.033–1.273)	.010
Stage (adjusted for histology, age and diagnostic period)			
Localized disease	1.000	1.252 (1.179–1.330)	<.001
Regional disease	1.000	1.112 (1.059–1.168)	<.001
Metastatic disease	1.000	1.103 (1.066–1.141)	<.001
Unknown	1.000	1.135 (1.045–1.233)	.003
Age (y) (adjusted for histology, stage and diagnostic period)			
0–49	1.000	1.169 (1.053–1.298)	.003
50–59	1.000	1.185 (1.117–1.257)	<.001
60–69	1.000	1.169 (1.119–1.220)	<.001
70–79	1.000	1.108 (1.064–1.154)	<.001
80 and over	1.000	1.095 (1.017–1.179)	.016
Diagnostic period (adjusted for histology, stage and age)			
1988–1992	1.000	1.100 (1.042–1.162)	.001
1993–1997	1.000	1.137 (1.081–1.196)	<.001
1998–2002	1.000	1.163 (1.110–1.218)	<.001
2003–2007	1.000	1.125 (1.076–1.175)	<.001

Relative risks of death within 5 y of diagnosis for men versus women stratified by histology, stage, age groups, and diagnostic periods.

Abbreviation: NOS, not otherwise specified.

From Sagerup CM, Smastuen M, Johannesen TB, Helland A, Brustugun OT. Sex-specific trends in lung cancer incidence and survival: a population study of 40,118 cases. Thorax. 2011;66(4):301-307.

analysis of the Surveillance, Epidemiology, and End Results database from 1975 to 1999 evaluated outcomes in 228,572 patients with primary lung cancer (35.8% female and 64.2% male).[109] Incidence rates peaked in men in 1984 and in women in 1991. However, the subsequent rate of decline in incidence rates in men exceeded that in women, resulting in a narrowing of the male/female incidence ratio over the study period, with a substantially lower ratio observed in younger patients. For every stage of cancer, survival rates for women were significantly higher than for men, with the greatest difference noted in local-stage disease. Multivariate analysis demonstrated that this sex-related survival advantage was independent of race, stage, histology, or treatment, and was particularly pronounced in older patients (≥50 years of age).

Similarly, a study of the US National Cancer Database comparing outcomes of lobectomy versus sublobar resection in 11,990 patients with Stage IA NSCLC over the period 2003 to 2006 demonstrated that female sex was independently associated with a 5-year survival advantage, with HR of death in women compared with men of 0.76 (95% CI 0.72–0.80, P<.0001).[110]

Sex may be a surrogate for other factors that influence prognosis. The higher prevalence in women of factors such as never-smoking status and positive *EGFR* mutational status may contribute to the survival benefit associated with female sex that has been consistently reported. Unfortunately, population database studies typically lack detailed information about intensity and duration of smoking exposure or comorbidities that may influence survival. Despite these limitations, the consistent observation across continents that women have better lung cancer survival in men merits much more investigation.

FINAL COMMENTS

Lung cancer now kills more women in industrialized nations than breast cancer. That grim trend is being recapitulated around the world, fueled overtly by continued manipulation of cigarette consumption by the tobacco industry, and insidiously by poorly understood carcinogenic factors to which women are differentially exposed in domestic and work environments. It is now clear that sex-related differences likely exist in every aspect of lung cancer, but our ability to answer fundamental questions even as basic as whether women are more susceptible to the carcinogenic effects of cigarette smoke remains limited. The WHO estimated that nearly 600,000 women died of lung cancer around the world in 2019, and that toll is rising.[111] Much more work needs to be dedicated to understanding mechanisms of carcinogenesis that influence the development of lung cancer in women and the factors that contribute to consistent observations of better female survival. That deeper understanding and its therapeutic implications have the potential to improve lung cancer outcomes for both women and men.

CLINICS CARE POINTS

- Lung cancer is the leading cause of cancer death in women in industrialized countries.
- The incidence of lung cancer in women in developing nations around the world is rising.
- Smoking is the most important risk factor for lung cancer in women.
- In the United States, 15-20% of lung cancers in women occur in never smokers. Around the world approximately half of all lung cancers in women occur in never smokers.
- Lung cancer outcomes in women are better than in men.
- A deeper understanding of the biology of lung cancer in women will improve lung cancer outcomes for both women and men.

REFERENCES

1. US Department of Health, Education, and Welfare. Smoking and health: report of the Advisory Committee to the Surgeon General of the Public Health Service. PHS publication No. 1103. Washington: US Department of Health, Education, and Welfare, Public health Service, Center for Disease Control; 1964.

2. US Department of Health and Human Services. The health consequences of smoking for women. A report of the Surgeon General. In: US Department of Health and Human Services PHS, Office of the Assistant Secretary for Health, Office on Smoking and Health, editors. Washington: US Department of Health and Human Services; 1980.

3. Siegel RL, Miller KD, Fuchs HE, et al. Cancer statistics, 2021. CA Cancer J Clin 2021;71:7–33.

4. IARC's Mission. Cancer research for cancer prevention. Available at: https://www.iarc.fr/about-iarc-mission/. Accessed January 2, 2021.

5. International Agency for Research on Cancer, World Health Organization. Cancer Today. Estimated age-standardized incidence rates (World) in 2020, all cancers, females, ages 30+. 2020. Available at: https://gco.iarc.fr/today/online-analysis-table. Accessed January 2, 2021.

6. International Agency for Research on Cancer, World Health Organization. Cancer Today. Estimated number of new cases in 2020, worldwide, both sexes, all ages. 2020. Available at: https://gco.iarc.fr/today/online-analysis-table. Accessed January 2, 2021.

7. Martin-Sanchez JC, Lunet N, Gonzalez-Marron A, et al. Projections in breast and lung cancer mortality among women: a bayesian analysis of 52 countries worldwide. Cancer Res 2018;78(15):4436–42.

8. Jemal A, Miller KD, Ma J, et al. Higher lung cancer incidence in young women than young men in the United States. N Engl J Med 2018;378(21):1999–2009.

9. Nelson DE, Mowery P, Tomar S, et al. Trends in smokeless tobacco use among adults and adolescents in the United States. Am J Public Health 2006;96(5):897–905.

10. Giovino GA, Villanti AC, Mowery PD, et al. Differential trends in cigarette smoking in the USA: is menthol slowing progress? Tob Control 2015;24(1):28–37.

11. Blot WJ, Cohen SS, Aldrich M, et al. Lung cancer risk among smokers of menthol cigarettes. J Natl Cancer Inst 2011;103(10):810–6.

12. Moyer VA, Force USPST. Screening for lung cancer: U.S. Preventive Services Task Force recommendation statement. Ann Intern Med 2014;160(5):330–8.

13. National Lung Screening Trial Research Team, Aberle DR, Adams AM, et al. Reduced lung-cancer mortality with low-dose computed tomographic screening. N Engl J Med 2011;365(5):395–409.

14. de Koning HJ, Meza R, Plevritis SK, et al. Benefits and harms of computed tomography lung cancer screening strategies: a comparative modeling study for the U.S. Preventive Services Task Force. Ann Intern Med 2014;160(5):311–20.

15. de Koning HJ, van der Aalst CM, de Jong PA, et al. Reduced lung-cancer mortality with volume CT screening in a randomized trial. N Engl J Med 2020;382(6):503–13.

16. Krist AH, Davidson KW, Mangione CM, et al. Screening for lung cancer: US preventive Services Task Force recommendation statement. JAMA 2021;325(10):962–70.

17. Jonas DE, Reuland DS, Reddy SM, et al. Screening for lung cancer with low-dose computed tomography: updated evidence report and systematic review for the US Preventive Services Task Force. JAMA 2021;325(10):971–87.

18. Meza R, Jeon J, Toumazis I, et al. Evaluation of the benefits and harms of lung cancer screening with low-dose computed tomography: modeling study for the US Preventive Services Task Force. JAMA 2021;325(10):988–97.

19. National Lung Screening Trial Research Team. Lung cancer incidence and mortality with extended follow-up in the national lung screening trial. J Thorac Oncol 2019;14(10):1732–42.

20. Rampinelli C, De Marco P, Origgi D, et al. Exposure to low dose computed tomography for lung cancer screening and risk of cancer: secondary analysis of trial data and risk-benefit analysis. BMJ 2017; 356:j347.

21. Office of the Surgeon General. The health consequences of smoking: a report of the Surgeon General. US Department of Health and Human Services. CDC publication No. 7829. Washington, DC: US Department of Health and Human Services; 2004.

22. Gallaway MS, Henley SJ, Steele CB, et al. Surveillance for cancers associated with tobacco use - United States, 2010-2014. MMWR Surveill Summ 2018;67(12):1–42.

23. Bernays E. Biography of an idea: memoirs of public relations Counsel Edward L. Bernays. New York: Simon and Schuster; 1965.

24. Brandt AM. Recruiting women smokers: the engineering of consent. J Am Med Womens Assoc 1996;51(1–2):63–6.

25. Amos A, Haglund M. From social taboo to "torch of freedom": the marketing of cigarettes to women. Tob Control 2000;9(1):3–8.

26. Cornelius ME, Wang TW, Jamal A, et al. Tobacco product Use among adults - United States, 2019. MMWR Morb Mortal Wkly Rep 2020;69(46): 1736–42.

27. Osann KE, Anton-Culver H, Kurosaki T, et al. Sex differences in lung-cancer risk associated with cigarette smoking. Int J Cancer 1993;54(1):44–8.

28. Harris RE, Zang EA, Anderson JI, et al. Race and sex differences in lung cancer risk associated with cigarette smoking. Int J Epidemiol 1993; 22(4):592–9.

29. Zang EA, Wynder EL. Differences in lung cancer risk between men and women: examination of the evidence. J Natl Cancer Inst 1996;88(3–4):183–92.

30. McDuffie HH, Klaassen DJ, Dosman JA. Female-male differences in patients with primary lung cancer. Cancer 1987;59(10):1825–30.

31. Risch HA, Howe GR, Jain M, et al. Are female smokers at higher risk for lung cancer than male smokers? A case-control analysis by histologic type. Am J Epidemiol 1993;138(5):281–93.

32. Powell HA, Iyen-Omofoman B, Hubbard RB, et al. The association between smoking quantity and lung cancer in men and women. Chest 2013; 143(1):123–9.

33. Bain C, Feskanich D, Speizer FE, et al. Lung cancer rates in men and women with comparable histories of smoking. J Natl Cancer Inst 2004;96(11): 826–34.

34. Prescott E, Osler M, Hein HO, et al. Gender and smoking-related risk of lung cancer. The Copenhagen Center for Prospective Population Studies. Epidemiology 1998;9(1):79–83.

35. Health NCfCDPaHPUOoSa, editor. The health consequences of smoking - 50 Years of Progress. A report of the Surgeon general. US Department of health and human Services. Public health Service. Office of the Surgeon general. Atlanta, GA: Centers for Disease Control and Prevention; 2014.

36. Pelosof L, Ahn C, Gao A, et al. Proportion of never-smoker non-small cell lung cancer patients at three diverse institutions. J Natl Cancer Inst 2017;109(7): djw295.

37. Sun S, Schiller JH, Gazdar AF. Lung cancer in never smokers–a different disease. Nat Rev Cancer 2007;7(10):778–90.

38. Parkin DM, Bray F, Ferlay J, et al. Global cancer statistics, 2002. CA Cancer J Clin 2005;55(2): 74–108.

39. Jindal SK, Malik SK, Dhand R, et al. Bronchogenic carcinoma in Northern India. Thorax 1982;37(5): 343–7.

40. Badar F, Meerza F, Khokhar RA, et al. Characteristics of lung cancer patients–the Shaukat Khanum Memorial experience. Asian Pac J Cancer Prev 2006;7(2):245–8.

41. Barta JA, Powell CA, Wisnivesky JP. Global epidemiology of lung cancer. Ann Glob Health 2019; 85(1). https://doi.org/10.5334/aogh.2419.

42. Toh CK, Gao F, Lim WT, et al. Never-smokers with lung cancer: epidemiologic evidence of a distinct disease entity. J Clin Oncol 2006;24(15):2245–51.

43. Shimizu H, Tominaga S, Nishimura M, et al. Comparison of clinico-epidemiological features of lung cancer patients with and without a history of smoking. Jpn J Clin Oncol 1984;14(4):595–600.

44. Tammemagi CM, Neslund-Dudas C, Simoff M, et al. Smoking and lung cancer survival: the role

of comorbidity and treatment. Chest 2004;125(1): 27–37.

45. Nordquist LT, Simon GR, Cantor A, et al. Improved survival in never-smokers vs current smokers with primary adenocarcinoma of the lung. Chest 2004; 126(2):347–51.

46. Cufari ME, Proli C, De Sousa P, et al. Increasing frequency of non-smoking lung cancer: Presentation of patients with early disease to a tertiary institution in the UK. Eur J Cancer 2017;84:55–9.

47. Wakelee HA, Chang ET, Gomez SL, et al. Lung cancer incidence in never smokers. J Clin Oncol 2007;25(5):472–8.

48. Mitsudomi T, Yatabe Y. Mutations of the epidermal growth factor receptor gene and related genes as determinants of epidermal growth factor receptor tyrosine kinase inhibitors sensitivity in lung cancer. Cancer Sci 2007;98(12):1817–24.

49. Lynch TJ, Bell DW, Sordella R, et al. Activating mutations in the epidermal growth factor receptor underlying responsiveness of non-small-cell lung cancer to gefitinib. N Engl J Med 2004;350(21): 2129–39.

50. Sharma SV, Bell DW, Settleman J, et al. Epidermal growth factor receptor mutations in lung cancer. Nat Rev Cancer 2007;7(3):169–81.

51. Paez JG, Janne PA, Lee JC, et al. EGFR mutations in lung cancer: correlation with clinical response to gefitinib therapy. Science 2004;304(5676):1497–500.

52. Yang SY, Yang TY, Chen KC, et al. EGFR L858R mutation and polymorphisms of genes related to estrogen biosynthesis and metabolism in never-smoking female lung adenocarcinoma patients. Clin Cancer Res 2011;17(8):2149–58.

53. Yang P-C. National lung cancer screening program in Taiwan: the TALENT study. WCLC 2020, Plenary Presentation. Singapore: World Conference on Lung Cancer; 2021.

54. Pinsky PF, Church TR, Izmirlian G, et al. The National Lung Screening Trial: results stratified by demographics, smoking history, and lung cancer histology. Cancer 2013;119(22):3976–83.

55. Thun MJ, Lally CA, Flannery JT, et al. Cigarette smoking and changes in the histopathology of lung cancer. J Natl Cancer Inst 1997;89(21): 1580–6.

56. Brownson RC, Chang JC, Davis JR. Gender and histologic type variations in smoking-related risk of lung cancer. Epidemiology 1992;3(1):61–4.

57. Janssen-Heijnen ML, Coebergh JW, Klinkhamer PJ, et al. Is there a common etiology for the rising incidence of and decreasing survival with adenocarcinoma of the lung? Epidemiology 2001;12(2):256–8.

58. Cheng YW, Chen CY, Lin P, et al. DNA adduct level in lung tissue may act as a risk biomarker of lung cancer. Eur J Cancer 2000;36(11):1381–8.

59. Reid ME, Santella R, Ambrosone CB. Molecular epidemiology to better predict lung cancer risk. Clin Lung Cancer 2008;9(3):149–53.

60. Wiencke JK. DNA adduct burden and tobacco carcinogenesis. Oncogene 2002;21(48):7376–91.

61. Mollerup S, Ryberg D, Hewer A, et al. Sex differences in lung CYP1A1 expression and DNA adduct levels among lung cancer patients. Cancer Res 1999;59(14):3317–20.

62. Kure EH, Ryberg D, Hewer A, et al. p53 mutations in lung tumours: relationship to gender and lung DNA adduct levels. Carcinogenesis 1996;17(10): 2201–5.

63. Ou SH. Lung cancer in never-smokers. Does smoking history matter in the era of molecular diagnostics and targeted therapy? J Clin Pathol 2013; 66(10):839–46.

64. Ahrendt SA, Decker PA, Alawi EA, et al. Cigarette smoking is strongly associated with mutation of the K-ras gene in patients with primary adenocarcinoma of the lung. Cancer 2001;92(6):1525–30.

65. Dogan S, Shen R, Ang DC, et al. Molecular epidemiology of EGFR and KRAS mutations in 3,026 lung adenocarcinomas: higher susceptibility of women to smoking-related KRAS-mutant cancers. Clin Cancer Res 2012;18(22):6169–77.

66. Shaw AT, Yeap BY, Mino-Kenudson M, et al. Clinical features and outcome of patients with non-small-cell lung cancer who harbor EML4-ALK. J Clin Oncol 2009;27(26):4247–53.

67. Solomon B, Varella-Garcia M, Camidge DR. ALK gene rearrangements: a new therapeutic target in a molecularly defined subset of non-small cell lung cancer. J Thorac Oncol 2009;4(12):1450–4.

68. Hsu LH, Chu NM, Kao SH. Estrogen, estrogen receptor and lung cancer. Int J Mol Sci 2017;18(8): 1713.

69. Zhang G, Liu X, Farkas AM, et al. Estrogen receptor beta functions through nongenomic mechanisms in lung cancer cells. Mol Endocrinol 2009; 23(2):146–56.

70. Stabile LP, Siegfried JM. Estrogen receptor pathways in lung cancer. Curr Oncol Rep 2004;6(4): 259–67.

71. Schwartz AG, Prysak GM, Murphy V, et al. Nuclear estrogen receptor beta in lung cancer: expression and survival differences by sex. Clin Cancer Res 2005;11(20):7280–7.

72. Siegfried JM, Stabile LP. Estrongenic steroid hormones in lung cancer. Semin Oncol 2014;41(1): 5–16.

73. Weinberg OK, Marquez-Garban DC, Fishbein MC, et al. Aromatase inhibitors in human lung cancer therapy. Cancer Res 2005;65(24):11287–91.

74. Wakelee HA, Dahlberg SE, Brahmer JR, et al. Differential effect of age on survival in advanced NSCLC in women versus men: analysis of recent

Eastern Cooperative Oncology Group (ECOG) studies, with and without bevacizumab. Lung Cancer 2012;76(3):410–5.

75. Brinton LA, Gierach GL, Andaya A, et al. Reproductive and hormonal factors and lung cancer risk in the NIH-AARP Diet and Health Study cohort. Cancer Epidemiol Biomarkers Prev 2011;20(5): 900–11.

76. Baik CS, Strauss GM, Speizer FE, et al. Reproductive factors, hormone use, and risk for lung cancer in postmenopausal women, the Nurses' Health Study. Cancer Epidemiol Biomarkers Prev 2010; 19(10):2525–33.

77. Heiss G, Wallace R, Anderson GL, et al. Health risks and benefits 3 years after stopping randomized treatment with estrogen and progestin. JAMA 2008;299(9):1036–45.

78. Chlebowski RT, Schwartz AG, Wakelee H, et al. Oestrogen plus progestin and lung cancer in postmenopausal women (Women's Health Initiative trial): a post-hoc analysis of a randomised controlled trial. Lancet 2009;374(9697):1243–51.

79. Hulley S, Furberg C, Barrett-Connor E, et al. Non-cardiovascular disease outcomes during 6.8 years of hormone therapy: heart and Estrogen/progestin Replacement Study follow-up (HERS II). JAMA 2002;288(1):58–66.

80. Slatore CG, Chien JW, Au DH, et al. Lung cancer and hormone replacement therapy: association in the vitamins and lifestyle study. J Clin Oncol 2010;28(9):1540–6.

81. Clague J, Reynolds P, Sullivan-Halley J, et al. Menopausal hormone therapy does not influence lung cancer risk: results from the California Teachers Study. Cancer Epidemiol Biomarkers Prev 2011;20(3):560–4.

82. Chlebowski RT, Anderson GL, Gass M, et al. Estrogen plus progestin and breast cancer incidence and mortality in postmenopausal women. JAMA 2010;304(15):1684–92.

83. Chlebowski RT, Anderson GL, Manson JE, et al. Lung cancer among postmenopausal women treated with estrogen alone in the women's health initiative randomized trial. J Natl Cancer Inst 2010;102(18):1413–21.

84. Kabat GC, Miller AB, Rohan TE. Reproductive and hormonal factors and risk of lung cancer in women: a prospective cohort study. Int J Cancer 2007; 120(10):2214–20.

85. Schabath MB, Wu X, Vassilopoulou-Sellin R, et al. Hormone replacement therapy and lung cancer risk: a case-control analysis. Clin Cancer Res 2004;10(1 Pt 1):113–23.

86. Greiser CM, Greiser EM, Doren M. Menopausal hormone therapy and risk of lung cancer- Systematic review and meta-analysis. Maturitas 2010;65(3):198–204.

87. Health Effects of Exposure to Radon. Beir VI. Washington, DC: National Academy Press. National Academy of Sciences.; 1999.

88. EPA Assessment of Risks from Radon in Homes. Office of Radiation and Indoor Air. United States Environmental Protection Agency. . Washington, DC 204602003.

89. Kurmi OP, Arya PH, Lam KB, et al. Lung cancer risk and solid fuel smoke exposure: a systematic review and meta-analysis. Eur Respir J 2012;40(5):1228–37.

90. Barone-Adesi F, Chapman RS, Silverman DT, et al. Risk of lung cancer associated with domestic use of coal in Xuanwei, China: retrospective cohort study. BMJ 2012;345:e5414.

91. Dores GM, Metayer C, Curtis RE, et al. Second malignant neoplasms among long-term survivors of Hodgkin's disease: a population-based evaluation over 25 years. J Clin Oncol 2002;20(16):3484–94.

92. Travis LB, Gospodarowicz M, Curtis RE, et al. Lung cancer following chemotherapy and radiotherapy for Hodgkin's disease. J Natl Cancer Inst 2002; 94(3):182–92.

93. Gilbert ES, Stovall M, Gospodarowicz M, et al. Lung cancer after treatment for Hodgkin's disease: focus on radiation effects. Radiat Res 2003;159(2): 161–73.

94. Foss Abrahamsen A, Andersen A, Nome O, et al. Long-term risk of second malignancy after treatment of Hodgkin's disease: the influence of treatment, age and follow-up time. Ann Oncol 2002; 13(11):1786–91.

95. Taylor C, Correa C, Duane FK, et al. Estimating the risks of breast cancer radiotherapy: evidence from modern radiation doses to the lungs and heart and from previous randomized trials. J Clin Oncol 2017; 35(15):1641–9.

96. The 2007 Recommendations of the International Commission on Radiological Protection. ICRP Publication 103. . Vol Annals of the ICRP; 37, Nos. 2-4: Elsevier; 2007.

97. Lahham A, Masri HAL, Kameel S. Estimation of female radiation doses and breast cancer risk from chest CT examinations. Radiat Prot Dosim 2018; 179(4):303–9.

98. Yilmaz MH, Albayram S, Yasar D, et al. Female breast radiation exposure during thorax multidetector computed tomography and the effectiveness of bismuth breast shield to reduce breast radiation dose. J Comput Assist Tomogr 2007; 31(1):138–42.

99. National Research Council. Health risks from exposure to low levels of ionizing radiation: BEIR VII phase 2. Washington, DC: National Research Council. The National Academies Press; 2006.

100. Frank L, Christodoulou E, Kazerooni EA. Radiation risk of lung cancer screening. Semin Respir Crit Care Med 2013;34(6):738–47.

101. Bach PB, Mirkin JN, Oliver TK, et al. Benefits and harms of CT screening for lung cancer: a systematic review. JAMA 2012;307(22):2418–29.

102. Mettler FA Jr, Huda W, Yoshizumi TT, et al. Effective doses in radiology and diagnostic nuclear medicine: a catalog. Radiology 2008;248(1):254–63.

103. Osei EK, Darko J. A survey of organ equivalent and effective doses from diagnostic radiology procedures. ISRN Radiol 2013;2013:204346.

104. National Council on radiation protection and measurements. Ionizing radiation exposure of the population of the United States. National Council on radiation protection and measurements. NCRP report 160. Bethesda, MD: National Council on Radiation Protection and Measurements.; 2009.

105. Bolus N. NCRP report 160 and what it means for medical imaging and nuclear medicine. J Nucl Med Technol 2013;41:255–60.

106. Mettler FA Jr, Thomadsen BR, Bhargavan M, et al. Medical radiation exposure in the US in 2006: preliminary results. Health Phys 2008;95(5):502–7.

107. Sagerup CM, Smastuen M, Johannesen TB, et al. Sex-specific trends in lung cancer incidence and survival: a population study of 40,118 cases. Thorax 2011;66(4):301–7.

108. Kinoshita FL, Ito Y, Morishima T, et al. Sex differences in lung cancer survival: long-term trends using population-based cancer registry data in Osaka, Japan. Jpn J Clin Oncol 2017;47(9):863–9.

109. Fu JB, Kau TY, Severson RK, et al. Lung cancer in women: analysis of the national Surveillance, Epidemiology, and End Results database. Chest 2005;127(3):768–77.

110. Speicher PJ, Gu L, Gulack BC, et al. Sublobar resection for clinical stage IA non-small-cell lung cancer in the United States. Clin Lung Cancer 2016;17(1):47–55.

111. World Health Organization. The global health observatory. Global health estimates: life expectancy and leading causes of death and disability 2020. Available at: https://www.who.int/data/gho/data/themes/mortality-and-global-health-estimates. Accessed January 8, 2021.

Pulmonary Considerations for Pregnant Women

Nicholas Nassikas, MD[a], Isabelle Malhamé, MD, MSc[b], Margaret Miller, MD[c], Ghada Bourjeily, MD[d,e],*

KEYWORDS

• Pulmonary disease • Pregnancy • Imaging • Pharmacotherapy • Preconception counseling

KEY POINTS

• Respiratory conditions are common in pregnancy and may contribute to significant maternal morbidity.
• Pregnancy is associated with dynamic and profound physiologic changes that impact disease presentation, outcomes, and management.
• Most chest diagnostic studies are justified in pregnancy with nuances.
• Pharmacotherapy needs to weigh the impact of the untreated condition on the health of the mother and her unborn child against the risk of a medication.
• Preconception counseling is a key component of the care of reproductive age women and needs to be performed periodically during a woman's reproductive years.

INTRODUCTION

Pregnant and postpartum women with pulmonary conditions represent a unique and complex population group, with some respiratory disorders occurring frequently in this population. For instance, asthma, the most commonly diagnosed respiratory condition in pregnancy, occurs in up to 13% of pregnant women.[1–3] Sleep-disordered breathing, although infrequently diagnosed and coded in the pregnant population,[4,5] is identified in 9% of low-risk pregnancies screened for the disorder, but in up to 70% of pregnancies complicated by gestational diabetes, obesity, hypertension, and small for gestational age.[6–8]

Several pulmonary conditions may be first diagnosed during pregnancy (eg, obstructive sleep apnea and pulmonary embolism) or may be exacerbated by pregnancy (eg, asthma and pulmonary hypertension). Respiratory conditions such as pulmonary sepsis, pulmonary embolism, or pulmonary edema are a frequent cause of severe maternal morbidity[9,10] and an important contributor to maternal mortality.[9] Furthermore, pulmonary diseases are associated with a higher risk of adverse perinatal outcomes, including low

Funding: Dr G. Bourjeily has received funding from the National Heart, Lung, and Blood Institute (NHLBI) R01HL130702 and National Institute of Child Health and Human Development (NICHD) R01HD078515.
[a] Department of Medicine, Pulmonary and Critical Care Medicine Fellowship, Lifespan Hospitals, Alpert Medical School of Brown University, 593 Eddy Street, Providence, RI 02903, USA; [b] Department of Medicine, Obstetric Medicine Division, McGill University Health Center and Research Institute of the McGill University Health Center, 1001 Decarie Boulevard, D05.5839.3, Montreal, Quebec H4A 3J1, Canada; [c] Department of Medicine, Division of Obstetric Medicine, Lifespan Hospitals, Alpert Medical School of Brown University, 146 West River Street, Suite 11C, Providence, RI, USA; [d] Department of Medicine, Division of Pulmonary, Critical Care and Sleep Medicine, Lifespan Hospitals, Warren Alpert Medical School of Brown University, 146 West River Street, Suite 1F, Providence, RI 02904, USA; [e] Department of Medicine, Division of Obstetric Medicine, Lifespan Hospitals, Warren Alpert Medical School of Brown University, 146 West River Street, Suite 1F, Providence, RI 02904, USA
* Corresponding author. Department of Medicine, Division of Pulmonary, Critical Care and Sleep Medicine, Lifespan Hospitals, Warren Alpert Medical School of Brown University, 146 West River Street, Suite 1F, Providence, RI 02904.
E-mail address: Ghada_Bourjeily@brown.edu

Clin Chest Med 42 (2021) 483–496
https://doi.org/10.1016/j.ccm.2021.04.008
0272-5231/21/© 2021 Elsevier Inc. All rights reserved.

birth weight, preterm birth, and neonatal mortality.[1,5,11–14] Understanding the impact of pulmonary diseases on pregnancy and the impact of pregnancy on the natural course of pulmonary diseases is, therefore, essential for pulmonary care providers.

Physiologic changes in pregnancy and fetal considerations may lead to modifications in investigative approaches and treatment modalities. Indeed, a nuanced approach is required when interpreting certain laboratory values and imaging findings altered by pregnancy physiology, and these pharmacodynamic and pharmacokinetic changes should be accounted for when prescribing in pregnancy.[15,16] In addition, fetal safety must be taken into consideration when planning for radiologic testing and choosing from available therapeutic options, without compromising the care of the mother.

Thus, a review of general principles to apply when caring for pregnant and postpartum women is of paramount importance to avoid the pitfalls related to substandard maternal care owing a lack of pregnancy-specific considerations and fear of fetal harm. We hereby propose an overview of pregnancy physiology as well as imaging and medication prescription in pregnancy and highlight the need for periodic preconception counseling in reproductive age women.

PULMONARY PHYSIOLOGY IN PREGNANCY

Pregnancy is associated with changes in respiratory physiology that involve the nasopharynx, the lungs, and the chest wall, and often result from hormonal alterations and increasing abdominal distention.

Upper Airway

Mucosa in both the nasopharynx and oropharynx undergoes histologic changes that include increased phagocytic activity, increased mucopolysaccharides, leakage of plasma into the stroma, and glandular hyperactivity.[17,18] These changes likely occur in response to estrogen, progesterone, placental growth factor, and interleukins, as well as in response to an effect on histamine receptors.[17,19] The histologic changes translate into a mucosa that is edematous and friable, impacting the ease of intubation and nasogastric tube insertion, and increasing the risk of epistaxis.[20] In addition, one-fifth of pregnant women develop gestational rhinitis, a diagnosis characterized by nasal congestion that resolves soon after delivery.[19]

Apart from nasal congestion, other upper airway changes are relevant to the pathogenesis of sleep-disordered breathing, including a decrease in the oropharyngeal junction area and the mean pharyngeal area in pregnant women compared with nonpregnant women.[21] Mallampati scores have also been shown to increase during pregnancy[22] and 34% more women have Mallampati grade 4 in late pregnancy compared with early pregnancy.[22]

Chest Wall and Diaphragm

The chest wall undergoes changes during pregnancy as well. Owing to increases in the abdominal component of the chest wall by the third trimester, chest wall volume increases by 4.46 L.[23] Chest wall compliance decreases late in pregnancy as a result of increasing uterine size and possibly an increase in breast size, although lung compliance does not change.[24,25]

In addition, the subcostal angle of the thorax (the angle of the lower ribs at the level of the xiphoid process), increases along with the anterior–posterior and mediolateral measurements and cross-sectional area of the rib cage. However, the total volume of the rib cage remains constant.[23] The widening of the subcostal angle occurring early in pregnancy cannot be entirely explained by the enlarging uterus. Accordingly, these changes may partly occur owing to the hormone relaxin, which is known to cause relaxation of the pelvic ligaments in pregnancy as well as remodeling in bones and muscle[26–28] and may also cause relaxation of the lower rib cage ligaments.[18]

The diaphragm moves cranially 1.5 to 4.0 cm during pregnancy.[23] Despite the cranial shift of abdominal contents, the thickness of the diaphragm and the excursion of the diaphragmatic dome remain similar to nulliparous women over the course of pregnancy.[23] The muscle function of the respiratory system remains normal.[29]

Lung Function

Spirometry does not change significantly over the course of pregnancy. The forced expiratory volume in 1 second, peak expiratory flow, and the ratio of forced expiratory volume in 1 second to forced vital capacity remain within normal values throughout pregnancy.[30–32] Although studies vary, with some suggesting an increase in forced vital capacity,[33] there is likely no significant change in forced vital capacity during pregnancy.[31,32,34]

Elevation of the diaphragm, decreased outward recoil of the chest wall, and decreased downward tension of the abdomen during pregnancy lead to a 14% to 27% decrease (400–1000 mL) in functional residual capacity (FRC) between the postpartum period and the third trimester, with the percent change varying according to technique.[32,35] This decreased in the FRC is exacerbated further in the supine position.[18,36] There is also a decrease in expiratory reserve volume of approximately 200 mL[29,30,34,35] and a small to nonsignificant decrease in the residual volume.[29,30] Total lung capacity, which is a function of FRC and inspiratory capacity, remains the same throughout pregnancy because inspiratory capacity increases at a rate proportional to the decreasing FRC.[30,37] Closing capacity, which provides an assessment of small airway closure, is lower during pregnancy compared with the postpartum period.[21] There is no change in static lung recoil pressure and lung compliance.[30,34,38] The diffusion capacity for carbon monoxide, also known as the transfer factor, is highest in the first trimester and decreases to a lowest mean value between 24 to 27 weeks of gestation before increasing again postpartum.[39] Despite the presence of factors that typically increase airway resistance, such as upper airway edema and a decreased FRC, airflow rates remain the same during pregnancy likely owing to hormonally mediated dilatory effects on bronchial smooth muscle late in pregnancy.[36,37]

The respiratory rate does not change during pregnancy, yet minute ventilation increases by up to 30% to 50% owing to an increase in tidal volumes.[31,34,40,41] Compared with nonpregnant women, in whom the tidal volume is mostly a function of diaphragmatic movement, the tidal volume in pregnant women is determined by both diaphragmatic movement and intercostal accessory muscle use.[20,35] Hyperventilation in pregnancy occurs in response to increased levels of progesterone, the increased metabolic rate, and increased CO_2 production. Progesterone increases the sensitivity to CO_2; stimulates regions in the brain responsible for controlling ventilation such as the medulla oblongata, thalamus, and hypothalamus; and increases the peripheral ventilatory response to hypoxia via stimulation of the carotid body.[42,43] Estrogen may act synergistically with progesterone, possibly potentiating some of these effects.[44] The results of studies examining dead space ventilation in pregnancy have been conflicting. Although physiologic dead space is expected to decrease in pregnancy owing to increases in cardiac output and perfusion of lung apices, dead space ventilation may in fact increase, maintaining a similar dead space to tidal volume ratio to the nonpregnant population.[41,45] There is an increase in dead space ventilation, likely owing to an increase in alveolar dead space rather than anatomic dead space, although the mechanism for this change is unclear.[18,41] Hyperventilation

related to pregnancy leads to decreased Pa_{CO_2} levels and increased Pa_{O_2} levels, with a resulting mild respiratory alkalosis that is renally compensated.[30,45]

The clinical implications of respiratory physiologic changes include a less patent upper airway, increasing the risk for sleep-disordered breathing, nasal congestion, epistaxis, and a more difficult airway intubation. Changes in upper airways, hormone levels, and gastroesophageal reflux may increase the risk of asthma exacerbations in pregnancy. Immunologic changes may increase the risk[46] and the severity of viral infections,[47,48] and possibly impact the natural history of inflammatory conditions. The anatomic chest wall changes and the increased oxygen demands may increase the risk for ventilatory insufficiency in patients at risk.

CARDIAC PHYSIOLOGY IN PREGNANCY
Blood Volume

Blood volume increases rapidly around 6 weeks of gestation[49] and, in the third trimester, blood volume peaks between 4800 mL in singleton pregnancies and 5800 mL in twin pregnancies, accounting for a 50% increase.[50] Red blood cell mass increases by 17% to 40% in response to hormonal influences on erythropoiesis by progesterone, placental chorionic somatomammotropin, and possibly prolactin.[51] A simultaneous increase in plasma volume outpaces the increase in red cell mass, thus resulting in lower hemoglobin concentrations, termed physiologic anemia of pregnancy.

Hemodynamics

The heart rate increases gradually over the course of pregnancy, before returning to baseline, 14 to 17 weeks postpartum.[52] Cardiac output increases by 30% to 47% over the course of pregnancy, with the most substantial increase early in the first trimester before peaking between 25 and 32 weeks of gestation.[53–57] In twin pregnancies, cardiac output is 20% higher as compared with singleton pregnancies.[58] Early in gestation, cardiac output is mostly influenced by an increase in stroke volume, whereas later in gestation, the heart rate is the primary driver of increased cardiac output, because the stroke volume remains constant or slightly decreased in the third trimester.[56,57] Cardiac output is also influenced by body position— cardiac output decreases in the supine position owing to decreased venous return, which is most decreased in the third trimester.[59]

Although there is no change in pulmonary capillary wedge pressure and central venous pressure, systemic vascular resistance and pulmonary vascular resistance decrease.[60] The mean arterial blood pressure decreases early in pregnancy then increases again during the third trimester and postpartum period.[52,61]

Oxygen uptake and CO_2 output increase in the first 8 to 11 weeks of pregnancy and continue to increase over the rest of the pregnancy to a peak of 20% to 30% above baseline near term.[20,51,62] In early pregnancy, the increase in oxygen consumption is balanced with an increase in cardiac output to meet the demands during the critical period of organogenesis. Later in pregnancy, oxygen consumption outpaces the increase in cardiac output, resulting in a widening in the arteriovenous oxygen levels. Although total red cell mass increases during pregnancy leading to an increase in oxygen-carrying capacity, the arterial O_2 content is actually lower owing to physiologic anemia.[40]

Thus, cardiovascular physiologic changes may lead to a worsening in hemodynamics in patients with pulmonary hypertension, cardiomyopathy, arrhythmias, or valvular heart disease. Changes in blood volume, in conjunction with alterations in the balance of oncotic and hydrostatic pressures, increase the risk of pulmonary edema in pregnancy and in the postpartum period.

CHANGES IN PHYSIOLOGY DURING LABOR AND DELIVERY

Physiologic changes within the respiratory and cardiovascular systems during pregnancy are then followed by another series of rapid and significant changes during labor, delivery, and the postpartum period.

Respiratory Physiology during Labor and Delivery

There is dramatic variability in tidal volumes (330–2250 mL) and minute ventilation (7–90 L/min) during labor and delivery.[63] Hyperventilation is common during labor and delivery, likely as a result of pain; narcotic analgesics have been shown to decrease hyperventilation during labor and delivery.[18,63]

Cardiovascular Physiology during Labor and Delivery

Cardiac output increases substantially as a result of both an increase in stroke volume and heart rate during labor, 30% to 50% above baseline at term and 50% above baseline during labor.[64,65] This increase in cardiac output is potentiated by an increase in catecholamines and by cyclic autotransfusions from uterine contractions.[66,67] In the early postpartum period, there is a further increase in cardiac output of 60% to 80% compared with prelabor levels from an increase in preload with approximately 500 mL of blood owing to release of aortocaval compression by the gravid uterus, diversion away from uteroplacental vascular bed, and mobilization of extracellular fluid.[18,51,57,68]

Understanding the physiologic changes during labor and delivery can assist clinicians in planning for this event. Most women with mild to moderate respiratory insufficiency tolerate pregnancy and labor and delivery well, with certain modifications. The additional strain on the respiratory system during labor and delivery may place women at a higher risk from increased intrathoracic pressures, hyperventilation, respiratory muscle fatigue, or ventilatory insufficiency. Thus, discussions with the anesthesiology team regarding specific airway intubation strategies or anesthetic considerations in women with sleep-disordered breathing, women with restrictive physiology, or women with significant airway obstruction, for instance, with deliberate plans for the event, is essential. Similarly, the strain on the cardiovascular system and sympathetic activation may increase the risk of cardiovascular complications. The risk of complications can be mitigated with careful planning in collaboration with the obstetric and anesthesiology teams to adapt delivery and pain management strategies while optimizing cardiac output.

Return to Baseline

Pregnancy-related physiologic changes return to baseline over variable timeframes during the postpartum period. In the upper airway, pregnancy rhinitis resolves within 2 weeks of delivery.[19]

By 24 weeks postpartum, the chest wall returns to baseline; however, the subcostal angle remains 20% larger than at baseline.[29] Decompression of the diaphragm and lungs after delivery results in normalization of static lung volumes.[18] FRC, which is a function of expiratory reserve volume and residual volume, increases along with expiratory reserve volume in the postpartum period compared with the third trimester of pregnancy.[35] Although studies disagree on whether the forced vital capacity increases or remains constant during pregnancy, one study found increases in forced vital capacity that persisted at 6 months postpartum and suggest that changes in the forced vital capacity may be permanent in parous women as compared with nulliparous women.[33]

In the cardiovascular system, after the significant increase in cardiac output during labor and delivery, cardiac output quickly decreased postpartum[65] and returns to the prepregnancy level 2 weeks after delivery.[68] Left ventricular wall thickness, which increases along with left ventricular mass during pregnancy,[53] is often back to baseline by 24 weeks after delivery.[20]

RADIOLOGIC TESTING IN PREGNANT WOMEN WITH PULMONARY DISEASES

In a study of 3.5 million pregnancies in the United States and Ontario, Canada, the use of ionizing radiation during the course of pregnancy has increased nearly 4-fold in the United States and 2-fold in Ontario, between 1996 and 2016.[69] Although the use of most chest imaging modalities is mostly justifiable in pregnant women for the right indications, understanding the use of imaging studies in pregnancy is key.

Fetal Adverse Effects with Pulmonary Diagnostic Imaging

Two types of fetal adverse effects can arise from ionizing radiation. First, deterministic effects from damage to cell tissue may bear fetal consequences at a given radiation dose threshold.[70] These teratogenic effects depend on the dose and gestational age at the time of radiation, and no teratogenicity has been reported with doses of less than 50 mGy, which is well above the current radiation doses used for most routine diagnostic radiologic chest examinations (Table 1).[70–72] In the first 2 weeks after conception, fetal loss can occur with exposure to high doses of radiation.[71,72] The majority of teratogenic effects take place between 2 and 15 weeks after fertilization.[71,73] During organogenesis, between 2 and 8 weeks after conception, congenital skeletal, ocular, and genital anomalies, as well as growth restriction, have been observed.[10] Between 8 and 15 weeks after conception, microcephaly and severe intellectual disability have also been reported.[72] A low risk of severe intellectual disability

may persist between 16 and 25 weeks after conception.[72]

Second, stochastic effects from damage to as little as a single cell, can have fetal consequences in the absence of any predictable threshold.[70] These effects include oncogenicity with the induction of cancer in childhood and hereditary diseases in future generations.[70] The oncogenic risk after exposure to radiation is thought to be proportional to the radiation dose received and is estimated to be significant when occurring after 3 to 4 weeks of fertilization as opposed to before implantation.[70] Beyond the first month after conception, oncogenesis does not seem to be influenced by gestational age at the time of radiation.[70] In terms of risk estimation, childhood cancer may be doubled with a dose of 25 mGy, as reflected by an increase in absolute excess childhood cancer risk of 1 in 13,000 per mGy in the UK.[70] Overall, the lifetime risk of malignancy per 20 mGy of radiation is estimated at 40 per 5000 infants, representing a cumulative incidence of about 0.8%.[71] Accordingly, more than 99% of infants are expected to be as healthy as other children after exposure to medically required diagnostic testing during pregnancy.[71]

Using alternative diagnostic modalities, when feasible, and optimizing the radiation dose via several techniques can minimize fetal risk. Scattered radiations from imaging outside of the abdomen and pelvis represent very low doses and thus negligible fetal risk (see Table 1).[71] Measures to minimize the radiation dose received by the fetus include limiting the number of images captured and restricting radiation to the area of interest, as well as improvements in imaging equipment.[71] For nuclear medicine procedures, decreased administered activity accompanied by increased radiopharmaceutical excretion, as well as increased scanner efficiency and image reconstitution techniques can further optimize this risk.[71] In general terms, most diagnostic chest imaging modalities are justifiable in pregnancy. The

Table 1
Estimated ionizing radiation doses per chest imaging

Type of Examination	Estimated Fetal Dose (mGy)
Chest radiograph	0.0005–0.01
Chest CT scan or CT pulmonary angiography	0.01–0.66
Low-dose perfusion scintigraphy	0.1–0.5
Perfusion/ventilation scan	0.32–0.74

As defined by the American College of Obstetricians and Gynecologists (ACOG),[122] and the American Thoracic Society (ATS)/Society of Thoracic Radiology (STR).[123]

involvement of a medical physicist and the radiology department to implement protocol modifications and minimize radiation exposure allow for diagnostic procedures to be performed safely, without delaying or withholding care from this population.

Although iodine-based contrast agents can cross the placental barrier, they have not been associated with teratogenic or oncogenetic effects.[71,72,74] Moreover, the theoretic risk of contrast-induced neonatal hypothyroidism has been dismantled by several studies, which included a total of more than 480 neonates of mothers who had received intravenous iodinated contrast for computed tomography (CT) scan testing.[75–77] With thyroid testing being part of routine newborn screening in many countries, no additional neonatal measures need to be routinely undertaken after delivery. However, given that pregnancy physiology impacts stroke volume and plasma volume, the dose or protocol of contrast agents may need to be modified to optimize enhancement.

Choosing between Chest Imaging Modalities to Rule Out Pulmonary Embolism

Although both CT pulmonary angiography (CTPA) and ventilation perfusion (VQ) scans deliver minimal doses of radiation to the fetus (see **Table 1**), CTPA delivers a higher dose of radiation to the proliferating breast tissue than does a VQ scan (20–35 mGy for CTPA vs 0.28 mGy for a VQ scan).[78] Despite this finding, in a population-based study with longitudinal follow-up, neither a CT scan of the chest nor a VQ scan led to a detectable short-term excess risk of maternal breast cancer.[79] In addition, in a systematic review, both imaging modalities were associated with low false-negative rates and comparable nondiagnostic testing rates.[80] However, nondiagnostic CTPA testing rates may be considerably decreased by using a protocol adapted to the hemodynamic effects of pregnancy.[80] Thus, from a maternal and fetal standpoint, both imaging modalities are reasonable options to rule out pulmonary embolism. VQ single photon emission CT (VQ-SPECT) imaging is another potential diagnostic modality that is thought to have superior diagnostic accuracy to planar VQ scintigraphy in the general population.[81] This imaging modality has not been adopted widely. VQ-SPECT scan use has been reported in pregnancy in the diagnosis of pulmonary embolism and may offer some advantages. VQ-SPECT scans seem to have the same diagnostic yield as CTPA; however, they are associated with a lower radiation dose to

the maternal breasts.[82] Because the estimated fetal dose differs by the proximity of the fetus to the radiation source in imaging studies such as CT scans, a recent study found that, in the first and second trimesters, the radiation dose was lower to the fetus when using CTPA compared with a VQ-SPECT scan, but higher in the third trimester for CTPA.[83]

The lack of ionizing radiation with MRI is an advantage compared with other imaging modalities. MRI has been used for fetal imaging without an apparent negative impact.[84] Although an MRI does not expose fetuses to ionizing radiation, the safety of gadolinium-based contrast media has not been well-established. Owing to its high molecular weight, only a small fraction of this contrast medium is believed to pass from maternal blood to fetal tissue.[85] However, the total duration of fetal exposure to the media is not known because gadolinium excreted into amniotic fluid eventually reenters the fetal circulation.[72,85] In a case series of 26 women who received either periconceptional or first trimester gadolinium-based contrast media with an MRI examination, 23 had a term delivery, 2 had a miscarriage, and 1 patient underwent elective abortion.[86] Among women with term delivery, 1 patient had a baby with an intracranial hemangioma.[86] Owing to this small sample size, firm conclusions could not be drawn. The largest population-based study on adverse effects from gadolinium contrast media included more than 1 million pregnancies in the province of Ontario in Canada.[87] The adjusted risk ratio for a composite of stillbirths and neonatal death among women exposed to gadolinium was 3.70 (95% confidence interval, 1.55–8.85) when compared with women unexposed to any MRI testing.[87] Moreover, despite no increased risk of nephrogenic systemic fibrosis in the newborn, investigators found a slightly higher risk of rheumatologic, inflammatory, or infiltrative skin conditions in newborns exposed in utero (hazard ratio, 1.36; 95% confidence interval, 1.09–1.69).[87] It remains possible that poorer fetal outcomes may have been, in fact, due to residual confounding by indication from the underlying clinical condition leading to imaging by gadolinium-enhanced MRI.[88] In light of these results and an absence of better safety data, gadolinium contrast should only be given when truly warranted by maternal indications and is expected to change management, and after appropriate counseling.[71,72] Similar to any management decision in pregnancy, a risk assessment of the use of a diagnostic or therapeutic modality examining the risk of the untreated or poorly managed disease against the risk of the procedure or treatment helps to guide clinical management decisions. If used, only gadolinium-based contrast agents associated with the lowest risk of nephrogenic systemic fibrosis should be administered.[75]

PRESCRIBING FOR THE PREGNANT AND THE BREASTFEEDING WOMAN
Prescribing in Pregnancy

Prescribing medications in pregnant and lactating women poses a unique challenge for clinicians. Concerns include the potential toxicity of drugs to the fetus and breastfeeding infant, and alterations in pharmacokinetics that may require changes in dosing.[89] Despite studies showing an increase in medication use in pregnancy in the United Stgates,[90] there is a significant lack of clinical trials and limited understanding of effects of medications on the long-term health of infants and mothers.[91] As a result, discontinuing a medication in pregnancy may seem like the safest course. However, untreated or undertreated conditions most often pose a greater risk to the pregnant woman and her baby than medication use.

Faced with this dilemma, many clinicians have heavily relied on the US Food and Drug Administration (FDA) drug categories for pregnancy (ABCDX). However, in 2015, the FDA retired this system. After a lengthy process of review, the FDA concluded that the letter categories were flawed for several reasons: (1) they were almost exclusively derived from animal data, (2) they were perceived as a simple gradient of risk that failed to differentiate severity and range of adverse outcomes, (3) they failed to address the importance of dose, route, and gestational timing, and (4) they did not consider the indication for the drug or have a mechanism that weighs the risk of the drug against the risk of the untreated condition. In addition, there was no requirement for updating the categories. The conclusion of the FDA was that the pregnancy categories were often misinterpreted and misused. In 2015, the ABCDX categories were replaced by the FDA Pregnancy and Lactation Labeling Rule.[92] This new ruling requires narrative text that will provide prescribers with relevant information for critical decision-making when treating pregnant or lactating women. The FDA Pregnancy and Lactation Labeling Rule includes a more complete statement of the known risks based on the best available data. The new format will encourage the consideration of the untreated disease, will present animal data in the context of human exposure, and explicitly state when human data are available and when no data are available. The new rule includes 3 categories: (1) pregnancy including labor and birth, (2) lactation, and (3) females and males of reproductive potential. The goal of the FDA Pregnancy and Lactation Labeling Rule is to provide prescribers with relevant information for decision-making when treating pregnant or lactating women. In all cases of prescribing in pregnancy, the clinician must weigh the potential risk of medication with the risk of untreated disease (**Fig. 1**). A shared decision-making approach is important. Clinicians must provide women with accurate safety information about medication use in pregnancy, but also be sensitive to the patients and families' concerns about risk of medication use in pregnancy.

Useful online resources for information on drugs in pregnancy include Reprotox[93] and MotherToBaby.[94]

Prescribing in Breastfeeding Women

A large body of medical literature has long established that human milk is the best nutrition for infants. Exclusive breastfeeding for a minimum of 6 months provides many short- and long-term benefits to the mother and her infant.[95] However, women are often advised to discontinue breastfeeding when medications are prescribed. Although nearly all medications transfer into human milk to some degree, it is almost always in very low amounts and is unlikely to result in a clinically relevant dose to the infant. The American Academy of Pediatrics advises that "most drugs likely to be prescribed to the nursing mother should have no effect on milk supply or on infant well-being."[96]

Factors that influence risk to the breastfed infant include the concentration of drug in the breastmilk, as well as the bioavailability, lipid solubility, and protein binding of the drug.[97] The mother's plasma level is the most important factor impacting the level of the drug in breastmilk. The concentration in breastmilk will increase and decrease as a function of the maternal plasma level. A few drugs may be trapped in the breastmilk owing to the low pH of human milk. Drugs with a high pKa (such as barbiturates) are generally avoided if an alternative drug is available. Iodines are pumped into breastmilk in a similar way that iodine is pumped into the thyroid.[98]

Once a drug has entered the breastmilk and has been ingested by the infant, the bioavailability of the drug plays a significant role in determining the final dose in the infant. Drugs may be destroyed by proteolytic enzymes and acids in the infant's gut or fail to be absorbed through the gut wall or rapidly picked up by the liver, all of which generally leads to a decreased effect of the drug on the infant.

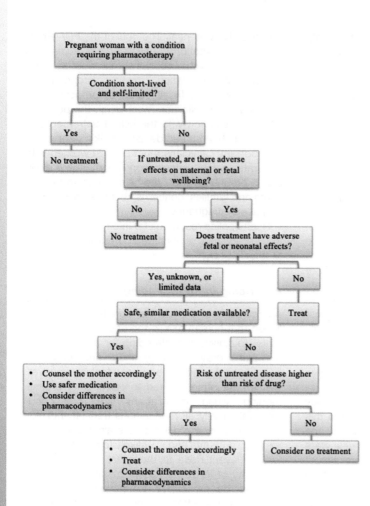

Fig. 1. Approach to pharmacotherapy for the pregnant and breastfeeding woman. (*Adapted from* Miller, M. A., Mehta, N., Clark-Bilodeau, C., & Bourjeily, G. (2020). Sleep Pharmacotherapy for Common Sleep Disorders in Pregnancy and Lactation. Chest, 157(1), 184–197.With permission.)

Drugs with high lipid solubility transfer into milk in higher concentrations. For example, central nervous system–active drugs nearly always have the unique characteristics required to enter milk. Although significant levels can be expected in milk, they are nearly always still subclinical.

Protein binding also plays a role in transfer into breastmilk. It is the unbound portion of the drug that transfers; therefore, drugs with high maternal protein binding (warfarin, nonsteroidal anti-inflammatory drugs) have low milk levels.

In addition to the characteristics of the drug, the timing of the exposure and infant characteristic play a role in decisions about drug use during breastfeeding. During the first 72 hours postpartum, large gaps between mammary alveolar cells allow most drugs to transfer easily into breastmilk. By the end of the first week postpartum, prolactin levels increase and cause the alveolar cells to swell, closing the intracellular gaps and reducing transfer. Although drugs may penetrate at higher levels during the early colostrum production period, the minimal volume of colostrum produced means

the absolute dose transferred is generally quite low. Infant characteristics such as age and health status should also be considered. A premature or medically unstable infant may be susceptible to even low doses of a medication.[99]

Helpful references for medications in breastfeeding include Thomas Hale's *Medication and Mother's Milk*[100] and the Drugs and Lactation Database (LactMed), a free online database from the National Library of Medicine.[101]

PRECONCEPTION COUNSELING

Aside from caring for women with lung disease during pregnancy, preparing women with chronic lung disease for a successful pregnancy is just as important. An American College of Obstetricians and Gynecologists committee opinion piece defined the goal of prepregnancy care as one that decreased the risk of adverse health effects for the woman, the fetus, and the neonate by working with the patient to optimize her health, provide education about a healthy pregnancy, and address modifiable risk factors.[102] Because the health of an individual varies throughout their lifespan, preconception counseling needs to occur multiple times during the course of a woman's reproductive years. Women should be counseled to seek care ideally before they attempt to get pregnant, and as soon as they find out they are pregnant. This effort will aid in devising a monitoring plan for the course of pregnancy and the postpartum period.

A multinational survey on family planning for women of childbearing age has shown that medical specialists often fail to adequately communicate with and support women with chronic conditions, citing suboptimal communication between specialists, leading to inconsistent advice and information.[103]

Preconception counseling is a key feature of the care of a woman of reproductive age with chronic lung disease. Reproductive age women with chronic lung disease who are sexually active, have a partner, and those who have children need to have conversations regarding the possibility of a pregnancy and the implications of pregnancy.[104] Because nearly one-half of all pregnancies are unplanned and given that control of chronic lung disease may vary over the years, these conversations need to occur repeatedly throughout the reproductive years. A significant relay of information is necessary when it comes to meeting the challenges related to pregnancy and parenting. The aim of preconception counseling would be to assist in planning an optimal timing of pregnancy and to improve management before conception and throughout pregnancy and the postpartum period.[105] Women may prefer preconception conversations to happen in the presence of a partner.

Preconception counseling in women with chronic illnesses should focus on the importance of avoiding unplanned pregnancies and the potential maternal and fetal risks associated with such pregnancies.[102] Counseling on and routinely visiting birth control methods with these women can help to prevent unplanned pregnancies. In general, women with active disease and disease that is poorly controlled should practice effective birth control until the condition is better controlled.

Risk assessment includes the examination of the risk of the chronic disease on pregnancy and perinatal outcomes, as well as the risks of the pregnancy on the chronic condition.[106] Understanding and counseling patients on the risk of worsening of certain common conditions such as asthma or sleep apnea, or rare conditions such as pulmonary hypertension or lymphangioleiomyomatosis during pregnancy can paint a clearer picture of expectations for the pregnant woman and assist her in making informed decisions about

management and medication choices.[102] In other circumstances, reviewing the risk of recurrence of a condition such as venous thromboembolism and the implications of that risk such as the use of subcutaneous injections for the duration of pregnancy and a planned labor and delivery help to set the appropriate expectations with patients and their families. Because pregnancy physiology may modify or worsen certain preexisting conditions, women must be made aware that the frequency of monitoring, testing, and follow-up visits will likely increase in pregnancy as well. For instance, women with cystic fibrosis or asthma likely need more frequent monitoring during the course of pregnancy, although no specific guidelines exist for the use of pulmonary function testing in pregnancy. In contrast, women need to be informed of the risk of a treated or untreated chronic condition on the health of the pregnancy and the fetus and newborn. This understanding of risk can guide decision-making regarding therapy choices.

Another aim of preconception counseling is to review the risk of medications prescribed to control or treat a chronic condition.[102,107] Ideally, women would enter pregnancy on medications that are nonteratogenic. However, this scenario may not occur for various reasons. Given the status of pregnancy drug trials and the systematic exclusion of pregnant women from many interventional trials, many drugs remain poorly examined for safety and efficacy in pregnancy. Indeed, in 2011 and 2012, pregnant women were excluded from 95% of phase IV interventional industry-sponsored trials.[108] Further, 98% of the 172 drugs approved in the United States between 2000 and 2010 lacked data or had insufficient data to determine the risk of developmental toxicity in humans.[109] For this reason, many first-line medications may not be the safest alternative in pregnancy.[110] To complicate matters further, nearly 85% of all couples will get pregnant within 1 year if they have regular sex and do not use contraceptive methods[111]; however, the time span from intention to conception varies by couple. Hence, deciding on the optimal timing to withdraw a medication that is treating and keeping a chronic condition optimally controlled in anticipation of pregnancy may be challenging.

Genetic counseling should also be considered in women with a respiratory genetic disorder so that proper evaluation be performed and the expectant mother and her family are informed about potential risk of transmission of the disorder and clarify expectations, as well as the implications for the management at the time of delivery and in neonatal to adult life.

Women with respiratory diseases anticipating or planning pregnancy should also receive general recommendations regarding lifestyle changes that could improve their overall health.[102] Smoking is associated with a higher risk of infertility, ectopic pregnancy, miscarriage, growth restriction, and preterm birth, among other complications.[112] Most animal studies suggest that electronic cigarette smoking is associated with potential danger to the developing fetus primarily because nicotine consumption has multiple effects on the immune system, neural development, lung function, and cardiac function.[113,114] Hookah smoking, also known as waterpipe smoking, has been associated with adverse obstetric outcomes such as low birthweight,[115–117] low Apgar scores,[117,118] and pulmonary complications at birth. Smoking cessation before pregnancy would be ideal and likely yields the greatest benefits to the fetus.[119] However, smoking cessation at any time during pregnancy still bears significant benefits.[120] In addition to obesity-related pulmonary complications, women with obesity have an increased risk of pregnancy-related complications, including higher rates of gestational diabetes, hypertensive disorders of pregnancy, macrosomia, venous thromboembolism, and congenital anomalies.[121] Because weight loss is not recommended during pregnancy, women with obesity should be advised to seek weight management recommendations before conception.

SUMMARY

The management of pregnant women with chronic lung diseases should be performed by a multidisciplinary team consisting of a pulmonologist, an obstetric medicine physician, and a specialist obstetrician in high-risk conditions, with open communications with the primary care physician, as well as an anesthesiologist in later pregnancy. Involving the patient and her family in the decision-making is key to setting expectations and clarifying the intensity and frequency of monitoring.

CLINICS CARE POINTS

- Withholding diagnostic studies or therapeutic interventions in pregnant women may be more harmful than administering them.
- Preconception counseling may be an opportunity to plan a future pregnancy and optimize the care of women during pregnancy.

CONFLICTS OF INTEREST

All authors have no conflicts of interest to report.

REFERENCES

1. Clifton VL, Engel P, Smith R, et al. Maternal and neonatal outcomes of pregnancies complicated by asthma in an Australian population. Aust N Z J Obstet Gynaecol 2009;49:619–26.
2. Kwon HL, Triche EW, Belanger K, et al. The epidemiology of asthma during pregnancy: prevalence, diagnosis, and symptoms. Immunol Allergy Clin North Am 2006;26:29–62.
3. Mendola P, Laughon SK, Männistö TI, et al. Obstetric complications among US women with asthma. Am J Obstet Gynecol 2013;208:127.e1-8.
4. Bin YS, Cistulli PA, Ford JB. Population-based study of sleep apnea in pregnancy and maternal and infant outcomes. J Clin Sleep Med 2016;12: 871–7.
5. Bourjeily G, Danilack VA, Bublitz MH, et al. Obstructive sleep apnea in pregnancy is associated with adverse maternal outcomes: a national cohort. Sleep Med 2017;38:50–7.
6. Bublitz MH, Monteiro JF, Caraganis A, et al. Obstructive sleep apnea in gestational diabetes: a pilot study of the role of the hypothalamic-pituitary-adrenal axis. J Clin Sleep Med 2018;14: 87–93.
7. Fung AM, Wilson DL, Lappas M, et al. Effects of maternal obstructive sleep apnoea on fetal growth: a prospective cohort study. PLoS One 2013;8: e68057.
8. Reutrakul S, Zaidi N, Wroblewski K, et al. Interactions between pregnancy, obstructive sleep apnea, and gestational diabetes mellitus. J Clin Endocrinol Metab 2013;98:4195–202.
9. Centers for Disease Control and Prevention, Division of Reproductive Health, National Center for Chronic Disease Prevention and Health Promotion. Pregnancy Mortality Surveillance System 2020. Available at: https://www.cdc.gov/reproductivehealth/maternal-mortality/pregnancy-mortality-surveillance-system. htm [Accessed September 8, 2020].
10. Rojas-Suarez J, Bello-Munoz C, Paternina-Caicedo A, et al. Maternal mortality secondary to acute respiratory failure in Colombia: a population-based analysis. Lung 2015;193:231–7.
11. Doyle TJ, Goodin K, Hamilton JJ. Maternal and neonatal outcomes among pregnant women with 2009 pandemic influenza A(H1N1) illness in Florida, 2009-2010: a population-based cohort study. PLoS One 2013;8:e79040.
12. Sliwa K, van Hagen IM, Budts W, et al. Pulmonary hypertension and pregnancy outcomes: data from the Registry of Pregnancy and Cardiac Disease

(ROPAC) of the European Society of Cardiology. Eur J Heart Fail 2016;18:1119–28.

13. Bublitz MH, Bourjeily G. Sleep disordered breathing in pregnancy and adverse maternal outcomes-a true story? US Respir Pulm Dis 2017; 2:19–20.

14. Bourjeily G, Danilack VA, Bublitz MH, et al. Maternal obstructive sleep apnea and neonatal birth outcomes in a population based sample. Sleep Med 2020;66:233–40.

15. Weinberger SE, Weiss ST, Cohen WR, et al. Pregnancy and the lung. Am Rev Respir Dis 1980; 121:559–81.

16. Bourjeily G, Levinson A. Pulmonary disease and critical illness in pregnancy. Semin Respir Crit Care Med 2017;38:121–2.

17. Philpott CM, Conboy P, Al-Azzawi F, et al. Nasal physiological changes during pregnancy. Clin Otolaryngol Allied Sci 2004;29:343–51.

18. Hegewald MJ, Crapo RO. Respiratory physiology in pregnancy. Clin Chest Med 2011;32:1–13.

19. Ellegard EK. The etiology and management of pregnancy rhinitis. Am J Respir Med 2003;2: 469–75.

20. Crapo RO. Normal cardiopulmonary physiology during pregnancy. Clin Obstet Gynecol 1996;39:3–16.

21. Izci B, Vennelle M, Liston WA, et al. Sleep-disordered breathing and upper airway size in pregnancy and post-partum. Eur Respir J 2006;27:321–7.

22. Pilkington S, Carli F, Dakin MJ, et al. Increase in Mallampati score during pregnancy. Br J Anaesth 1995;74:638–42.

23. LoMauro A, Aliverti A, Frykholm P, et al. Adaptation of lung, chest wall, and respiratory muscles during pregnancy: preparing for birth. J Appl Physiol (1985) 2019;127:1640–50.

24. Marx GF, Murthy PK, Orkin LR. Static compliance before and after vaginal delivery. Br J Anaesth 1970;42:1100–4.

25. Campbell LA, Klocke RA. Implications for the pregnant patient. Am J Respir Crit Care Med 2001;163: 1051–4.

26. MacLennan AH. The role of relaxin in human reproduction. Clin Reprod Fertil 1983;2:77–95.

27. Unemori EN, Amento EP. Relaxin modulates synthesis and secretion of procollagenase and collagen by human dermal fibroblasts. J Biol Chem 1990;265:10681–5.

28. Dehghan F, Haerian BS, Muniandy S, et al. The effect of relaxin on the musculoskeletal system. Scand J Med Sci Sports 2014;24:e220–9.

29. Contreras G, Gutierrez M, Beroiza T, et al. Ventilatory drive and respiratory muscle function in pregnancy. Am Rev Respir Dis 1991;144:837–41.

30. Jensen D, Webb KA, Davies GA, et al. Mechanical ventilatory constraints during incremental cycle exercise in human pregnancy: implications for respiratory sensation. J Physiol 2008;586:4735–50.

31. Kolarzyk E, Szot WM, Lyszczarz J. Lung function and breathing regulation parameters during pregnancy. Arch Gynecol Obstet 2005;272:53–8.

32. Garcia-Rio F, Pino-Garcia JM, Serrano S, et al. Comparison of helium dilution and plethysmographic lung volumes in pregnant women. Eur Respir J 1997;10:2371–5.

33. Grindheim G, Toska K, Estensen ME, et al. Changes in pulmonary function during pregnancy: a longitudinal cohort study. BJOG 2012;119: 94–101.

34. McAuliffe F, Kametas N, Costello J, et al. Respiratory function in singleton and twin pregnancy. BJOG 2002;109:765–9.

35. Gilroy RJ, Mangura BT, Lavietes MH. Rib cage and abdominal volume displacements during breathing in pregnancy. Am Rev Respir Dis 1988;137: 668–72.

36. Bourjeily G, Mazer J, Levinson A. Chapter 97: pulmonary disorders and pregnancy. In: Grippi MA, Elias JA, Fishman JA, et al, editors. Fishman's pulmonary diseases and disorders. 5th edition. New York: McGraw-Hill Education; 2015. p. 1479–96.

37. LoMauro A, Aliverti A. Respiratory physiology of pregnancy: physiology masterclass. Breathe (Sheff) 2015;11:297–301.

38. Gee JB, Packer BS, Millen JE, et al. Pulmonary mechanics during pregnancy. J Clin Invest 1967;46: 945–52.

39. Milne JA, Mills RJ, Coutts JR, et al. The effect of human pregnancy on the pulmonary transfer factor for carbon monoxide as measured by the single-breath method. Clin Sci Mol Med 1977;53: 271–6.

40. Bobrowski RA. Pulmonary physiology in pregnancy. Clin Obstet Gynecol 2010;53:285–300.

41. Pernoll ML, Metcalfe J, Kovach PA, et al. Ventilation during rest and exercise in pregnancy and postpartum. Respir Physiol 1975;25:295–310.

42. Jensen D, Wolfe LA, Slatkovska L, et al. Effects of human pregnancy on the ventilatory chemoreflex response to carbon dioxide. Am J Physiol Regul Integr Comp Physiol 2005;288:R1369–75.

43. Bayliss DA, Millhorn DE. Central neural mechanisms of progesterone action: application to the respiratory system. J Appl Physiol (1985) 1992; 73:393–404.

44. Hannhart B, Pickett CK, Moore LG. Effects of estrogen and progesterone on carotid body neural output responsiveness to hypoxia. J Appl Physiol (1985) 1990;68:1909–16.

45. Templeton A, Kelman GR. Maternal blood-gases, PAo2–Pao2), physiological shunt and VD/VT in normal pregnancy. Br J Anaesth 1976;48:1001–4.

46. Esmonde TF, Herdman G, Anderson G. Chicken-pox pneumonia: an association with pregnancy. Thorax 1989;44:812–5.

47. Mosby LG, Rasmussen SA, Jamieson DJ. 2009 pandemic influenza A (H1N1) in pregnancy: a systematic review of the literature. Am J Obstet Gynecol 2011;205:10–8.

48. Siston AM, Rasmussen SA, Honein MA, et al. Pandemic 2009 influenza A(H1N1) virus illness among pregnant women in the United States. JAMA 2010;303:1517–25.

49. Hytten FE, Paintin DB. Increase in plasma volume during normal pregnancy. J Obstet Gynaecol Br Emp 1963;70:402–7.

50. Pritchard JA. Changes in the blood volume during pregnancy and delivery. Anesthesiology 1965;26:393–9.

51. Ouzounian JG, Elkayam U. Physiologic changes during normal pregnancy and delivery. Cardiol Clin 2012;30:317–29.

52. Mahendru AA, Everett TR, Wilkinson IB, et al. A longitudinal study of maternal cardiovascular function from preconception to the postpartum period. J Hypertens 2014;32:849–56.

53. Mabie WC, DiSessa TG, Crocker LG, et al. A longitudinal study of cardiac output in normal human pregnancy. Am J Obstet Gynecol 1994;170:849–56.

54. Vered Z, Poler SM, Gibson P, et al. Noninvasive detection of the morphologic and hemodynamic changes during normal pregnancy. Clin Cardiol 1991;14:327–34.

55. Bader RA, Bader ME, Rose DF, et al. Hemodynamics at rest and during exercise in normal pregnancy as studies by cardiac catheterization. J Clin Invest 1955;34:1524–36.

56. Robson SC, Hunter S, Boys RJ, et al. Serial study of factors influencing changes in cardiac output during human pregnancy. Am J Physiol 1989;256:H1060–5.

57. Sanghavi M, Rutherford JD. Cardiovascular physiology of pregnancy. Circulation 2014;130:1003–8.

58. Kametas NA, McAuliffe F, Krampl E, et al. Maternal cardiac function in twin pregnancy. Obstet Gynecol 2003;102:806–15.

59. Yeomans ER, Gilstrap LC 3rd. Physiologic changes in pregnancy and their impact on critical care. Crit Care Med 2005;33:S256–8.

60. Clark SL, Cotton DB, Lee W, et al. Central hemodynamic assessment of normal term pregnancy. Am J Obstet Gynecol 1989;161:1439–42.

61. Rebelo F, Farias DR, Mendes RH, et al. Blood pressure variation throughout pregnancy according to early gestational BMI: a Brazilian cohort. Arq Bras Cardiol 2015;104:284–91.

62. Gazioglu K, Kaltreider NL, Rosen M, et al. Pulmonary function during pregnancy in normal women

and in patients with cardiopulmonary disease. Thorax 1970;25:445–50.

63. Cole PV, Nainby-Luxmoore RC. Respiratory volumes in labour. Br Med J 1962;1:1118.

64. Fujitani S, Baldisseri MR. Hemodynamic assessment in a pregnant and peripartum patient. Crit Care Med 2005;33:S354–61.

65. Robson SC, Dunlop W, Boys RJ, et al. Cardiac output during labour. Br Med J (Clin Res Ed) 1987;295:1169–72.

66. Lee W, Rokey R, Miller J, et al. Maternal hemodynamic effects of uterine contractions by M-mode and pulsed-Doppler echocardiography. Am J Obstet Gynecol 1989;161:974–7.

67. Nisell H, Hjemdahl P, Linde B. Cardiovascular responses to circulating catecholamines in normal pregnancy and in pregnancy-induced hypertension. Clin Physiol 1985;5:479–93.

68. Hunter S, Robson SC. Adaptation of the maternal heart in pregnancy. Br Heart J 1992;68:540–3.

69. Kwan ML, Miglioretti DL, Marlow EC, et al. Trends in medical imaging during pregnancy in the United States and Ontario, Canada, 1996 to 2016. JAMA Netw Open 2019;2:e197249.

70. Health Protection Agency, The Royal College of Radiologists and the Royal College of Radiographers. Protection of pregnant patients during diagnostic medical exposures to ionising radiation: Health Protection Agency, Radiation, Chemical and Environmental Hazards. 2009. Available at: http://www.who.int/tb/advisory_bodies/impact_measurement_taskforce/meetings/prevalence_survey/imaging_regnant_hpa.pdf [Accessed October 12, 2020].

71. American College of Radiology, Committee on Drugs and Contrast Media. Manual on contrast media. version 10.3 2017. Available at: https://www.acr.org/Clinical-Resources/Contrast-Manual [Accessed October 12, 2020].

72. Committee Opinion No. 723: guidelines for diagnostic imaging during pregnancy and lactation. Obstet Gynecol 2017;130:e210–6.

73. Gjelsteen AC, Ching BH, Meyermann MW, et al. CT, MRI, PET, PET/CT, and ultrasound in the evaluation of obstetric and gynecologic patients. Surg Clin North Am 2008;88:361–90, vii.

74. Puac P, Rodriguez A, Vallejo C, et al. Safety of contrast material use during pregnancy and lactation. Magn Reson Imaging Clin N Am 2017;25:787–97.

75. Bourjeily G, Chalhoub M, Phornphutkul C, et al. Neonatal thyroid function: effect of a single exposure to iodinated contrast medium in utero. Radiology 2010;256:744–50.

76. Kochi MH, Kaloudis EV, Ahmed W, et al. Effect of in utero exposure of iodinated intravenous contrast on neonatal thyroid function. J Comput Assist Tomogr 2012;36:165–9.

77. Rajaram S, Exley CE, Fairlie F, et al. Effect of antenatal iodinated contrast agent on neonatal thyroid function. Br J Radiol 2012;85:e238–42.

78. Chan WS, Rey E, Kent NE, et al. Venous thromboembolism and antithrombotic therapy in pregnancy. J Obstet Gynaecol Can 2014;36:527–53.

79. Burton KR, Park AL, Fralick M, et al. Risk of early-onset breast cancer among women exposed to thoracic computed tomography in pregnancy or early postpartum. J Thromb Haemost 2018;16:876–85.

80. Ridge CA, Mhuircheartaigh JN, Dodd JD, et al. Pulmonary CT angiography protocol adapted to the hemodynamic effects of pregnancy. AJR Am J Roentgenol 2011;197:1058–63.

81. Gutte H, Mortensen J, Jensen CV, et al. Comparison of V/Q SPECT and planar V/Q lung scintigraphy in diagnosing acute pulmonary embolism. Nucl Med Commun 2010;31:82–6.

82. Gruning T, Mingo RE, Gosling MG, et al. Diagnosing venous thromboembolism in pregnancy. Br J Radiol 2016;89:20160021.

83. Rafat Motavalli L, Hoseinian Azghadi E, Miri Hakimabad H, et al. Pulmonary embolism in pregnant patients: assessing organ dose to pregnant phantom and its fetus during lung imaging. Med Phys 2017;44:6038–46.

84. Kanal E, Barkovich AJ, Bell C, et al. ACR guidance document for safe MR practices: 2007. AJR Am J Roentgenol 2007;188:1447–74.

85. Webb JA, Thomsen HS, Morcos SK, et al. The use of iodinated and gadolinium contrast media during pregnancy and lactation. Eur Radiol 2005;15:1234–40.

86. De Santis M, Straface G, Cavaliere AF, et al. Gadolinium periconceptional exposure: pregnancy and neonatal outcome. Acta Obstet Gynecol Scand 2007;86:99–101.

87. Ray JG, Vermeulen MJ, Bharatha A, et al. Association between MRI exposure during pregnancy and fetal and childhood outcomes. JAMA 2016;316:952–61.

88. Potts J, Lisonkova S, Murphy DT, et al. Gadolinium magnetic resonance imaging during pregnancy associated with adverse neonatal and postneonatal outcomes. J Pediatr 2017;180:291–4.

89. Koren G, Pariente G. Pregnancy- associated changes in pharmacokinetics and their clinical implications. Pharm Res 2018;35:61.

90. Mitchell AA, Gilboa SM, Werler MM, et al. Medication use during pregnancy, with particular focus on prescription drugs: 1976-2008. Am J Obstet Gynecol 2011;205:51.e1-e8.

91. Illamola SM, Bucci-Rechtweg C, Costantine MM, et al. Inclusion of pregnant and breastfeeding women in research - efforts and initiatives. Br J Clin Pharmacol 2018;84:215–22.

92. US Food and Drug Administration, HHS. Content and format of labeling for human prescription drug and biological products requirements for pregnancy and lactation labeling 2014. Available at: https://www.fda.gov/media/90279/download [Accessed October 14, 2020].

93. Reproductive Toxicology Center. Available at: www.reprotox.org [Accessed October 20, 2020].

94. MotherToBaby. Available at: https://mothertobaby.org [Accessed October 20, 2020].

95. Bartick MC, Schwarz EB, Green BD, et al. Suboptimal breastfeeding in the United States: maternal and pediatric health outcomes and costs. Matern Child Nutr 2017;13:e12366.

96. Transfer of drugs and other chemicals into human milk. Pediatrics 2001;108:776–89.

97. Anderson PO, Sauberan JB. Modeling drug passage into human milk. Clin Pharmacol Ther 2016;100:42–52.

98. Mattsson S, Johansson L, Leide Svegborn S, et al. Annex D. Recommendations on breast-feeding interruptions. ICRP publication 128 In: Clement CH, Hamada N, editors. Annals of the ICRP. Radiation dose to patients from radiopharmaceuticals: a compendium of current information related to frequently used substances: the International Commission on Radiological Protection. Ottawa, Ontario, Canada, 2015. p. 7–321.

99. Newton ER, Hale TW. Drugs in breast milk. Clin Obstet Gynecol 2015;58:868–84.

100. Hale TW. Hale's medications & mothers' milk (TM) 2021: a manual of lactational pharmacology. New York: Springer Pub Co Inc; 2020.

101. National Library of Medicine, National Institutes of Health. Drugs and Lactation Database (LactMed). Available at: https://www.ncbi.nlm.nih.gov/books/NBK501922/ [Accessed October 14, 2020].

102. ACOG Committee Opinion No. 762: prepregnancy counseling. Obstet Gynecol 2019;133:e78–89.

103. Chakravarty E, Clowse ME, Pushparajah DS, et al. Family planning and pregnancy issues for women with systemic inflammatory diseases: patient and physician perspectives. BMJ Open 2014;4:e004081.

104. Wexler ID, Johannesson M, Edenborough FP, et al. Pregnancy and chronic progressive pulmonary disease. Am J Respir Crit Care Med 2007;175:300–5.

105. Skogsdal Y, Fadl H, Cao Y, et al. An intervention in contraceptive counseling increased the knowledge about fertility and awareness of preconception health-a randomized controlled trial. Ups J Med Sci 2019;124:203–12.

106. Johnson K, Posner SF, Biermann J, et al. Recommendations to improve preconception health and health care–United States. A report of the CDC/ATSDR preconception care work group and the

select panel on preconception care. MMWR Recomm Rep 2006;55:1–23.

107. Lanik AD. Preconception counseling. Prim Care 2012;39:1–16.

108. Shields KE, Lyerly AD. Exclusion of pregnant women from industry-sponsored clinical trials. Obstet Gynecol 2013;122:1077–81.

109. Adam MP, Polifka JE, Friedman JM. Evolving knowledge of the teratogenicity of medications in human pregnancy. Am J Med Genet C Semin Med Genet 2011;157c:175–82.

110. Cox M, Whittle MJ, Byrne A, et al. Prepregnancy counselling: experience from 1,075 cases. Br J Obstet Gynaecol 1992;99:873–6.

111. Trussell J, Wynn LL. Reducing unintended pregnancy in the United States. Contraception 2008; 77:1–5.

112. Einarson A, Riordan S. Smoking in pregnancy and lactation: a review of risks and cessation strategies. Eur J Clin Pharmacol 2009;65:325–30.

113. Whittington JR, Simmons PM, Phillips AM, et al. The use of electronic cigarettes in pregnancy: a review of the literature. Obstet Gynecol Surv 2018;73: 544–9.

114. Glover M, Phillips CV. Potential effects of using non-combustible tobacco and nicotine products during pregnancy: a systematic review. Harm Reduct J 2020;17:16.

115. Tamim H, Yunis KA, Chemaitelly H, et al. Effect of narghile and cigarette smoking on newborn birthweight. BJOG 2008;115:91–7.

116. Bachir R, Chaaya M. Maternal smoking: determinants and associated morbidity in two areas in Lebanon. Matern Child Health J 2008;12:298–307.

117. Nuwayhid IA, Yamout B, Azar G, et al. Narghile (hubble-bubble) smoking, low birth weight, and other pregnancy outcomes. Am J Epidemiol 1998;148:375–83.

118. Rachidi S, Awada S, Al-Hajje A, et al. Risky substance exposure during pregnancy: a pilot study from Lebanese mothers. Drug Healthc Patient Saf 2013;5:123–31.

119. Murin S, Rafii R, Bilello K. Smoking and smoking cessation in pregnancy. Clin Chest Med 2011;32: 75–91.

120. Xaverius PK, O'Reilly Z, Li A, et al. Smoking cessation and pregnancy: timing of cessation reduces or eliminates the effect on low birth weight. Matern Child Health J 2019;23:1434–41.

121. Poston L, Caleyachetty R, Cnattingius S, et al. Preconceptional and maternal obesity: epidemiology and health consequences. Lancet Diabetes Endocrinol 2016;4:1025–36.

122. Committee Opinion No. 723 summary: guidelines for diagnostic imaging during pregnancy and lactation. Obstet Gynecol 2017;130:933–4.

123. Leung AN, Bull TM, Jaeschke R, et al. An official American Thoracic Society/Society of Thoracic Radiology clinical practice guideline: evaluation of suspected pulmonary embolism in pregnancy. Am J Respir Crit Care Med 2011;184:1200–8.

Unique Aspects of Asthma in Women

Casper Tidemandsen, MD[a],[*],[1], Erik Soeren Halvard Hansen, MD[b],[1],
Soeren Malte Rasmussen, MD[b], Charlotte Suppli Ulrik, MD, DMSci[a],
Vibeke Backer, MD, DMSci[b]

KEYWORDS

- Asthma • Women • Estrogen • Hormones • Clinical management • Pregnancy • Fertility

KEY POINTS

- Asthma is more common in women and expresses unique aspects compared with men.
- Asthma affects fertility and therapy with female sex hormones affect asthma.
- Pregnant women with asthma should be managed by an asthma specialist.

INTRODUCTION

Asthma is one of the most common chronic conditions among women in Western society.[1,2] Many patients with asthma have characteristic symptoms in common, for example, wheeze, chest tightness, dyspnea, and cough together with triggers like physical activity, allergens, and environmental irritants.[3] However, the underlying mechanisms driving these symptoms often vary between men and women. Until recently, asthma has been considered a homogenous disease; however, in this era of precision medicine, immunologic endotyping and phenotyping are becoming part of the general diagnostic workup for asthma, and asthma is now truly recognized as a heterogeneous disease. Accordingly, it is becoming clear that there are several unique aspects to asthma in women. First, women develop asthma at different ages than men with many women being diagnosed around the age of menarche, pregnancy, and menopause, whereas men are typically diagnosed with asthma before puberty in close association with the atopic march.[4–6] Second, asthma among women is often severe, leading to women being more often prescribed biological therapies compared with men. Obesity has been linked to the onset of asthma,

especially in adult women developing asthma around and after menopause.[7] Last, it is becoming clear that both intrinsic and extrinsic female sex hormones influence human lung tissue. However, recent and former observational studies investigating the role of estrogens in general are interestingly ambiguous and it is yet undetermined whether the major types of estrogens (estrone), estradiol, estriol, and estetrol) should be considered friends or foes.[8–11] Nevertheless, in an era of precision medicine, the heterogeneity in women's asthma makes management of the disease challenging. Uncontrolled asthma is closely associated with decreased quality of life and socioeconomic burden; therefore, it is vital for both general practitioners and pulmonologists to understand the clinical presentations, clinical management, and treatable traits throughout the lifespan of women with asthma.[12,13] Thus, this review aims to explore the unique aspects of asthma in women.

EPIDEMIOLOGY

It is estimated that 4.3% (>300 million people) of the worlds' population has asthma and the overall prevalence of asthma is around 20% higher in women than in men.[1,3,14] In the younger ages

[a] Department of Respiratory Medicine, Hvidovre University Hospital, Denmark; [b] Centre for Physical Activity Research, Rigshospitalet, Copenhagen University Hospital, Blegdamsvej 9, 2100 Copenhagen, Denmark
[1] Shared first authorship.
* corresponding author.
E-mail address: casper.tidemandsen.02@regionh.dk

Clin Chest Med 42 (2021) 497–506
https://doi.org/10.1016/j.ccm.2021.04.009

(<15 years), boys have a higher incidence of allergy, asthma, and asthma-related hospitalizations and exacerbations than girls.[6,15] However, around puberty there is a shift and new-onset asthma becomes more common among girls.[4] Severe asthma and nonallergic asthma are especially frequent among younger and adult women.[4,10] Among adults over 65 years of age, the prevalence of asthma has been estimated to somewhere between 7.5% and 12.5%, with a female predominance.[16]

DIAGNOSIS

The Global Initiative for Asthma[14] recommends that asthma be diagnosed based on a medical history with 1 or more characteristic symptoms (**Box 1**) and a positive asthma test documenting airflow variability or airway hyperresponsiveness.[17] Generally, symptoms present as a group, are often worse at night or in the morning, and are often triggered by exercise, laughter, cold air, and viral infections. Evidence of airflow variability can easily be performed in general practice, but this test cannot exclude asthma. Therefore, referral to a pulmonary physician can be necessary in the evaluation of a potential asthma diagnosis. Further testing focuses on airway hyperresponsiveness to direct and indirect bronchial challenges with different compounds.[18,19]

COMMON DIFFERENTIAL DIAGNOSES IN WOMEN

When failing to establish a diagnosis of asthma or the effect of treatment is insufficient, it is important to consider asthma with concomitant diseases or other diagnoses mimicking asthma.

Vocal Cord Dysfunction

Among women aged 12 to 39 years, vocal cord dysfunction is more commonly seen among women than men with treatment resistant symptoms combined with severe symptoms while exercising. The symptoms resembles asthma with the most pronounced difference being that symptoms often are most distinct during the inspiratory phase.[14] Further, it is not uncommon that vocal cord dysfunction coexists with asthma and should be considered in patients having severe symptoms, despite moderate to high doses of inhaled corticosteroids (ICS) and long-acting beta-agonists.

Dysfunctional Breathing

Another common reason for treatment resistant asthma in women is dysfunctional breathing.[20] Although the mechanisms of dysfunctional breathing are still under review, it is becoming clear that biomechanical and psychophysiological aspects of breathing can impact asthma symptoms and disease control.[21]

Chronic Cough

Chronic cough can occur in both patients with and without asthma. Patients with chronic cough are often women over 65 years of age.[22] It is important that chronic cough is not neglected as an acceptable symptom of asthma and should be evaluated thoroughly. Causes of chronic cough that range from undertreated asthma to malignant diseases and bronchiectasis should be considered, especially when the cough is resistant to treatment with asthma medications.

Cardiac Disease

Patients with asthma and other obstructive pulmonary diseases have an increased risk of cardiac disease. Thus, in patients with difficult-to-control asthma, cardiac reasons for dyspnea should be considered.[23]

PATHOPHYSIOLOGY, PHENOTYPES, AND ENDOTYPES
Type 2-Mediated Asthma

In type 2-mediated asthma, inflammation is facilitated by several cell types, including eosinophils, mast cells, macrophages, T lymphocytes, and epithelial cells.[24] Asthma can present as allergic or nonallergic, where the nonallergic eosinophilic endotype is mediated through type 2 innate

---

Box 1
Characteristic of asthma

Classic symptoms

- Shortness of breath
- Wheeze
- Chest tightness
- Cough
- Nighttime awakenings

Triggers

- Physical activity
- Allergens
- Smoke/pollution
- Cold and moist air
- Respiratory tract infections

lymphoid[3] cells. Androgens have been shown to decrease type 2 innate lymphoid signaling and could be one of the drivers of the sex difference in asthma and explain the shift in incidence around puberty.[25] One-way to differentiate is the presence or absence of IgE antibodies to aeroallergens. Both allergic and nonallergic asthma are characterized by infiltration with T-helper cells in the airways, which stimulates the secretion of IL-4, IL-5, and IL-13.[26] All these cytokines attract eosinophils, stimulate mast cells, encourage leukocytosis, and increase B-cell IgE production, which subsequently leads to eosinophilic inflammation of the airways. Eosinophilic cell counts of 3% or higher in sputum are regarded as eosinophilic inflammation of the airways and a blood eosinophilic cell count of more than 0.3×10^9/L is regarded as systemic eosinophilic inflammation.[27–29]

Long-term type 2 inflammation often induces hypertrophy of the smooth muscle fibers in the airways, hyperplasia, and edema.[30] Permanent changes in the airways have been reported, including subepithelial edema and thickening of the subbasement, as well as blood vessel proliferation and dilation, airway smooth muscle hypertrophy, and mucus hypersecretion.[31]

Non–Type 2-Mediated Asthma

In non–type 2-mediated asthma the airway epithelium is often dominated by neutrophilic inflammation, defined as a neutrophilic cell count with thresholds ranging from 41% to 61% of the total cell count in sputum samples.[32] Unlike blood eosinophilia, blood neutrophilic cell count cannot be used as differential between type 2 or non–type 2 inflammation in asthma. Evidence suggests that T-helper 17 cell may play an important role in pathophysiology of non–type 2-mediated asthma.[33] T-helper 17 cells secret the cytokines IL-17A, IL-17F, IL-21, and IL-22. These cytokines have been recognized in both biopsies from the bronchial tree and in bronchioalveolar lavage fluids.[34,35]

In patients with more severe, non–type 2-mediated asthma, neutrophils are increased in the sputum and bronchioalveolar lavage fluid. Often, these patients do not respond well to corticosteroid treatments.[36] Increased neutrophils in the airway are driven by increased IL-17A–secreting and/or interferon-γ–secreting cells, including T-helper 17 cells, T-helper 1, and natural killer cells.[37]

Childhood and Menarche

Early-onset asthma is driven by several factors. It has been suggested that exposure to allergens, viruses, and bacteria could be triggering factors of asthma development as well as nonbiologic factors as smoking, pollution, and other environmental factors.[38,39] Regardless of exposure, atopy, IgE and probably eosinophilic inflammation are common features among children with asthma.[3,40] Genome studies have found that polymorphisms in several genes involved in the adaptive immune response and epithelial function are associated with an increased risk of asthma.[3] Determining endotypes in childhood asthma reveals that childhood asthma is typically a type 2–mediated disease. Studies in young women have shown that early menarche and obesity are associated with an increased risk of developing asthma.[4,41]

Female Sex Hormones Effect on Type 2-Mediated Asthma and Non–Type 2-Mediated Asthma

The effect of the female sex hormones (estrone, estradiol, estriol, and estetrol) on asthma in humans is still unclear. However, in murine models comparing male and female mice with allergic asthma mice who underwent ovalbumin or house dust mite induction, eosinophils were elevated in bronchioalveolar lavage fluid in both male and female mice. Female mice had elevated levels of IL-5 and, IL-13 in the lungs and elevated levels of serum IgE compared with male mice.[42,43] In female mice who had undergone surgical removal of the ovaries, levels of eosinophils, IL-5, and total IgE were found to be lower compared with hormonally intact mice. This finding shows that ovarian hormones probably play an important role in inducing allergic airway inflammation.[43] However, this claim remains to be verified thoroughly in mechanistic studies in humans.

Neutrophils and cytokines like IL-17 are increased in the airway epithelium in patients with non–type 2-mediated asthma.[34,35] Further, in women, studies have found that 17β-estradiol and progesterone were essential for enhancing T-helper 17 cell differentiation, production of IL-17A, and IL-17A–mediated airway inflammation.[44] It has also been shown that estrogen and progesterone play a role in airway mucus production and mucocilliary clearance and that airway epithelial cells express estrogen and progesterone receptors.[45] In mice, studies have shown that 17β-estradiol increases mucus production.[45]

During and after menopause, estrogen seemingly plays a role in asthma pathology. Menopause has been suggested as both protective against asthma and harmful with decreasing lung function.[46,47] In line with this finding, the role of exogenous estrogen in menopause with hormonal replacement therapy on asthma is still under review. Exogenous estrogen has revealed to improve airway hyperresponsiveness in mice, increase lung function in older women, and decrease the use of corticosteroids as well as decrease asthma exacerbations.[48–50] If this finding is confirmed, it is not surprising that decreasing estrogen levels in women have been linked to increased asthma severity and that mice experiencing a loss of estrogen develop increased airway hyperresponsiveness.[51,52] However, previous questionnaire-based studies have suggested that exogenous estrogen is linked to new asthma incidence in women by a risk ratio of 1.3 to 2.4.[9,53,54] Further, hormonal replacement therapy has also been linked to increased admission rates owing to asthma exacerbations[55]

CLINICAL PRESENTATIONS OF ASTHMA IN WOMEN
Adolescents and Young Adults

As stated elsewhere in this article, asthma in childhood is found mainly in boys. However, around the time of menarche there is a shift toward a female predominance. Asthma in the premenstrual phase is often severe and these patients are more likely to be obese and to have aspirin-induced symptoms. Further, their transition into physical adulthood is often impacted by more severe symptoms of dysmenorrhea, short menstrual cycles, and mood changes compared with girls without premenstrual asthma.[14,56,57]

Across childhood, symptoms of asthma vary. In young children (<5 years of age), asthma often starts with recurrent wheezing in relation to upper and lower respiratory tract infections.[14] Some children only experience wheezing without having asthma (happy wheezers), which makes the differential diagnostics challenging. Eczema and allergic rhinitis are common features among children with asthma. Further, family history with asthma and/or atopy are often present.[14]

Adulthood

Fertile women experience changes in ovarian hormone concentrations each month (**Fig. 1**). Early studies reported worsening of asthma symptoms, decreased peak flow rates, and increased use of rescue medications in women with asthma during the premenstrual or perimenstrual phase of the cycle corresponding to low progesterone and estrogen levels (see **Fig. 1**).[58] Sputum eosinophils and fractional exhaled nitric oxide are reported to be increased significantly during the premenstrual phase when compared with immediately after the menstrual phase, indicating a cyclic variation in the inflammation.[59] Further, menstruation has

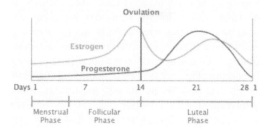

Fig. 1. Female sex hormone cycle. (Illustration by Casper Tidemandsen.)

been linked to emergency department visits and a higher use of corticosteroids.[60] However, the evidence is ambiguous. Some studies have found no difference in asthma control during the menstrual cycle, whereas other studies find that asthma symptoms increase during menstruation, but that medication use and lung function do not change.[61–63]

Menopause and after Menopause

Women with an onset of severe and/or difficult-to-treat asthma around the time of menopause often have low eosinophilic inflammation, a high level of symptoms, obesity, and a poor treatment effect of ICS.[64] Allergy and atopy are less frequent and triggers initiating the development of asthma remain largely unidentified. This phenotype typically has a non–type 2 endotype in their airway pathology. It is believed that T-helper 17 cells are involved in the pathogenesis of late-onset, noneosinophilic asthma with a predominantly neutrophilic infiltration of the airways. However, comorbidities in the lungs as well as infections have been discussed as possible causes for this predominance.[3] Elderly people have been shown to be poor perceivers of asthma as their awareness of bronchoconstriction is lower compared with younger individuals.[16] Further, they less often recognize their dyspnea as part of disease, but attribute these symptoms to a natural part of getting older.

Clinical Management and Treatable Traits

To date, there are no real differences in the clinical management or treatment of women with asthma compared with men. Traditionally a stepwise approach has been used. Currently, the Global Initiative for Asthma guidelines from 2020 are recommended (**Fig. 2**).[65] The cornerstone of treatment for asthma is ICS with relief therapy either being ICS with long-acting beta-agonists or short acting beta-agonists.

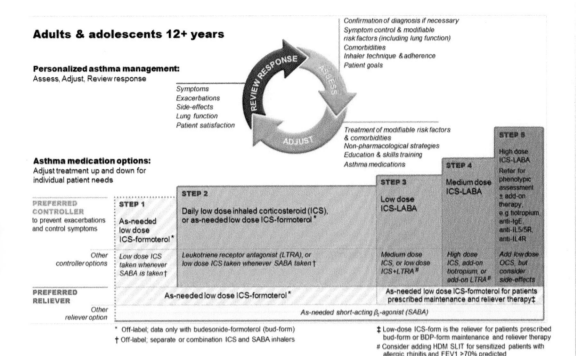

Fig. 2. BDP, FEV, forced expiratory volume; HDM, LABA, long-acting beta-agonists; SLIT. BDP, beclometasone dipropionate; HDM, house dust mite; SLIT, sublingual immunotherapy; ICS, inhaled corticosteroid; LABA, long-acting beta2 -agonist; IgE, immunoglobulin-E; IL5, interleukin-5; IL4R, interleukin-4 receptor; SABA, short-acting beta2 -agonist; LTRA, leukotriene receptor antagonist; BDP, beclomethasone dipropionate; HDM, house dust mite; SLIT, sublingual immunotherapy; FEV1, forced expiratory volume in 1 second. (©2020 Global Initiative for Asthma, reprinted with permission. Available from www.ginasthma.org.)

The monitoring of treatment effect is done most efficiently by medical history, including asthma control questionnaires and clinical examinations with measurements of lung function and exhaled nitric oxide.[66]

In recent years, a new approach called "treatable traits," has emerged. It is hypothesized to be a promising tool in difficult-to-treat asthma. Treatable traits are divided into 3 main categories: pulmonary, extrapulmonary, and behavioral/psychosocial (**Fig. 3**). Identified traits are subsequently evaluated and assessed as clinically relevant, measurable, and/or treatable (**Table 1**).[67]

The identification of treatable traits facilitates an individualized precision medicine strategy for the management of asthma that seems to be promising compared with the traditional one-size-fits-all stepwise strategy.[68,69]

DISEASE COMPLICATIONS AND SPECIAL CIRCUMSTANCES IN WOMEN
Infertility

Although still quite novel, evidence is emerging to support that asthma affects fertility in women. It has recently been shown that women with asthma

have prolonged time to pregnancy and a tendency toward a greater number of pregnancy losses owing to spontaneous abortions.[70–72] Further, a study including women with asthma who recently had given birth to a full-term child and a control cohort, found that asthma was associated with longer time to pregnancy.[73] Another study showed an increased need for fertility treatment among women with asthma compared with women without asthma.[74] To date, there is no clear explanation for the link between female asthma and a decrease in fertility. However, it is well-known that changes in the inflammatory environment both systemically and locally in the endometrium can affect fertility negatively with a decreased likelihood of implantation of the embryo.[71]

The endometrium is a dynamic structure that continuously changes in response to hormonal stimulation and inflammatory changes. A small offset in the inflammatory level of the endometrium can have implications for implantation and, thereby, fertility. A study found an imbalance in the inflammatory environment of the uterine endometrium at the time of implantation in women with asthma.[75] This change likely interferes negatively with the immune processes required for a

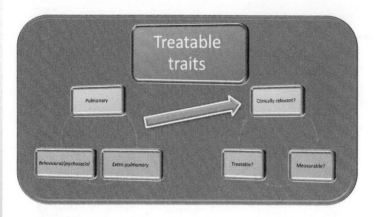

Fig. 3. Treatable traits: Main categories and defining domains. (Illustration by Casper Tidemandsen.)

Table 1
"Treatable traits": Possible traits to target

Domains	Traits
Pulmonary treatable traits	Airflow limitation
	Airway smooth muscle contraction
	Airway mucosal edema
	Eosinophilic airway inflammation
	Loss of elastic recoil (emphysema)
	Chronic bronchitis
	Airway bacterial colonization
	Cough reflex hypersensitivity
	Bronchiectasis
	Arterial hypoxemia
Extrapulmonary treatable traits	Deconditioning
	Obesity
	Obstructive sleep apnea syndrome
	Cardiovascular disease
	Cachexia
	Gastroesophageal reflux disease
	Upper airway diseases: rhinosinusitis with and without nasal polyps
	Vocal cord dysfunction
	Psychiatric disorders: depression
	Upper airway diseases: inducible laryngeal obstruction
	Psychiatric disorders: anxiety/other behavioral aspects including breathing pattern disorders
	Persistent systemic inflammation
Behavioral and psychosocial treatable traits	Smoking and other exposures
	Exposure to sensitizing agents/pollution
	Side effects of other treatments
	Inhaler device polypharmacy
	Symptom perception
	Adherence to controller therapy
	Poor inhalation technique
	Family and social support

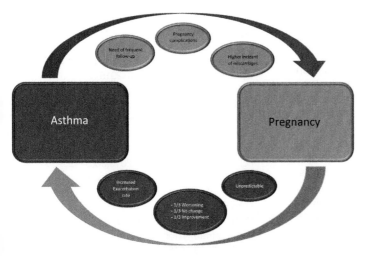

Fig. 4. The effect of pregnancy on asthma and the effect of asthma on pregnancy. (Illustrations by Casper Tidemandsen.)

successful conception as high levels of vascular endothelial growth factor are associated with successful implantation as well as twin pregnancies.[75] An imbalance in the inflammatory cytokines might lead to a less receptive endometrium and thereby a decreased rate of implantation in women with asthma, which could explain the lower fertility reported from studies of women with asthma.

The Effect of Pregnancy on Asthma and the Effect of Asthma on Pregnancy

Asthma during pregnancy has been an area of interest for decades. Several aspects are important for describing the effect of pregnancy on asthma, such as asthma severity, comorbidities, and the physiologic changes that occur during pregnancy.[76] It is estimated that approximately one-third of pregnant women with asthma experience a symptomatic worsening, one-third remain the same, and one-third experience a symptomatic improvement[77,78] (**Fig. 4**). Further, a study showed that 6% of women with asthma experienced an asthma exacerbation during pregnancy.[79] This finding is further supported by another study also describing a high exacerbation rate during pregnancy.[80] Several factors play a role in the improvement or worsening in asthma during pregnancy, but the final mechanism are largely unexplained making the course of asthma during pregnancy quite unpredictable.[79]

Studies investigating the association between maternal asthma or exacerbations of asthma and adverse maternal and perinatal outcomes have revealed conflicting evidence. Several studies have shown that uncontrolled maternal asthma is associated with a higher risk of pregnancy complications, such as gestational hypertension, pre-eclampsia, gestational diabetes, and a small for gestational age infant.[81–84] Further, there is also a tendency toward a greater number of pregnancy losses owing to spontaneous abortions.[72] However, a number of studies have found no association between asthma in pregnancy and adverse outcomes.[85–88] One explanation for the conflicting evidence could be the big variation between the studies with regard to population characteristics, asthma severity, and treatment. Because the course is difficult to predict, it is of vital importance that treatment is optimized as much as possible; women should be monitored closely and adherence to controller therapy is encouraged during pregnancy[84] (see **Fig. 4**).

SUMMARY

All stages of a woman's life affect asthma in different ways. Additionally, because it is becoming clear that asthma affects fertility and female sex hormones in various forms affect asthma, further mechanistic and epidemiologic research into this field is highly warranted. Last, because pregnant women are at high risk of adverse outcomes of asthma and pregnancy, they should be followed by an asthma specialist.

CLINICS CARE POINTS

- Different stages of a woman's lifeexpress unique aspects of asthma.
- Asthma affects the fertility.
- Hormone therapy affects asthma.
- The course of asthma during pregnancy is unpredictable.

CONFLICTS OF INTEREST

Dr ESH Hansen has no relevant conflicts of interest to declare. Dr C. Tidemandsen has no relevant conflicts of interest to declare. Dr SM Rasmussen has no relevant conflicts of interest to declare. Professor V. Backer has received an unrestricted grant for an asthma and fertility study by Novartis, has been part of advisory boards concerning asthma therapy by GSK, Teva, Chiesi, MSD, Novartis, AZ. Professor CS Ulrik has received personal fees for lectures, advisory board meetings, and so one, from AstraZeneca, Novartis, Chiesi, TEVA, GSK, ALK-Abello, Boehringer-Ingelheim, Mundipharma, Actelion, Orion Pharma, Sanofi and Mylan.

ACKNOWLEDGMENTS

The Center for Physical Activity Research (CFAS) is supported by TrygFonden (grants ID 101390 and ID 20045).

REFERENCES

1. Global Asthma Network. The global asthma report 2018 2018.
2. World Health Organisation (WHO). "Asthma, fact sheet, WHO," asthma fact sheet 2017. Available at: https://www.who.int/news-room/fact-sheets/detail/ asthma. Accessed October 30, 2019.
3. Papi A, Brightling C, Pedersen SE, et al. Asthma. Lancet 2018;391(10122):783–800.
4. Lieberoth S, Gade EJ, Brok J, et al. Age at menarche and risk of asthma: systematic review and meta-analysis. J Asthma 2014;51(6):559–65.
5. Leynaert B, Sunyer J, Garcia-Esteban R, et al. Gender differences in prevalence, diagnosis and incidence of allergic and non-allergic asthma: a population-based cohort. Thorax 2012;67(7): 625–31.
6. Wijga A, Tabak C, Postma DS, et al. Sex differences in asthma during the first 8 years of life: the Prevention and Incidence of Asthma and Mite Allergy (PIAMA) birth cohort study. J Allergy Clin Immunol 2011;127(1):275–7.
7. Thomsen SF, Ulrik CS, Kyvik KO, et al. Association between obesity and asthma in a twin cohort. Allergy Eur J Allergy Clin Immunol 2007;62(10): 1199–204.
8. Nwaru BI, Sheikh A. Hormonal contraceptives and asthma in women of reproductive age: analysis of data from serial National Scottish Health Surveys. J R Soc Med 2015;108(9):358–71.
9. Lange P, Parner J, Prescott E, et al. Exogenous female sex steroid hormones and risk of asthma and asthma-like symptoms: a cross sectional study of the general population. Thorax 2001;56(8):613–6.
10. Matheson MC, Burgess JA, Lau MYZ, et al. Hormonal contraception increases risk of asthma among obese but decreases it among nonobese subjects: a prospective, population-based cohort study. ERJ Open Res 2015;1(2):00026–2015.
11. Macsali F, Svanes C, Bjørge L, et al. Respiratory health in women: from menarche to menopause. Expert Rev Respir Med 2012;6(2):187–202.
12. O'Toole J, Mikulic L, Kaminsky DA. Epidemiology and pulmonary physiology of severe asthma. Immunol Allergy Clin North Am 2016;36(3):425–38.
13. Loftus PA, Wise SK. Epidemiology and economic burden of asthma. Int Forum Allergy Rhinol 2015; 5(April):S7–10.
14. Global Initiative for Asthma. 2019 GINA report: global strategy for asthma management and prevention 2019 2018.
15. Blanche Dawson GH, Maturity, Raymond Illsley RM. Survey of childhood asthma in Aberdeen. Paediatr Res Soc 1962;1:135–6.
16. Gillman A, Douglass JA. Asthma in the elderly. Asia Pac Allergy 2012;2:101–8.
17. Graham BL, Steenbruggen I, Barjaktarevic IZ, et al. Standardization of spirometry 2019 update an official American Thoracic Society and European Respiratory Society technical statement. Am J Respir Crit Care Med 2019;200(8):E70–88.
18. Hallstrand TS, Leuppi JD, Joos G, et al. ERS technical standard on bronchial challenge testing: pathophysiology and methodology of indirect airway challenge testing. Eur Respir J 2018;52(5):1–18.
19. Coates AL, Wanger J, Cockcroft DW, et al. ERS technical standard on bronchial challenge testing: general considerations and performance of methacholine challenge tests. Eur Respir J 2017; 49(5):1–17.
20. Sedeh FB, Von Bülow A, Backer V, et al. The impact of dysfunctional breathing on the level of asthma control in difficult asthma. Respir Med 2020;163: 105894.
21. Courtney R. Breathing training for dysfunctional breathing in asthma: taking a multidimensional approach. ERJ Open Res 2017;3(4):00065–2017.
22. Mathur A, Liu-Shiu-Cheong PSK, Currie GP. The management of chronic cough. QJM 2019;112(9):651–6.
23. Ingebrigtsen TS, Marott JL, Vestbo J, et al. Coronary heart disease and heart failure in asthma, COPD and asthma-COPD overlap. BMJ Open Respir Res 2020;7(1):1–11.
24. Oliphant CJ, Barlow JL, Mckenzie ANJ. Insights into the initiation of type 2 immune responses. Immunology 2011;134(4):378–85.
25. Laffont S, Blanquart E, Savignac M, et al. Androgen signaling negatively controls group 2 innate lymphoid cells. J Exp Med 2017;214(6):1581–92.
26. Papi A, Brightling C, Pedersen SE, et al. Seminar: asthma. Lancet 2018;391:783–800.

27. Flood-Page P, Swenson C, Faiferman I, et al. A study to evaluate safety and efficacy of mepolizumab in patients with moderate persistent asthma. Am J Respir Crit Care Med 2007;176(11):1062–71.

28. Carr TF, Zeki AA, Kraft M. Eosinophilic and noneosinophilic asthma. Am J Respir Crit Care Med 2018; 197(1):22–37.

29. Westerhof GA, Korevaar DA, Amelink M, et al. Biomarkers to identify sputum eosinophilia in different adult asthma phenotypes. Eur Respir J 2015;46(3): 688–96.

30. Kroegel C, Foerster M, Workalemahu G, et al. Asthmatic airway inflammation. Zeitschrift für ärztliche Fortbildung 2001;95(10):677–83.

31. Pałgan K, Dziedziczko A, Bartuzi Z. Remodeling of the basement membrane and airway epithelium in patients with asthma. Pol Merkur Lek 2005;19(112): 553–5.

32. Hastie AT, Hatton RD, Mangan PR, et al. Analyses of asthma severity phenotypes and inflammatory proteins in subjects stratified by sputum granulocytes. J Allergy Clin Immunol 2010;125(5):1028–36.e13.

33. Park H, Li Z, Yang XO, et al. A distinct lineage of CD4 T cells regulates tissue inflammation by producing interleukin 17. Nat Immunol 2005;6(11):1133–41.

34. Harrington LE, Hatton RD, Mangan PR, et al. Interleukin 17-producing CD4+ effector T cells develop via a lineage distinct from the T helper type 1 and 2 lineages. Nat Immunol 2005;6(11):1123–32.

35. Bhakta NR, Woodruff PG. Human asthma phenotypes: from the clinic, to cytokines, and back again. Immunol Rev 2011;242(1):220–32.

36. American Lung Association. Trends in asthma morbidity and mortality. Am Lung Assoc Epidemiol Stat 2012;1–28.

37. Fuseini H, Newcomb DC. Mechanisms driving Gender differences in asthma. Curr Allergy Asthma Rep 2017;17(3).

38. de Benedictis FM, Attanasi M. Asthma in childhood. Eur Respir Rev 2016;25(139):41–7.

39. Konradsen JR, Nordlund B, Lidegran M, et al. Problematic severe asthma: a proposed approach to identifying children who are severely resistant to therapy. Pediatr Allergy Immunol 2011;22(1 PART 1):9–18.

40. Fitzpatrick AM, Teague WG, Meyers DA, et al. Heterogeneity of severe asthma in childhood: confirmation by cluster Analysis of children in the NIH/NHLBI severe asthma research program (SARP). J Allergy Clin Immunol 2012;127(2):382–9.

41. Castro-Rodríguez JA, Holberg CJ, Morgan WJ, et al. Increased incidence of asthmalike symptoms in girls who become overweight or obese during the school years. Am J Respir Crit Care Med 2001;163(6):1344–9.

42. Hayashi T, Adachi Y, Hasegawa K, et al. Less sensitivity for late airway inflammation in males than females in BALB/c Mice. Scand J Immunol 2003; 57(6):562–7.

43. Riffo-Vasquez Y, Ligeiro De Oliveira AP, Page CP, et al. Role of sex hormones in allergic inflammation in mice. Clin Exp Allergy 2007;37(3):459–70.

44. Newcomb DC, et al. Estrogen and progesterone decrease let-7f microRNA expression and increase IL-23/IL-23 receptor signaling and IL-17A production in patients with severe asthma. J Allergy Clin Immunol 2015;136(4):1025–1034e11.

45. Tam A, Wadsworth S, Dorscheid D, et al. Estradiol increases mucus synthesis in bronchial epithelial cells. PLoS One 2014;9(6).

46. Real FG, et al. Lung function, respiratory symptoms, and the menopausal transition. J Allergy Clin Immunol 2008;121(1).

47. Zein JG, Erzurum SC. Asthma is different in women. Curr Allergy Asthma Rep 2015;15(6):1–16.

48. Kos-Kudła B, Ostrowska Z, Marek B, et al. Effects of hormone replacement therapy on endocrine and spirometric parameters in asthmatic postmenopausal women. Gynecol Endocrinol 2001;15(4):304–11.

49. Carlson CL, Cushman M, Enright PL, et al. Hormone replacement therapy is associated with higher FEV1 in elderly women. Am J Respir Crit Care Med 2001; 163(2):423–8.

50. Dimitropoulou C, Drakopanagiotakis F, Chatterjee A, et al. Estrogen replacement therapy prevents airway dysfunction in a murine model of allergen-induced asthma. Lung 2009;187(2):116–27.

51. Keselman A, Heller N. Estrogen signaling modulates allergic inflammation and contributes to sex differences in asthma. Front Immunol 2015;6:568.

52. Carey MA, Card JW, Bradbury JA, et al. Spontaneous airway hyperresponsiveness in estrogen receptor-α- deficient mice. Am J Respir Crit Care Med 2007;175(2):126–35.

53. Gómez Real F, Svanes C, Björnsson EH, et al. Hormone replacement therapy, body mass index and asthma in perimenopausal women: a cross sectional survey. Thorax 2006;61(1):34–40.

54. Barr RG, Wentowski CC, Grodstein F, et al. Prospective study of postmenopausal hormone Use and newly diagnosed asthma and chronic obstructive pulmonary disease. Arch Intern Med 2004;164(4): 379–86.

55. Bønnelykke K, Raaschou-Nielsen O, Tjønneland A, et al. Postmenopausal hormone therapy and asthma-related hospital admission. J Allergy Clin Immunol 2015;135(3):813–6.e5.

56. Ensom MH, Chong E, Carter D. Premenstrual symptoms in women with premenstrual asthma. Pharmacotherapy 1999;19(4 CC-Airways):374–82.

57. Sánchez-Ramos JL, Pereira-Vega AR, Alvarado-Gómez F, et al. Risk factors for premenstrual asthma: a systematic review and meta-analysis. Expert Rev Respir Med 2017;11(1):57–72.

58. Thornton J, Lewis J, Lebrun CM, et al. Clinical characteristics of women with menstrual-linked asthma. Respir Med 2012;106(9):1236–43.

59. Oguzulgen IK, Turktas H, Erbas D. Airway inflammation in premenstrual asthma. J Asthma 2002;39(6): 517–22.

60. Rao CK, Moore CG, Bleecker E, et al. Characteristics of perimenstrual asthma and its relation to asthma severity and control: data from the Severe Asthma Research Program. Chest 2013;143(4): 984–92.

61. Zimmerman JL, Woodruff PG, Clark S, et al. Relation between phase of menstrual cycle and emergency department visits for acute asthma. Am J Respir Crit Care Med 2000;162(2 I):512–5.

62. Brenner BE, Holmes TM, Mazal B, et al. Relation between phase of the menstrual cycle and asthma presentations in the emergency department. Thorax 2005;60(10):806–9.

63. Juniper EF, Kline PA, Roberts RS, et al. Airway responsiveness to methacholine during the natural menstrual cycle and the effect of oral contraceptives. Am Rev Respir Dis 1987;135(5):1039–42.

64. Haldar P, Pavord ID, Shaw DE, et al. Europe PMC funders group cluster analysis and clinical asthma phenotypes. Am J Respir Crit Care Med 2014; 178(3):218–24.

65. Bateman ED, Hurd SS, Barnes PJ, et al. Global iniciative for asthma. GINA Appendix 2019 2019. https://doi.org/10.1183/09031936.00138707.

66. Skappak C, Saude EJ. Monitoring asthma status. Curr Opin Allergy Clin Immunol 2011;11(3):174–80.

67. Agusti A, Bel E, Thomas M, et al. Treatable traits: toward precision medicine of chronic airway diseases. Eur Respir J 2016;47(2):410–9.

68. McDonald VM, Hiles SA, Godbout K, et al. Treatable traits can be identified in a severe asthma registry and predict future exacerbations. Respirology 2019;24(1):37–47.

69. McDonald VM, Clark VL, Cordova-Rivera L, et al. Targeting treatable traits in severe asthma: a randomised controlled trial. Eur Respir J 2020;55(3).

70. Gade EJ, Thomsen SF, Lindenberg S, et al. Asthma affects time to pregnancy and fertility: A register-based twin study. In: European Respiratory Journal 2014. https://doi.org/10.1183/09031936.00148713.

71. Gade EJ, Thomsen SF, Lindenberg S, et al. Fertility outcomes in asthma: a clinical study of 245 women with unexplained infertility. Eur Respir J 2016;47(4): 1144–51.

72. Blais L, Kettani FZ, Forget A. Relationship between maternal asthma, its severity and control and abortion. Hum Reprod 2013. https://doi.org/10.1093/humrep/det024.

73. Grzeskowiak LE, Smithers LG, Grieger JA, et al. Asthma treatment impacts time to pregnancy:

74. evidence from the international SCOPE study. Eur Respir J 2018. https://doi.org/10.1183/13993003.02035-2017.

74. Vejen Hansen A, Ali Z, Malchau SS, et al. Fertility treatment among women with asthma: a case-control study of 3689 women with live births. Eur Respir J 2019. https://doi.org/10.1183/13993003.00597-2018.

75. Gade EJ, Thomsen SF, Lindenberg S, et al. Lower values of VEGF in endometrial secretion are a possible cause of subfertility in non-atopic asthmatic patients. J Asthma 2015. https://doi.org/10.3109/02770903.2014.966915.

76. Gluck JC. The change of asthma course during pregnancy. Clin Rev Allergy Immunol 2004;26(3): 171–80.

77. Rey A, Jassem E, Chelminska M. Evaluation of asthma course in pregnancy. Ginekol Pol 2019; 90(8):464–9.

78. Gluck JC, Gluck PA. The effect of pregnancy on the course of asthma. Immunol Allergy Clin North Am 2006;26(1):63–80.

79. Ali Z, Ulrik CS. Incidence and risk factors for exacerbations of asthma during pregnancy. J Asthma Allergy 2013;6:53–60.

80. Murphy VE, Gibson P, Talbot PI, et al. Severe asthma exacerbations during pregnancy. Obstet Gynecol 2005;106(5):1046–54.

81. Johnston S, Said J. Perinatal complications associated with maternal asthma during pregnancy. Obstet Med 2012;5(1):14–8.

82. Martel MJ, Rey É, Beauchesne MF, et al. Use of inhaled corticosteroids during pregnancy and risk of pregnancy induced hypertension: nested case-control study. Br Med J 2005;330(7485):230–3.

83. Baghlaf H, Spence AR, Czuzoj-Shulman N, et al. Pregnancy outcomes among women with asthma. J Matern Neonatal Med 2019;32(8):1325–31.

84. Ali Z, Nilas L, Ulrik CS. Low risk of adverse obstetrical and perinatal outcome in pregnancies complicated by asthma: a case control study. Respir Med 2016;120:124–30.

85. Enriquez R, Griffin MR, Carroll KN, et al. Effect of maternal asthma and asthma control on pregnancy and perinatal outcomes. J Allergy Clin Immunol 2007;120(3):625–30.

86. Clifton VL, Engel P, Smith R, et al. Maternal and neonatal outcomes of pregnancies complicated by asthma in an Australian population. Aust N Z J Obstet Gynaecol 2009;49(6):619–26.

87. Murphy VE, Clifton VL, Gibson PG. Asthma exacerbations during pregnancy: incidence and association with adverse pregnancy outcomes. Thorax 2006;61(2):169–76.

88. Dombrowski MP, et al. Asthma during pregnancy. Obstet Gynecol 2004;103(1):5–12.

Lung Diseases Unique to Women

Rachel N. Criner, MD[a,1], Abdullah Al-abcha, MD[b,1], Allison A. Lambert, MD, MHS[c,d], MeiLan K. Han, MD, MS[e,*]

KEYWORDS

- Women • Lymphangioleiomyomatosis • Endometriosis • Sirolimus

KEY POINTS

- Several lung diseases are unique to women. An in-depth understanding of the mechanisms of these diseases is important to guide diagnosis and management.
- Lymphangioleiomyomatosis is a rare, diffuse cystic lung disease seen almost exclusively in women.
- Treatment with a mammalian target of rapamycin can help to stabilize lung function and may improve survival.
- Thoracic endometriosis syndrome—inclusive of catamenial pneumothorax, hemothorax, hemoptysis and pulmonary nodules—is an uncommon and underdiagnosed disorder.
- Although the temporal relationship of symptoms with menses provokes clinical suspicion, invasive modalities such as -assisted thoracoscopic surgery, are often required for diagnosis.

INTRODUCTION

The differences in the respiratory system between women and men begin in utero. As discussed elsewhere in this issue, biologic sex plays a critical role in fetal development, airway anatomy, inhalational exposures, and inhaled particle deposition of the respiratory system, thus leading to differences in risk for disease, as well as clinical manifestations, morbidity and mortality. In this article, we focus on those respiratory diseases unique to females: lymphangioleiomyomatosis (LAM) and thoracic endometriosis syndrome (TES).

LYMPHANGIOLEOMYOMATOSIS

LAM is a rare, diffuse cystic lung disease seen nearly exclusively in women (5 per million).[1–3] In addition to cystic destruction of the lung parenchyma, LAM can also cause axial lymphatic cystic masses called lymphangioleiomyomas (39%) and/ or benign abdominal tumors called angiomyolipomas (40%–80%), typically found in the kidneys.[1,2,4–6] Management includes mammalian target of rapamycin (mTOR) inhibitors, which stabilize lung function and improve survival in transplant and nontransplanted patient, supportive care in the form of oxygen therapy, pulmonary rehabilitation, and/or bronchodilators, and lung transplantation for progressive and debilitating disease.[7–10] This review explores the epidemiology, pathophysiology, clinical presentation, current treatment recommendations, and ongoing and future studies for LAM.

Epidemiology

LAM can either occur secondary to tuberous sclerosis complex (TSC), an autosomal-dominant condition associated with cerebral calcifications, cognitive impairment, seizures, and hamartomatous lesions in several organs, or can occur

[a] Division of Pulmonary, Allergy and Critical Care, University of Pennsylvania, Philadelphia, PA, USA; [b] Department of Internal Medicine, Michigan State University, East Lansing, MI, USA; [c] Department of Pulmonary and Critical Care Medicine, University of Washington, Seattle, WA, USA; [d] Providence Medical Research Center, Spokane, WA, USA; [e] Division of Pulmonary and Critical Care Medicine, University of Michigan, Ann Arbor, MI, USA
[1] Co-first authors.
* Corresponding author.
E-mail address: mrking@med.umich.edu

Clin Chest Med 42 (2021) 507–516
https://doi.org/10.1016/j.ccm.2021.04.014

sporadically.[1] Sporadic LAM affects roughly 5 in 1 million adults; secondary LAM occurs about one-third of women with TSC.[2,3,11] The average age at diagnosis is 35 years.[1,2,4] Sporadic LAM is rarely seen in men, but ranges from 13% to 38% in TSC-associated LAM.[4] Children are rarely affected.[2]

Pathophysiology

Both sporadic and TSC-associated LAM are secondary to mutations in the tuberous sclerosis gene TSC1, which leads to functional loss of the protein product hamartin, or in TSC2, leading to functional loss of tuberin.[1] The mutations in TSC-associated LAM are autosomal dominant, whereas the mutations in sporadic LAM occur somatically.[12]

Mutations in the hamartin/tuberin heterotrimer leads to continuous activation of the mTOR signaling pathway, resulting in continuous cell growth and proliferation of migrating abnormal smooth-muscle like cells, known as LAM cells.[1,13] These LAM cells lead to cystic destruction in the lung parenchyma and infiltrate lymphatic channels, lymph nodes, and the thoracic duct, resulting in lymphangioleiomyomas and chylous fluid in the pleural and peritoneal spaces.[14]

Clinical Manifestations

Patients on average have respiratory symptoms for 2 to 6 years and experience 2.2 pneumothoraces before a definitive LAM diagnosis.[4,11] Most common symptoms include progressive dyspnea with daily activities (>70%), recurrent pneumothoraces (50%), chylous pleural effusions, hemoptysis, and hypoxia requiring supplemental oxygen.[1–5] Rarely, patients present may also present with bleeding angiomyolipomas.[15] Angiomyolipomas are more common in TSC-LAM (95.7%) than in sporadic LAM (41.3%), whereas lymphangioleiomyomas and chylous effusions are more common in sporadic LAM (38% and 20%, respectively) than in TSC-LAM (12.8% and 13.8%, respectively).[16]

Depending on a patients' degree of disease, pulmonary function studies may be normal or show obstruction and/or reduced diffusion capacity for carbon monoxide (DLCO).[3,8,17] The DLCO may be a more sensitive indicator of early disease because it is often abnormal before the forced expiratory volume in 1 second (FEV_1) decreases.[7]

Diagnosis

There are 3 main pillars for definite clinical LAM diagnosis, which include typical clinical history, characteristic high-resolution computed tomography (HRCT) scan findings in the chest, and 1 or more of various supporting characteristics, from laboratory, histopathology, and additional clinical manifestations.[17]

The clinical history should include young to middle-aged women with dyspnea, pneumothorax, and/or chylothorax.[17] A patient being considered for a LAM diagnosis should not have clinical characteristics and/or manifestations that are compatible with other diffuse cystic lung diseases, such as history of significant smoking, sicca symptoms, connective tissue disease, and personal or family history of non–TSC-related facial skin lesions and/or renal tumors.[7,17]

Features on HRCT chest compatible with LAM include thin-walled, air-filled round cysts of more than 10 in number, uniform in shape, and diffusely distributed throughout the lungs. Outside of these characteristic cystic changes, the lung parenchyma is typically normal.[17,18] Expert radiologists have demonstrated an ability to recognize LAM on HRCT in the absence of additional clinical data. In a retrospective review of 89 patients referred to the LAM Foundation Clinics at the University of Cincinnati, expert radiologists identified LAM upon review of HRCT alone in 91% of patients with LAM and were able to exclude LAM in 98% of patients without LAM. These numbers decreased when HRCTs were reviewed by expert pulmonologists, pulmonary fellows, and general pulmonologists. The data suggest that HRCT can diagnose LAM accurately 72% to 91% of the time.[19–21] As a result, despite the capability of expert radiologists and appeal of noninvasive expedient diagnostic testing, the American Thoracic Society (ATS) does not recommend use of HRCT alone for LAM diagnosis.[17]

In addition to supporting clinical history and HRCT chest, LAM diagnosis requires 1 or more of the following findings: (1) TSC diagnosis, (2) renal angiomyolipoma(s), (3) lymphangioleiomyomas, (4) a serum vascular endothelial growth factor-D (VEGF-D) of greater than or equal to 800 pg/mL, (5) chylous pleural and/or ascites effusions, (6) the presence of LAM cells and/or cell clusters on cytologic examination of effusions and/or lymph nodes, and/or (7) biopsy of lung or retroperitoneal and/or pelvic masses showing histopathologic evidence of LAM.[17]

In the absence of TSC and pleural/ascitic fluid, serologic evaluation with VEGF-D level is commonly performed first owing to the noninvasive nature of sampling. VEGF-D is a lymphangiogenic growth factor expressed by LAM cells that forms lymphatic vessels and is involved in the spread of tumor cells to lymph nodes.[1,2] It is now used as a diagnostic serum biomarker because levels of 574 pg/mL or greater are associated with LAM diagnosis with a specificity of 91% and sensitivity of 86%. The current cut-off value for LAM diagnosis must be 800 pg/mL or greater.[17] If VEGF-D is unrevealing, a noncontrast CT or MRI of the abdomen/pelvis can be used to assess for renal angiomyolipomas or lymphangioleiomyomas.

Asymptomatic patients with compatible clinical history and HRCT findings of mild cystic changes can be considered probable LAM and do not require further invasive diagnostic testing, given that a definitive LAM diagnosis will not impact management.[5] Instead, these patients are monitored with repeat pulmonary function tests every 3 to 12 months, with the frequency depending on whether there are changes concerning for disease progression.[5,17] Patients who become symptomatic or demonstrate disease progression on surveillance pulmonary function tests should undergo further workup to definitively confirm or exclude LAM diagnosis.[17] If abdominopelvic imaging, VEGF-D testing, and/or aspirates of chylous fluid, lymph nodes, or abdominopelvic masses are indeterminate or not applicable, then a lung biopsy should be pursued.[17] Despite a diagnostic yield of only about 50%, a transbronchial lung biopsy should be considered before -assisted thoracoscopic surgery (VATS)–guided lung biopsy because a transbronchial lung biopsy is minimally invasive with a lower complication rate and cost.[17]

Management: Pharmacologic

Significant progress has been made for LAM treatment in the past decade, with the US Food and Drug Administration (FDA) approving sirolimus, otherwise known as rapamycin, in 2015 as the first FDA-approved LAM therapy.[22] Sirolimus is an mTOR inhibitor, which in turn blocks activation of downstream kinases, restoring normal cellular processes, such as growth, motility, and survival in cells with TSC mutations.[2,7] Support for sirolimus is largely the result of the Multicenter International LAM Efficacy of Sirolimus (MILES) trial, which was a 2011 double-blinded, randomized, placebo-controlled, parallel group trial that evaluated 12 months of oral sirolimus 2 mg/d or matched placebo in adult women with LAM with an FEV_1 of 70% or less of predicted (n = 89), with an additional 12-month off-treatment observation period.[7] More patients treated with sirolimus demonstrated improvements in their FEV_1 from baseline to 12 months (46% sirolimus vs 12% in placebo group; $P<.001$).[7] Furthermore, the sirolimus group had stabilization of lung function during treatment whereas the control group had continued monthly lung function decline

(FEV_1 1 ± 2 mL/mo for sirolimus vs −12 ± 2 mL/mo for placebo [$P<.001$]; FVC 8 ± 3 mL/mo for sirolimus vs −11 ± 3 mL/mo for placebo [$P<.001$]).[7] After 12 months of treatment, participants treated with sirolimus had an average FEV_1 that was 152 mL higher than those treated with placebo ($P<.001$). Twelve months after treatment was withdrawn, the decrease in FEV_1 in the sirolimus arm was similar to the placebo arm (8 ± 2 mL/mo vs 14 ± 3 mL/mo, respectively [$P = .08$]).[7]

Sirolimus also significantly improved quality of life and self-reported functional performance, and significantly lowered mean VEGF-D levels at 6 and 12 months, as compared with the placebo group.[7] Adverse events during the treatment period, including mucositis, diarrhea, nausea, elevated cholesterol, acneiform rash, and lower extremity swelling, were more common in the sirolimus arm than placebo; however, serious adverse events were similar between the 2 arms.[7] Because of the outcomes of this study, the ATS/ERC issued a 1A recommendation in 2016 for sirolimus initiation in patients with LAM with an FEV_1 of less than 70% predicted.[2]

Sirolimus is also recommended by the ATS/ERS for patients with LAM with chylous effusions or ascites based on a 2011 observational study in which 12 patients with LAM had chylous effusions, including pleural and/or ascitic, and were observed for 2.5 years without sirolimus and then a subsequent 2.6 years with sirolimus.[7,13] After a range of 131 to 410 ± 61 to 111 days of sirolimus therapy, all 12 patients had either decreases in effusion size or complete resolution.[13] Therefore, the ATS/ERS recommend that mTOR inhibitors be used before pursuing invasive therapeutic fluid drainage.[2] Taveira-DaSilva et al[13] also observed that 11 of their patients with LAM with lymphangioleiomyomas had either complete resolution or size reductions; however, the ATS/JRS do not specifically recommend mTOR inhibitor initiation for this indication.[2]

An alternative mTOR inhibitor recommended by the ATS/JRS is everolimus, based on a 2015 phase IIA multicenter, open-label trial that enrolled 24 patients with LAM with an FEV_1 of 80% or less than predicted or an FEV_1 of less than 90% and a DLCO of less than 80%.[23] Goldberg and colleagues[23] found improvements in FEV_1 and 6-minute walk distance (mean change of 114 mL and 47 m, respectively), stabilization of FVC (mean change of 10 mL), and a decrease in serum VEGF-D levels with similar adverse events and rates to sirolimus compared with baseline after 6 months of therapy.

The efficacy of lower dose sirolimus (blood trough level of ≤5 ng/mL), rather than the conventional dose (5–15 ng/mL) used in the MILES trial,[7,24] has been evaluated in several observational studies. A Japanese retrospective, observational study of 15 patients with LAM treated with lower dose sirolimus for at least 6 months found resolution of chylous effusions in 6 of the 7 patients with effusions and significant improvement in annual change of FEV_1 and FVC in 9 of their patients without chylous effusions (FEV_1 before sirolimus, -115 ± 86 mL vs on sirolimus, 128 ± 290 mL [$P = .015$]; FVC before sirolimus, -101.0 ± 314 mL vs on sirolimus, 190 ± 246 mL [$P = .046$]).[24] This outcome is similar to the MILES trial, with the FEV_1 increasing by 19 ± 124 mL ($P<.001$) and the FVC increasing by 97 ± 260 ($P = .001$) after 12 months of conventional-dose sirolimus.[7]

However, a 2018 South Korean 5-year retrospective study compared lung function between 20 patients with LAM treated with low-dose sirolimus with 19 patients LAM treated with conventional dose sirolimus.[25] These authors observed significant monthly rate of FEV_1 improvement in the conventionally dosed sirolimus group but no change in FEV_1 in the low-dose sirolimus group (FEV_1 on low-dose therapy: before sirolimus, -0.08 ± 0.38 vs on sirolimus, 0.19 ± 0.51 [$P = .264$]; FEV_1 on conventional dose: before sirolimus, -0.26 ± 0.54 vs on sirolimus, 0.22 ± 0.38 [$P = .024$]).[25] Adverse event rates were similar between the 2 treatment groups.[25] This more recent study, albeit small and nonrandomized, suggests that lower dose sirolimus is inferior to the conventional dose for lung function improvement.[25] A definitive randomized controlled trial, the Multicenter Interventional Lymphangioleiomyomatosis Early Disease Trial (MILED) is being conducted to determine whether lower dose sirolimus can achieve similar efficacy to conventional dosing in patients with LAM (NCT03150914).

Based on resumption of FEV_1 decline in the sirolimus arm that paralleled the control group during the withdrawal period in the MILES trial, it is thought that sirolimus suppresses LAM and does not lead to remission, suggesting that sirolimus may need to be a lifelong therapy.[7,26] To better understand whether long-term mTOR inhibitor therapy is safe and effective, a subanalysis of 12 patients with LAM enrolled in a 2014 observational study were followed for 5.5 ± 3.3 years before sirolimus initiation and then followed for an additional 4.6 ± 1.8 years while on sirolimus.[15] Yao and colleagues[15] found significant yearly FEV_1 decrease over a 5-year period while patients were on sirolimus, compared with no therapy (FEV_1, 0.3 ± 0.4 on sirolimus vs FEV_1, -1.4 ± 0.2 before therapy initiation [$P = .025$]). The adverse effects of sirolimus therapy were similar to those reported by McCormack and colleagues[7] and Taveira-DaSilva et al,[13,15] and thought to be manageable.

Doxycycline and hormonal therapies have been explored in the past, but are not recommended for LAM.[2] Patients with LAM have increased levels of matrix metalloproteinases 2 and 9, which are proteolytic enzymes that degrade the extracellular matrix and are thought to induce lung cyst formation because they are particularly positioned near these cysts. Therefore, it was hypothesized that doxycycline, which is a tetracycline antibiotic that inhibits matrix metalloproteinase production and activity, may decrease lung parenchymal destruction in LAM.[27] However, a 2-year randomized placebo-controlled trial comparing 12 patients receiving doxycycline with 11 patients receiving placebo found no significant difference in mean FEV_1 (FEV_1 of -123 ± 246 mL/y in doxycycline vs FEV_1 of -90 ± 154 mL/y in placebo [$P = .35$]), FVC, DLCO, and quality of life.[27]

There are no randomized controlled trials evaluating hormonal therapies. However, there have been numerous case reports, case series, and observational trials studying serum estrogen response modulators, progesterone, gonadotropin-releasing hormone (GnRH) agonists, combination hormonal therapy, and oophorectomy because, anecdotally, LAM tends to worsen during pregnancy, menstruation, and after exposure to estrogen-containing drugs, but stabilize in the postmenopausal period.[2] Based on the existing data, hormonal therapy is not recommended for patients with LAM.[2]

Management: Surveillance and Supportive Care

Bronchodilators are recommended for patients with LAM with reversible obstruction on pulmonary function tests.[5,8] Furthermore, patients should be prescribed supplemental oxygen if they have evidence of resting and/or exertional desaturations.[8] Pulmonary rehabilitation is an important program for patients with LAM to participate in, particularly because their most common cause of death is respiratory failure.[11] Pulmonary rehabilitation in patients with LAM is associated with significant improvements in dyspnea, exercise capacity, muscle strength, and quality of life and should be considered in patients once demonstrating diminished physical activity.[9]

Given that angiomyolipomas can lead to spontaneous hemorrhage, patients with known angiomyolipoma are generally periodically monitored with CT scans or MRI and considered for treatment if angiomyolipoma size is 4 cm or greater.[5] Treatment with embolization or nephron-sparing surgery is generally considered.

Management: Pleurodesis

Spontaneous pneumothorax is a common initial presentation of LAM. A pooled analysis of case series and observational studies by the ATS/JRS in 2017 found a 57% pneumothorax rate in patients with LAM, with recurrence rate ranging from 29% to 81%, and the recurrence rate per patient ranged from 3.2% to 5.0%.[17] The recurrence rate was decreased from about 65% for patients managed conservatively to 18% to 32% for patients managed with pleurodesis after initial pneumothorax.[17] Owing to this high risk for recurrence and the risk reduction with pleurodesis, ipsilateral pleurodesis after first pneumothorax is recommended for the management of pneumothorax in LAM.[17] Pleurodesis, as well as pleurectomy, are not contraindications to lung transplantation.[9]

Management: Lung Transplantation

Patients with an FEV_1 of 30% or less, a New York Heart Association functional class of III or IV with resting hypoxemia, or severe exercise capacity impairment should be referred for lung transplant evaluation.[5,28] A recent review of 138 patients with LAM who underwent lung transplant in the United States between 2003 and 2017 reported a 12-year median survival after lung transplantation and 1-, 5-, and 10-year survival rates at 94%, 73%, and 56%, respectively.[28] Although 81% of the patients underwent bilateral lung transplantation, there was no significant difference in the survival rate for single compared with bilateral transplantation.[28] In a retrospective cohort study of 410 patients with LAM with 10.4-year median observation time, independent predictors of decreased time to death or transplant were younger age at diagnosis, supplemental oxygen use, and increased weight loss.[11]

The most frequent causes of death within 1 year after transplantation were infection and graft failure (43%) and after 1 year after transplantation was bronchiolitis obliterans syndrome (27.2%), which are similar complications and complication rates compared with the general lung transplant population.[28]

The recurrence rate of LAM after transplantation is not well-studied, but thought to be rare.[5,10] In a 2019 retrospective analysis of 183 patients with LAM who underwent lung transplantation in the United States from 2003 to 2017, recurrent LAM occurred in 1 patient (0.72%).[28] The European Respiratory Society recommends against posttransplant LAM recurrence surveillance with biopsy owing to its low recurrence rate.[5]

Outcomes

Observational and registry data suggest the annual decrease in FEV_1 in untreated patients with LAM ranges from roughly 40 to 120 mL/y.[29–32] In randomized studies of doxycycline and sirolimus, the placebo groups experienced decline in the 90 to 134 mL/y range. The National Heart, Lung, and Blood Institute LAM registry reports an annual rate of decline of 89 mL/y.[33] Although early studies suggested the median survival was between 8 and 10 years from diagnosis, more recent data suggest that survival is likely longer. In the National Heart, Lung, and Blood Institute longitudinal LAM registry, the estimated 5-, 10-, 15- and 20-year transplant-free survival rates were 95%, 85%, 75%, and 64%, respectively.[33]

Conclusion and Future Directions

Significant progress has been made in the treatment of LAM over the past decade since the introduction of mTOR inhibitors. However, more data are still needed on the long-term impact of mTOR inhibitor therapy. The Multicenter International Durability and Safety of Sirolimus in LAM (MIDAS) trial is a longitudinal observational registry currently being conducted with the goal to enroll 600 patients with LAM who are either currently on or previously took mTOR inhibitors (either sirolimus or everolimus).[26] Enrolled patients are being observed for a 2-year period with particular attention focused on lung function test results and adverse events.[26] A recent study examining Reservatrol and Sirolimus in Lymphangioleiomyomatosis (RESULT) recently completed enrolling, but results are still pending (NCT03253913).

Immunotherapy in LAM represents a novel therapeutic approach that is under investigation. Human lung tissue from patients with LAM have increased expression of programmed death-ligand 1, which is a protein that leads to immune cell inactivation and thus can cause tumor proliferation.[34] Using murine models of LAM, in vivo treatment with anti–programmed death 1 antibody showed significant survival benefit with about 70% of anti–programmed death 1 treated mice surviving compared with about 30% of control isotype antibody mice surviving at day 55 ($P<.0001$).[34] Although no in vivo studies with immune checkpoint inhibitors have yet to be conducted on patients with LAM, these promising murine data suggest a future role for immunotherapy in LAM management.

Although a rare disease, significant research attention to LAM has led to improved prognosis and survival over the past decade, and the future for LAM management remains promising with the many active registries and studies devoted to better understanding the natural history of LAM, doses, and durations of mTOR inhibitors, as well as the role of novel immunotherapy.

THORACIC ENDOMETRIOSIS SYNDROME

Endometriosis is defined by the presence of endometrial-like tissue outside the uterine cavity.[35] It is estimated to involve 5% to 10% of women in their reproductive age[36]; however, it is reported to be underdiagnosed.[37] It most commonly involves the pelvic peritoneum, ovaries, and rectovaginal septum.[38] TES is a collection of clinical diseases related to ectopic endometrial tissue in the thoracic cavity; it includes catamenial hemothorax, catamenial pneumothorax, catamenial hemoptysis, and endometriotic lung nodules. Catamenial pneumothorax is the most common presentation of TES.[39] The peak incidence of TES is believed to be 5 years after the peak incidence of pelvic endometriosis.[40,41]

Pathophysiology

The pathogenesis of TES remains poorly understood. TES likely has a multifactorial etiology, because none of the theories can solely explain all of the clinical manifestations of the disease.[40] Sampson's theory of retrograde menstruation is the most accepted theory to explain TES, and is further validated because TES was found to be 9 times more likely to occur on the right than on the left hemidiaphragm.[42] It presumes that endometrial cells travel retrograde through the fallopian tubes and into the peritoneal cavity where an impaired clearance mechanism at the peritoneal level allows the survival, implantation, and proliferation of the endometrial tissue on peritoneal surfaces.[42] The peritoneal fluid containing the endometrial cells is presumed to follow a distinct pattern of movement within the peritoneal cavity. The falciform and phrenicocolic ligaments impose an obstruction of flow through the left hemidiaphragm, which results in a preferential flow of the cells from the pelvis through the right paracolic gutter via the right hemidiaphragm.[42] Once reaching the right subdiaphragmatic area, endometrial cells implant on the diaphragmatic surface or undergo transperitoneal–transdiaphragmatic migration to the pleural cavity where it may colonize the diaphragm or the pleural space. This migration is made possible through congenital diaphragmatic defects or acquired defects of the diaphragm called fenestrations.[42]

Another theory for the pathogenesis of TES hypothesizes that estrogen and other physiologic stimuli results in metaplasia of mesothelial cells into endometrial tissue.[43] This theory does not explain bronchopulmonary TES. Benign metastasis is another theory that might explain bronchopulmonary TES and is based on hematogenous or lymphatic dissemination of the endometrial tissue.[44,45]

Clinical Manifestations

TES has a wide range of presentations, from being asymptomatic to life-threatening hemoptysis. Catamenial pneumothorax is the most common presentation of TES. In a retrospective series of 112 patients, Joseph and colleagues[41] reported that 73% of the cases presented with catamenial pneumothorax, whereas 14% presented with hemothorax, 7% with hemoptysis, and 6% with lung nodules. The timing of these presentations is related to the onset of menses; it occurs between 24 hours before and 72 hours after the onset of menses, but not every menstrual cycle coincides with symptoms.[39,46] A patient's clinical presentation depends on the anatomic location of the disease; pleural disease can result in catamenial pneumothorax or hemothorax, and both can present with pleuritic chest pain, cough, and shortness of breath. In contrast, parenchymal disease can present with hemoptysis and lung nodules. The majority of these clinical manifestations are right sided, but left-sided and bilateral disease have been reported in the literature.[47–50] The temporal relationship with menses is what differentiates TES from other etiologies that presents in similar clinical manifestations. Other less common presentations have been proposed to be included under the umbrella of TES; Bobbio and colleagues[51] reported that catamenial chest pain, endometriosis-related diaphragmatic hernia, and endometriosis-related pleural effusion can be added to the classical manifestations of TES.

Diagnosis

The diagnosis of TES is often challenging. Noninvasive imaging modalities including chest radiograph, CT scan, and MRI offer nonspecific findings that can be useful for the diagnosis of TES, only when based on high clinical suspicious.[47,52,53] Invasive modalities including VATS and laparoscopy offer a superior assessment of the disease.[40,54]

A chest radiograph is the best initial imaging modality for most thoracic pathology. In TES, the chest radiograph can be normal, but common findings include pneumothorax, pleural effusion, pneumomediastinum, and, to a lesser extent, lung nodules.[47] In addition to the findings detected by a chest radiograph, a chest CT can detect ground glass opacities, parenchymal thin-walled cavities, and bullous formation.[52,55] MRI is beneficial for detecting diaphragmatic disease with a sensitivity of up to 83%.[56]

Bronchoscopy is mainly helpful in bronchopulmonary disease, and has the highest detection rate when performed at the time of menses. Bronchoscopic findings vary from normal airway appearance to the detection of red submucosal patches and white cystic lesions.[47,57,58] The yield of bronchoscopic biopsies and cytologic washing vary and is also related to the timing of menses. Brush cytology has a higher detection rate of ectopic endometrial cells than bronchoscopic biopsies.[59]

VATS is considered the gold standard modality for the diagnosis of TES, whereas laparoscopy is preferred for the diagnosis of diaphragmatic disease in TES.[39,40] VATS offers a superior visual detection and assessment of the lesions and is preferred over open thoracotomy because of lower rate of postoperative complications.[60–62]

Management

TES is a complex disease that require a multidisciplinary approach. Medical management is considered the initial therapy in TES and is similar to pelvic endometriosis.[40,47] It is based on the inhibition of endometrial tissue growth in the thorax. Different types of agents are available; the most common are the GnRH agonists.[40,63] Physiologically, GnRH binds to its receptors in the pituitary, which results in the release of gonadotropins; subsequently, estrogen release and endometrial tissue growth.[64] The long-term use of the long-acting GnRH agonists results in downregulating the GnRH receptors and pituitary desensitization, which results in a decreased production of estrogen and the inhibition of pelvic and ectopic endometrial tissue growth.[65] Three GnRH agonists are approved for endometriosis in the United States, namely, leuprolide, goserelin, and nafarelin. Treatment with GnRH agonists results in a hypoestrogen state and menopausal-like symptoms, including hot flashes, vaginal atrophy, decreased libido, osteoporosis, and, most important, infertility.[65] GnRH antagonists, the oral contraceptive danazol, and aromatase inhibitors are additional therapeutic options that have a similar efficacy to long-acting GnRH agonists.[40,65] Infertility, high cost, patient preference, and disease recurrence

after stopping the medications are the limiting factors to medical therapy in TES.

Surgical management is indicated in recurrent disease, failed medical management, and intolerance to medical therapy. A VATS procedure is considered the gold standard treatment modality of TES.[66–68] Superficial thoracic endometrial disease can be excised using different types of laser therapy,[40,69] whereas deep parenchymal nodules might require subsegmentectomy or lobectomy.[70,71] To prevent recurrence, concomitant medical therapy for 6 to 12 months after surgical treatment is recommended.[39] Pleurodesis is an alternative procedure for catamenial pneumothorax.[40] Bricelj and colleagues[39] reported that pleurodesis is the most common procedure performed for the treatment of catamenial pneumothorax. It can be performed using mechanical pleural abrasion with gauze, or chemically using talc, or tetracyclines derivates.[72] In cases were diaphragmatic endometrial lesions present, a VATS procedure combined with laparoscopy can be performed.[73] laparoscopy allows the visualization of the diaphragm, resection of the lesions, and repairing the diaphragm. Diaphragmatic repair can be done using endoscopic stapler for small defects, or synthetic mesh for larger lesions.[54,67]

SUMMARY

Lung diseases specific to women are rare, complex diseases. There have been significant achievements in the understanding and treatment of LAM since its first introduction to the medical literature in 1937.[74] Diagnosis is no longer as invasive as in the past, with lung biopsies only indicated if noninvasive means, including serum VEGF-D levels, are nondiagnostic. The discovery of mTOR inhibitors and their use in LAM was a monumental achievement for the LAM community because it was the first ever FDA-approved therapy for this condition. TES is a poorly understood disease that requires a high clinical suspicion of temporal relationship of symptoms with menses. Diagnosis is difficult and invasive modalities like VATS are often required for diagnosis and treatment. Medical management is widely available, but has limitations owing to cost and side effects.

CLINICS CARE POINTS

- Lymphangioleiomyomatosis is a rare, cystic lung disease seen almost exclusively in women.

- Treatment with rapamycin can help to stabilize lung function and may improve survival.
- Thoracic endometriosis syndrome is an uncommon but also underdiagnosed disorder.
- Although the temporal relationship of symptoms with menses provokes clinical suspicion, invasive modalities are often required to confirm the diagnosis.

DISCLOSURE

R.N. Criner, A. Al-abcha, A.A. Lambert have nothing to disclose. MeiLan Han receives funding from the NHLBI K24HL138188. Dr. Han has also received research funding from Novartis, Sunovion, Sanofi and Nuvaira. She has consulted for AstraZeneca, GlaxoSmithKline, Boehringer Ingelheim, Cipla, Chiesi, DevPro Pharma, Merck, Sanofi, Teva, Mylan and Verona.

REFERENCES

1. Torre O, Elia D, Caminati A, et al. New insights in lymphangioleiomyomatosis and pulmonary Langerhans cell histiocytosis. Eur Respir Rev 2017; 26(145):170042.
2. McCormack FX, Gupta N, Finlay GR, et al. Official American Thoracic Society/Japanese Respiratory Society Clinical Practice Guidelines: lymphangioleiomyomatosis diagnosis and management. Am J Respir Crit Care Med 2016;194(6):748–61.
3. Toledo do Nascimento EC, BG B, Mariana AW, et al. Immunohistological features related to functional impairment in lymphangioleiomyomatosis. Respir Res 2018;19(1):83.
4. Harari S, Torre O, Cassandro R, et al. The changing face of a rare disease: lymphangioleiomyomatosis. Eur Respir J 2015;46:1471–85.
5. Johnson SR, Cordier JF, Lazor R, et al. European Respiratory Society guidelines for the diagnosis and management of lymphangioleiomyomatosis. Eur Respir J 2010;35:14–26.
6. Avila NA, Kelly JA, Chu SC, et al. Lymphangioleiomyomatosis: abdominopelvic CT and US findings. Radiology 2000;216(1):147–53.
7. McCormack FX, Inoue Y, Moss J, et al. Efficacy and safety of sirolimus in lymphangioleiomyomatosis. N Engl J Med 2011;364(17):1595–606.
8. Ryu JH, Moss J, Beck GJ, et al. The NHLBI lymphangioleiomyomatosis registry: characteristics of 230 patients at enrollment. Am J Respir Crit Care Med 2006;173:105–11.
9. Araujo MS, Baldi BG, Freitas CSG, et al. Pulmonary rehabilitation in lymphangioleiomyomatosis: a controlled clinical trial. Eur Respir J 2016;47: 1452–60.
10. Kpodonu J, Massad MG, Chaer RA, et al. The US experience with lung transplantation for pulmonary lymphangioleiomyomatosis. J Heart Lung Transplant 2005;24:1247–53.
11. Oprescu N, McCormack FX, Byrnes S, et al. Clinical predictors of mortality and cause of death in lymphangioleiomyomatosis: a population-based registry. Lung 2013;19:35–42.
12. Carsillo T, Astrinidis A, Henske EP. Mutations in the tuberous sclerosis complex gene TSC2 are a cause of sporadic pulmonary lymphangioleiomyomatosis. Proc Natl Acad Sci U S A 2000;97(11): 6085–90.
13. Taveira-DaSilva AM, Hathaway O, Stylianou M, et al. Changes in lung function and chylous effusions in patients with lymphangioleiomyomatosis treated with sirolimus. Ann Intern Med 2011;154(12): 797–805. W-292-3.
14. Gupta R, Kitaichi M, Inoue Y, et al. Lymphatic manifestations of lymphangioleiomyomatosis. Lymphology 2014;47(3):106–17.
15. Yao J, Taveira-DaSilva AM, Jones AM, et al. Sustained effects of sirolimus on lung function and cystic lung lesions in lymphangioleiomyomatosis. Am J Respir Crit Care Med 2014;190(11): 1273–82.
16. Johnson SR, Taveira-DaSilva AM, Moss J. Lymphangioleiomyomatosis. Clin Chest Med 2016;37(3): 389–403.
17. Gupta N, Finlay GA, Kotloff RM, et al. Lymphangioleiomyomatosis diagnosis and management: high-resolution chest computed tomography, transbronchial lung biopsy, and pleural disease management. Am J Respir Crit Care Med 2017;196(10):1337–48.
18. Raoof S, Bondalapati P, Vydyula R, et al. Cystic lung diseases: algorithmic approach. Chest 2016;150(4): 945–65.
19. Gupta N, Meraj R, Tanase D, et al. Accuracy of chest high-resolution computer tomography in diagnosing diffuse cystic lung diseases. Eur Respir J 2015;46: 1196–9.
20. Bonelli FS, Hartman TE, Swensen SJ, et al. Accuracy of high-resolution CT in diagnosing lung diseases. AJR Am J Roentgenol 1998;170:1507–12.
21. Koyama M, Johkoh T, Honda O, et al. Chronic cystic lung disease: diagnostic accuracy of high-resolution CT in 92 patients. AJR Am J Roentgenol 2003;180: 827–35.
22. Danehy S. Pfizer's Rapamune (sirolimus) becomes first FDA-approved treatment for lymphangioleiomyomatosis (LAM), a rare progressive lung disease 2015. Available at: https://www.businesswire.com/news/home/20150529005131/en/Pfizer%E2%80%99s-RAPAMUNE%C2%AE-sirolimus-Becomes-First-FDA-Approved-Treatment-for-Lymphangioleiomyomatosis-LAM-A-Rare-Progressive-Lung-Disease.

23. Goldberg HJ, Harari S, Cottin V, et al. Everolimus for the treatment of lymphangioleiomyomatosis: a phase II study. Eur Respir J 2015;46:783–94.

24. Ando K, Kurihara M, Kataoka H, et al. The efficacy and safety of low-dose sirolimus for treatment of lymphangioleiomyomatosis. Respir Investig 2013;51: 175–83.

25. Yoon HY, Hwang JJ, Kim DS, et al. Efficacy and safety of low-dose sirolimus in lymphangioleiomyomatosis. Orphanet J Rare Dis 2018;13(1):204.

26. McCormack F. Safety and durability of sirolimus for treatment of LAM (MIDAS). N Engl J Med 2011; 364(17):1595-606.

27. Chang WYC, Cane JL, Kumaran M, et al. A 2-year randomised placebo-controlled trial of doxycycline for lymphangioleiomyomatosis. Eur Respir J 2014; 43:1114–23.

28. Khawar MU, Yazdani D, Zhu Z, et al. Clinical outcomes and survival following lung transplantation in patients with lymphangioleiomyomatosis. J Heart Lung Transplant 2019;38(9):949–55.

29. Urban T, Lazor R, Lacronique J, et al. Pulmonary lymphangioleiomyomatosis. A study of 69 patients. Groupe d'Etudes et de Recherche sur les Maladies "Orphelines" Pulmonaires (GERM"O"P). Medicine (Baltimore) 1999;78(5):321–37.

30. Johnson SR, Tattersfield AE. Decline in lung function in lymphangioleiomyomatosis: relation to menopause and progesterone treatment. Am J Respir Crit Care Med 1999;160(2):628–33.

31. Baldi BG, Salim C, Freitas G, et al. Clinical course and characterisation of lymphangioleiomyomatosis in a Brazilian reference centre. Sarcoidosis Vasc Diffuse Lung Dis 2014;31(2):129–35.

32. Hayashida M, Yasuo M, Hanaoka M, et al. Reductions in pulmonary function detected in patients with lymphangioleiomyomatosis: an analysis of the Japanese National Research Project on Intractable Diseases database. Respir Investig 2016;54(3): 193–200.

33. Gupta N, Lee HS, Ryu JH, et al. The NHLBI LAM registry: prognostic physiologic and radiologic biomarkers emerge from a 15-year prospective longitudinal analysis. Chest 2019;155(2):288–96.

34. Maisel K, Merrilees MJ, Atochina-Vasserman EN, et al. Immune checkpoint ligand PD-L1 is upregulated in pulmonary lymphangioleiomyomatosis. Am J Respir Cell Mol Biol 2018;59(6):723–32.

35. Vercellini P, Viganò P, Somigliana E, et al. Endometriosis: pathogenesis and treatment. Nat Rev Endocrinol 2014;10(5):261–75.

36. Zondervan KT, Becker CM, Koga K, et al. Endometriosis. Nat Rev Dis Prim 2018;4(1):9.

37. Nnoaham KE, Hummelshoj L, Webster P, et al. Impact of endometriosis on quality of life and work productivity: a multicenter study across ten countries. Fertil Steril 2011;96(2):366–73.e8.

38. Burney RO, Giudice LC. Pathogenesis and pathophysiology of endometriosis. Fertil Steril 2012; 98(3):511–9.

39. Bricelj K, Srpčič M, Ražem A, et al. Catamenial pneumothorax since introduction of -assisted thoracoscopic surgery: a systematic review. Wien Klin Wochenschr 2017;129(19–20):717–26.

40. Nezhat CC, Lindheim SR, Backhus L, et al. Thoracic endometriosis syndrome: a review of diagnosis and management. J Soc Laparoendosc Surg 2019; 23(3). https://doi.org/10.4293/JSLS.2019.00029. e2019.00029.

41. Joseph J, Sahn SA. Thoracic endometriosis syndrome: new observations from an analysis of 110 cases. Am J Med 1996;100(2):164–70.

42. Vinatier D, Orazi G, Cosson M, et al. Theories of endometriosis. Eur J Obstet Gynecol Reprod Biol 2001;96(1):21–34.

43. Matsuura K, Ohtake H, Katabuchi H, et al. Coelomic metaplasia theory of endometriosis evidence from in vivo studies and an in vitro experimental model. Gynecol Obstet Invest 1999;47(Suppl 1):18–20. discussion 20-2.

44. Javert CT. Observations on the pathology and spread of endometriosis based on the theory of benign metastasis. Am J Obstet Gynecol 1951; 62(3):477–87.

45. Ueki M. Histologic study of endometriosis and examination of lymphatic drainage in and from the uterus. Am J Obstet Gynecol 1991;165(1): 201–9.

46. Korom S, Canyurt H, Missbach A, et al. Catamenial pneumothorax revisited: clinical approach and systematic review of the literature. J Thorac Cardiovasc Surg 2004;165(1):201–9.

47. Augoulea A, Lambrinoudaki I, Christodoulakos G. Thoracic endometriosis syndrome. Respiration 2008;75(1):113–9.

48. Gamaleldin H, Tetzlaff JE, Whalley D. Anesthetic implications of thoracic endometriosis. J Clin Anesth 2002;14(1):36–8.

49. Nezhat C, King LP, Paka C, et al. Bilateral thoracic endometriosis affecting the lung and diaphragm. J Soc Laparoendosc Surg 2012;16(1):140–2.

50. Fukuda S, Hirata T, Neriishi K, et al. Thoracic endometriosis syndrome: comparison between catamenial pneumothorax or endometriosis-related pneumothorax and catamenial hemoptysis. Eur J Obstet Gynecol Reprod Biol 2018;225: 118–23.

51. Bobbio A, Canny E, Mansuet Lupo A, et al. Thoracic endometriosis syndrome other than pneumothorax: clinical and pathological findings. Ann Thorac Surg 2017;104(6):1865–71.

52. Rousset P, Rousset-Jablonski C, Alifano M, et al. Thoracic endometriosis syndrome: CT and MRI features. Clin Radiol 2014;69(3):323–30.

53. Marchiori E, Zanetti G, Rodrigues RS, et al. Pleural endometriosis: findings on magnetic resonance imaging. J Bras Pneumol 2012;38(6):797–802.

54. Alifano M. Catamenial pneumothorax. Curr Opin Pulm Med 2010;16(4):381–6.

55. Ziedalski TM, Sankaranarayanan V, Chitkara RK. Thoracic endometriosis: a case report and literature review. J Thorac Cardiovasc Surg 2004;127(5): 1513–4.

56. Rousset P, Gregory J, Rousset-Jablonski C, et al. MR diagnosis of diaphragmatic endometriosis. Eur Radiol 2016;26(11):3968–77.

57. L'Huillier JP, Salat-Baroux J. A patient with pulmonary endometriosis. Rev Pneumol Clin 2002;58(4 Pt 1):233–6.

58. Yu Z, Fleischman JK, Rahman HM, et al. Catamenial hemoptysis and pulmonary endometriosis: a case report. Mt Sinai J Med 2002;69(4):261–3.

59. Kuo PH, Wang HC, Liaw YS, et al. Bronchoscopic and angiographic findings in tracheobronchial endometriosis. Thorax 1996;51(10):1060–1.

60. Inderbitzi RGC, Leiser A, Furrer M, et al. Three years' experience in -assisted in thoracic surgery (VATS) for spontaneous pneumothorax. J Thorac Cardiovasc Surg 1994;107(6):1410–5.

61. Waller DA, Forty J, Morritt GN. -assisted thoracoscopic surgery versus thoracotomy for spontaneous pneumothorax. Ann Thorac Surg 1994;58(2):372–6. discussion 376-7.

62. Al-Tarshihi M. Comparison of the efficacy and safety of -assisted thoracoscopic surgery with the open method for the treatment of primary pneumothorax in adults. Ann Thorac Med 2008;3(1):9–12.

63. Koizumi T, Inagaki H, Takabayashi Y, et al. Successful use of gonadotropin-releasing hormone agonist in a patient with pulmonary endometriosis. Respiration 1999;66(6):544–6.

64. Desforges JF, Conn PM, Crowley WF. Gonadotropin-releasing hormone and its analogues. N Engl J Med 1991;324(2):93–103.

65. Ferrero S, Evangelisti G, Barra F. Current and emerging treatment options for endometriosis. Expert Opin Pharmacother 2018;19(10):1109–25.

66. Marshall MB, Ahmed Z, Kucharczuk JC, et al. Catamenial pneumothorax: optimal hormonal and surgical management. Eur J Cardiothorac Surg 2005; 27(4):662–6.

67. Alifano M, Roth T, Camilleri Broët S, et al. Catamenial pneumothorax: a prospective study. Chest 2003; 124(3):1004–8.

68. Alifano M, Trisolini R, Cancellieri A, et al. Thoracic endometriosis: current knowledge. Ann Thorac Surg 2006;81(2):761–9.

69. Corson SL, Woodland M, Frishman G, et al. Treatment of endometriosis with a Nd:YAG tissue-contact laser probe via laparoscopy. Int J Fertil 1989;34(4):284–8.

70. Terada Y, Chen F, Shoji T, et al. A case of endobronchial endometriosis treated by subsegmentectomy. Chest 1999;115(5):1475–8.

71. Kristiansen K, Fjeld NB. Pulmonary endometriosis causing haemoptysis: report of a case treated with lobectomy. Scand J Thorac Cardiovasc Surg 1993; 27(2):113–5.

72. Colt HG, Russack V, Chiu Y, et al. A comparison of thoracoscopic talc insufflation, slurry, and mechanical abrasion pleurodesis. Chest 1997;111(2):442–8.

73. Nezhat C, Nicoll LM, Bhagan L, et al. Endometriosis of the diaphragm: four cases treated with a combination of laparoscopy and thoracoscopy. J Minim Invasive Gynecol 2009;16(5):573–80.

74. Taylor JR, Ryu J, Colb TV, et al. Lymphangioleiomyomatosis: clinical course in 32 patients. N Engl J Med 1990;323(18):1254–60.

Challenges Faced by Women with Cystic Fibrosis

Raksha Jain, MD, MSCI[a],*, Traci M. Kazmerski, MD, MS[b],
Moira L. Aitken, MD, FRCP[c], Natalie West, MD, MHS[d],
Alexandra Wilson, MS, RDN, CDE[e], Kubra M. Bozkanat, MD[f],
Kristina Montemayor, MD, MHS[d], Karen von Berg, PT, DPT[g], Jacqui Sjoberg[h],
Maddie Poranski[i], Jennifer L. Taylor-Cousar, MD, MSCS[j,k]

KEYWORDS

- Cystic fibrosis • Sex differences • Puberty • Menopause • Hormones
- Sexual and reproductive health

KEY POINTS

- People with cystic fibrosis (CF) are living longer and healthier lives and women are more commonly living through their reproductive and even postmenopausal years without adequate information on topics unique to women with this chronic illness.
- Women with CF seek more information on topics, including the sex disparity in outcomes, puberty, contraception, fertility, pregnancy, menopause, osteoporosis, urinary incontinence, and body image, which have been understudied in the setting of CF.
- New therapies designed to treat the underlying protein defect in CF (CF transmembrane conductance regulator modulator therapies) may change and improve aspects of health, including fertility, osteoporosis, and even the sex disparity or gender gap.

INTRODUCTION

Women with cystic fibrosis (CF) face several unique and unaddressed concerns related to their health. Among these concerns is the long-standing observation that women with CF have worse health outcomes than men, with increasing evidence pointing to a role of sex hormones contributing to this phenomenon.[1,2] In addition, questions related to puberty, contraception, fertility, pregnancy, and menopause have been understudied in CF, leaving women with numerous unanswered questions about how to manage sexual and reproductive health (SRH) in the setting of CF. In addition, areas of concern such as body image, urinary incontinence, and early osteoporosis that affect women differently than men have

[a] Department of Medicine, University of Texas Southwestern, 5323 Harry Hines Boulevard, Dallas, TX 75390-8558, USA; [b] Department of Pediatrics, University of Pittsburgh School of Medicine, 120 Lytton Avenue Suite M060 University Center, Pittsburgh, PA 15213, USA; [c] Department of Medicine, University of Washington, 1959 NE Pacific Street - Room BB 1361, Seattle, WA 98195-6522, USA; [d] Department of Medicine, Johns Hopkins University, 1830 East Monument Street, 5th Floor, Baltimore, MD 21205, USA; [e] Department of Medicine, Cystic Fibrosis Clinical Research, National Jewish Health, 1400 Jackson Street, K333b, Denver, CO 80206, USA; [f] Department of Pediatrics, University of Texas Southwestern, 5323 Harry Hines Boulevard, Dallas, TX 75390-8558, USA; [g] Department of Physical Medicine and Rehabilitation, Johns Hopkins Hospital, 1800 Orleans Street, Baltimore, MD 21287, USA; [h] Adult with Cystic Fibrosis, 237 Russell Street, Oceanside, CA 92058, USA; [i] Adult with Cystic Fibrosis, 2700 University Avenue West Apartment 416, St Paul, MN 55114, USA; [j] Department of Medicine, National Jewish Health, 1400 Jackson Street; J318, Denver, CO 80206, USA; [k] Department of Pediatrics, National Jewish Health, 1400 Jackson Street; J318, Denver, CO 80206, USA
* Corresponding author.
E-mail address: raksha.jain@utsouthwestern.edu

Clin Chest Med 42 (2021) 517–530
https://doi.org/10.1016/j.ccm.2021.04.010
0272-5231/21/© 2021 Elsevier Inc. All rights reserved.

been void of literature and guidance for these women. Because CF is now largely diagnosed at birth, women cope with challenges related to hormonal shifts and SRH throughout their lives in the setting of this chronic illness (**Fig. 1**).

The current model of health care delivery in the CF setting inadequately addresses the needs of women, resulting in large gaps in SRH care use and knowledge and suboptimal health outcomes.[3–5] CF providers agree that they have a central role in the SRH care of these patients,[6] but most do not routinely address these topics in their practice, nor do most feel comfortable doing so.[7] Barriers to addressing topics unique to women's health in CF care include patient and provider discomfort discussing SRH, limited provider knowledge or expertise on this topic, and lack of time during CF clinic visits.[8] Because women with CF often view their CF provider as their main physician or de facto primary care provider,[9] recent models in CF have focused on embedding such topics into subspecialty care with the CF team acting as a broker for addressing SRH and referring to primary care or women's health providers.[10] Women with CF support this model and desire SRH patient educational resources and tailored discussions initiated by their CF team early and often.[6] Adolescent and adult women with CF and their parents have identified several general and disease-specific topics that are important to address in the CF care model and that highlight an important focus on improved patient-provider communication and shared decision making around SRH concerns.[11]

CONCERNS FROM WOMEN WITH CYSTIC FIBROSIS

Maddie, a 27-year-old single woman with CF, is currently working on her Masters of Public Health in epidemiology, and reports, "Sexual, reproductive, and general women's health care has been largely ignored by my CF teams. In my experience, CF teams are rarely comfortable with topics such as birth control and pregnancy. I am always told to consult a primary care doctor or obstetrician or gynecologist. These providers do not know enough about CF or the myriad of medications I take. They seem terrified to wade into the care of a woman with a chronic disease as complex as CF. Everything I have learned about safe and effective contraceptive options, pregnancy, and parenthood as a woman with CF has been acquired through my own research or by speaking with and listening to other women with CF. Until our caregivers can either collaborate or educate themselves on these issues, women with CF will continue to muddle through these topics, relying on each other to share our stories and give each other guidance and support."

Jacqui, a 42-year-old woman with CF, who has 2 boys aged 10 and 13 years states that, "The part I have found most frustrating is the lack of protocol coordination between specialty teams. I would

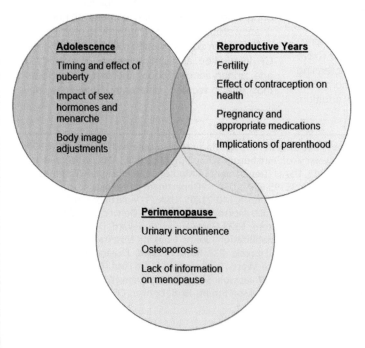

Fig. 1. A lifespan of overlapping challenges for women with CF.

like to see more universal protocols that are recognized and in place particularly by the obstetrics and gynecology community. I found it extremely frustrating trying to find clear answers to questions when various specialty team protocols do not line up exactly. For example, what birth control methods were available and most effective with the multitude of daily medications? What health parameters should be met in order to most safely start a family? What routine treatments and medications are safe during pregnancy? How to balance a diabetic diet with the CF diet requirements? How to manage daily life with children so the mother's health does not take a back seat?"

SEX DISPARITIES IN OUTCOMES OF PEOPLE WITH CYSTIC FIBROSIS

As an autosomal recessive inherited disease, the prevalence of CF at birth remains similar between men and women; however, women with CF have worse clinical outcomes across multiple domains.[1] Although survival has increased in both sexes over the years with advances in therapies, numerous epidemiologic studies have shown that female sex remains independently associated with risk of death, because women with CF have a median life expectancy nearly 3 years shorter than men.[1,12,13]

In addition to mortality, women with CF have worse clinical outcomes related to pulmonary exacerbations (PEx). PEx, commonly manifested by acute worsening of pulmonary symptoms and/or a decrease in lung function requiring treatment with antibiotic therapy, remain common occurrences in people with CF.[14,15] Researchers have shown that PEx are associated with lung function decline and reduced quality of life.[16–18] Notably, women with CF have more PEx per year compared with men[4] and female sex has been associated with a higher risk of failing to recover to baseline lung function after treatment of a PEx.[18]

Various sex differences related to lung anatomy, microbiology acquisition, and sex hormone–mediated effects have been evaluated as possible causes for the sex disparity seen in CF. Data have shown that girls have smaller lungs at birth and maintain smaller conducting airways into adulthood even when accounting for similar lung size and body morphometrics, potentially increasing women's susceptibility to pulmonary infections by hindering mucociliary airway clearance.[19]

Pseudomonas aeruginosa, a highly prevalent and virulent pathogen in CF, has been associated with a 2.6 times higher risk of death in people with CF.[20] Studies show that *P aeruginosa* with a mucoid phenotype commonly propagates biofilm development associated with increased antibiotic resistance associated with worse respiratory morbidity and mortality.[20–22] Data show that girls acquire *P aeruginosa* at an earlier age (median 9.5 years in girls and 11.2 years in boys) and was associated with an accelerated rate of decline of lung function.[21] Researchers also showed that women acquire other common pathogens earlier than men. Earlier acquisition combined with increased mortality in women has been associated with methicillin-resistant *Staphylococcus aureus*, *Achromobacter xylosoxidans*, *Burkholderia cepacia*, *Aspergillus* species, and nontuberculous mycobacterium infections.[1]

Researchers have also shown that women with CF have a significantly higher rate of PEx, which begins after puberty, suggesting female sex hormones may affect respiratory health.[22] Animal models show that estrogen affects mucus cell hyperplasia and upregulates mucus production while inhibiting chloride secretion, resulting in disturbances in mucociliary clearance.[23] Chotirmall and colleagues[24] showed that in vitro exposure of *P aeruginosa* to 17β-estradiol was associated with mucoid colony formation and proposed that estradiol levels correlated with pulmonary exacerbations in women with CF. Importantly, they observed that PEx occurred less frequently in women taking hormonal contraceptive pills.

Furthermore, data have shown that dehydroepiandrosterone-sulfate (DHEA-S) and testosterone, two circulating androgens with stable concentrations during the menstrual cycle, may enhance lung function in other chronic respiratory disease models.[16] DHEA-S inhibits airway smooth muscle cell migration and attenuates airway inflammation, whereas testosterone promotes airway smooth muscle relaxation.[16] DHEA-S levels are disproportionately low in women with CF.[25] Although testosterone levels in CF have not been extensively studied, higher levels of testosterone in female adolescents with asthma have been associated with higher lung function.[26]

Women with CF overall have increased respiratory morbidity and mortality compared with men. Significant research has been done to better understand the causes of this sex disparity, which are likely multifactorial. Although significant advances have been made, future work on the interplay of sex differences with CF is needed to improve the outcomes and survival of women with this condition.

PUBERTY AND MENARCHE

Puberty is commonly defined as physiologic and morphologic changes that occur within the growing child as the gonads change from an infantile to adult state.[27] Puberty in the healthy US population typically occurs between ages 10 and 14 years in girls and 12 to 16 years in boys. Formerly, CF was associated with delayed puberty. Older studies of CF reported delayed pubertal progression, age at menarche, skeletal maturity, and growth spurt.[28,29] Specifically, in 1 retrospective study from the 1990s, mean age at menarche for girls with CF was 14.9 ± 1.4 years, which was significantly later than healthy controls (13.0 ± 1 years).[30] Animal studies endorse these findings. CF S489X⁻/S489X⁻ knockout mice grew more slowly and had later onset of puberty than wild-type mice. These mice had chronic inflammation and gastrointestinal disease.[31] This finding was further confirmed in a CF F508del⁻/F508del⁻ knockout mouse model, which also had delayed pubertal timing.[31] CF care and therapies have significantly improved in the past 2 decades and the gap in pubertal onset has improved for most adolescents with CF, potentially because of improved nutrition and overall health.[32,33] In a retrospective study from 2014 using the US Cystic Fibrosis Foundation Patient Registry (CFFPR), the average age of puberty was found to be 13.2 ± 2.2 years in boys and 11.2 ± 2.0 years in girls. These investigators used peak height velocity to determine puberty onset, because menarche and Tanner staging are not available in the CFFPR.[22] The age ranges found in the CF population correlate with pubertal age reported in the healthy population.[34,35] Another French cohort study published in 2012 validates these findings, that age of onset of puberty and pubertal spurt in a CF population did not differ from healthy controls.[36] Studies in patients with CF-related diabetes and CF-related liver disease are limited; however, these populations are at risk of malnutrition and may also be at risk for abnormal pubertal development, and they therefore require careful consideration.[37]

Puberty may play a role in frequency of PEx in girls with CF. Sutton and colleagues[22] found that the rate of PEx increased in adolescent girls (1.17 ± 1.35 exacerbations per year) compared with boys (0.95 ± 1.27 exacerbations per year; $P<.001$) after undergoing puberty, with no differences found before pubertal onset. Note that physical and emotional changes associated with puberty can be challenging for all adolescents, and medical and psychosocial guidance is crucial in the prepubertal and pubertal periods for a healthy transition to adulthood.[38]

CONTRACEPTION

Limited data exist surrounding the use of contraception in CF.[39,40] The interplay of disease-specific risk factors, such as medication interactions, gastrointestinal absorption, CF-related liver disease, diabetes, bone health, and frequent use of intravenous access devices for antibiotics, may complicate contraception decisions for women with CF.

Types of combined hormonal contraceptives (containing estrogen and progesterone) include pills, patches, and vaginal rings. Such methods are also contraindicated in women with pulmonary hypertension and decompensated cirrhosis secondary to increased risk of thrombosis; however, such conditions rarely affect those with CF.[41,42] Standard preparations of the combined oral contraceptive pill are associated with a 2 to 3 times increased risk of venous thromboembolism, which is of particular importance for those with implantable vascular access devices (associated with a 5%–14% risk of venous thromboembolism alone).[42,43]

Medications commonly used in CF can interact with hormonal contraceptives. Liver enzyme-inducing drugs used for treatment of nontuberculous mycobacteria, including rifampicin and rifabutin, can interfere with the effectiveness of the hormonal contraceptives. Malabsorption of oral drugs caused by pancreatic enzyme insufficiency may theoretically decrease the effectiveness of oral contraceptive pills. Importantly, the cystic fibrosis transmembrane conductance regulator (CFTR) modulator lumacaftor/ivacaftor affects metabolism and reduces the efficacy of oral hormonal contraceptives, and product information recommends avoidance of all forms of hormonal contraception.[44] Other CFTR modulators, including ivacaftor, tezacaftor/ivacaftor, and elexacaftor/tezacaftor/ivacaftor, do not have this interaction.[45]

The hormonal injection, depot medroxyprogesterone acetate (DMPA), is associated with accelerated, but potentially reversible, loss of bone mineral density.[42] However, it has been noted that DMPA may be useful in the treatment of underweight women with CF.[46] Long-acting reversible contraceptives, such as copper and hormonal intrauterine devices (IUDs) and hormonal implants, are highly effective and reversible methods with increasing use in adolescents and nulliparous women.[42] For most women with CF, these methods are safe to use. Hormonal IUDs may be affected by use of lumacaftor/ivacaftor and, thus, are not recommended; however, the copper IUD is an effective option for women taking this medication.[44]

Evidence connecting female sex hormones and CF disease outcomes has prompted questions about the use of contraception as a treatment modality for women with CF. In a retrospective analysis of women attending a single CF center in the United Kingdom between 1981 and 2010, Kernan and colleagues[47] showed no difference in clinical outcome measures in 57 women exposed to combined hormonal contraceptive pills versus matched nonexposed controls over a 5-year period as well as no difference when analyzing intrapatient effect on women with CF who had exposure to the oral contraceptive pill followed by nonexposure over a 3-year period.[47] Another study showed an association with fewer PEx in women on oral contraceptives than in women who were not.[24] Data on the effect of various types of contraception on CF health are lacking and further research is ongoing.

Adolescent and young adult women with CF in the United States report lower rates of lifetime contraception use than the general population despite similar levels of sexual activity (55% vs 74%, $P<.0001$).[4] In addition, among young women who reported sex in the prior 3 months, 35% of adolescent and young adults with CF were not using any form of contraception compared with 26% of women in the general population ($P<.0001$). However, a higher percentage of women with CF reported the use of a long-acting reversible contraceptive method (IUD or implant) compared with US women without CF (17% vs 8%, $P<.0001$). In addition, fewer women with CF (17%) reported a history of emergency contraception use compared with women in the general US population (29%, $P<.0001$). Of note, these data were generated before the widespread use of highly effective therapies such as highly effective CFTR modulator therapy (HEMT) directed at correcting the basic protein defect in CF.

Women with CF report low rates of contraceptive counseling and rarely discuss this aspect of care in a CF setting.[5,48–50] Given the unique considerations outlined earlier, contraceptive choice should be discussed in the context of the CF care model and coordinated decisions with women's health providers to choose the best method for each individual woman with CF. Importantly, selection of a contraceptive method should take into consideration both the women's preferences and priorities and aspects of their CF disease.

FERTILITY

The structural anatomy of the reproductive system of a woman with CF is similar to that of a woman without CF; however, reproductive epithelial cells are subject to alterations secondary to mutations in the CFTR gene.[51,52] CFTR channels are present in the cervix.[53,54] Thus, their abnormal function in women with CF results in thick, dehydrated cervical mucus that is thought to impair penetration by sperm as well as create a pH-imbalanced uterine environment, resulting in failure of sperm capacitation and potential prevention of penetration and fertilization of the egg in some women with CF.[52] Although ovaries do not express CFTR, ovulatory disturbance may be related to redundant follicular cysts and reduced follicles.[51,52] Menarchal delay related to hormonal imbalances and amenorrhea caused by low body fat secondary to malnutrition can also result in subfertility.[51] In addition to these physiologic differences, Shteinberg and colleagues[55] found that 35% of women with CF report subfertility in a retrospective international study, which was associated with advanced age and pancreatic insufficiency.

Despite these concerns, most women with CF are able to conceive and carry a healthy pregnancy to term.[56] As mentioned earlier, sexually active women with CF report that they are less likely to use contraception than women without CF.[3,50] The decreased contraceptive use may be an indication that women with CF may underestimate their ability to conceive. Similar to the general US population, an online survey of 150 women with CF found that half of all pregnancies were unplanned.[57,58]

There are several reports indicating that women have a lack of knowledge regarding their fertility.[3,59–61] A pilot survey of 22 women with CF indicated confusion about how CF affects fertility and pregnancy, with women reporting they were infertile or have low fertility, which resulted in some women not using contraception.[59] This lack of understanding of female fertility in women with CF is further supported by the fact that 33% of a Polish cohort and 65% of an Australian cohort of women with CF indicated that they thought their fertility to be reduced.[3,60] Gage[61] concluded from a review of 9 studies (1995–2000 with 217 women) assessing SRH knowledge that women with CF are less likely to use contraception or engage in family planning when perceived risk of pregnancy is low.

Women with CF express a desire to be better informed about their fertility and the consequences of pregnancy.[61–63] A consistent theme in the literature is that women with CF think that access to SRH information is difficult and challenging to understand,[60,64] and is not discussed by CF care providers in sufficient quantity or quality.[59,61,62] Reports indicate that women and their families want SRH discussions to start in adolescence.[60,63,64] In addition, education regarding the safety of CF-related medications during pregnancy is desired.[62,64] Individualized discussion of these topics with CF care providers at regular intervals is required in order for women with CF to make well-informed decisions regarding the short-term and long-term effects of pregnancy and parenthood.[59,62]

Since 2019, with the era of access to highly effective CFTR modulators, which are hypothesized to improve fertility for most women with CF, it is increasingly important for women with CF to receive preconception counseling.[65–67] Twelve of 15 mothers with CF, 7 of whom thought they were infertile, experienced 13 pregnancies with an average time to conception of 3.2 months after starting CFTR treatment compared with 40 months of unprotected sexual intercourse without successful conception before starting treatment with a CFTR modulator.[68] The exact effect of CFTR modulators on fertility is not yet known, but they are thought to decrease viscosity and increase pH in cervical mucous secretions, promoting a fertile environment.[68]

RESPIRATORY SYMPTOMS DURING SEXUAL INTERCOURSE

Many adolescent and adult women with CF are involved in sexual relationships and engage in vaginal, anal, and/or oral sex similar to their counterparts without CF.[4] Sexual activity can cause an increase in heart rate and respiratory rate, which can result in shortness of breath and cough. In a recent survey of sexually active adolescent and young adult women with CF, 16% reported sexual functioning concerns and one-third reported cough during or after sexual intercourse.[4] In the general CF population, approximately 9.1% of people with CF reported hemoptysis over a 5-year period.[69] In survey referenced earlier, about 3% of adolescent and young adult women reported hemoptysis during or after sex.[4] To date, there is a paucity of evidence to help guide CF care teams in addressing respiratory symptoms during sexual activity in women with CF. To minimize cough and hemoptysis during sexual activity, it may be beneficial to recommend use of a short-acting bronchodilator 20 to 30 minutes before sex as well as completing airway clearance. In addition, positions that require less energy and decreased pressure on the chest and optimize breathing techniques may help decrease cough. Use of pillows to elevate the head and torso can be beneficial. In addition, although a cough is necessary to clear airway secretions, women with CF may prefer to wait to expel mucus until after sex. Practicing pursed lip breathing during sexual activity aids in the minimization of bronchoconstriction and therefore helps to suppress coughing. Given the lack of evidence-based literature on this topic, an opportunity exists to develop improved recommendations for women with CF on minimizing respiratory symptoms during or after sex.

PREGNANCY

The rate of pregnancy in women with CF continues to increase each year both in the United States (**Fig. 2**) and compared with historical rates around the world.[14] The first reported pregnancy of a woman with CF in the literature was in 1960.[70] Although the 20-year-old successfully delivered her preterm infant, she died 6 weeks after the infant's birth. Over subsequent years, several single-site retrospective case series that suggested that, although outcomes of pregnancy were worse in subgroups with low lung function and certain infections, pregnancy and motherhood could be successfully navigated by some women with CF.[71–76]

Although data in a more recent cohort study showed a decline in lung function and body mass index (BMI) associated with pregnancy in a cohort of 81 women with CF,[77] evaluation of data from the CFFPR from 1985 to 1997 showed that women with CF who became pregnant had similar long-term outcomes compared with women who never became pregnant.[78] Furthermore, Schechter and colleagues[79] analyzed data from pregnant women in a large CF epidemiologic study of 24,000 people with CF in the United States and Canada between 1994 and 2005. They found that women with CF who became pregnant (n = 119) had more illness-related visits and pulmonary exacerbations, including the need for intravenous antibiotics, and lower quality-of-life scores compared with women with CF who did not become pregnant. However, those women with CF who became pregnant did not have accelerated disease progression or increase in mortality compared with other women with CF. In contrast, Patel and colleagues[80] reviewed delivery-related discharges in a large national database and found that, although the incidence of adverse events was

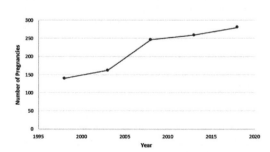

Fig. 2. Number of pregnancies reported in the United States Cystic Fibrosis Foundation (CFF) Patient Registry.

low, compared with women without CF, women with CF (n = 1119) were more likely to have cardiac conduction disorders, diabetes, asthma, thrombophilia, anemia, and death, and had longer postdelivery length of stay.

In addition to concern for maternal health during pregnancy for women with CF, the other major concern is the health of the infant. Jelin and colleagues[81] examined maternal and perinatal outcomes for women with CF in California using 4 state health databases. Compared with women without CF, infants of women with CF (n = 77) were more likely to be affected by congenital anomalies (14.3% vs 6.4%, $P = .005$; adjusted odds ratio, 2.6; confidence interval,1.4–5.0), have higher rates of jaundice (24.2% vs 15.3%, $P = .04$), be born via cesarean section (45% vs 29%, $P = .03$), and deliver at less than 37 weeks (18.2% vs 8.9%, $P = .008$).[81] These data suggest that infants of women with CF must be closely monitored and examined, and that neonatal intensive care units should be alerted at the time of labor and delivery for women with CF.

Another key factor for the health of the infants born of pregnant women with CF is related to in utero exposures of disease-specific medications. Expansion of the population of women with CF experiencing pregnancy is growing at least in part because of the availability of better chronic medications and the afforded increased quality and quantity of life. However, CF-specific therapies have not been formally tested in pregnant women with regard to safety for the fetus. Risks associated with medication exposure during pregnancy are evaluated by timing of administration during pregnancy, ability to cross the placenta, and the risk of teratogenesis. In the United States, preclinical, clinical, and postmarketing experiences often drive pregnancy classifications for drugs. Medication safety in women with CF has recently been reviewed,[82] and, in their statement on the management of reproduction and pregnancy in women with airway disease, the European Respiratory Society (ERS) and the Thoracic Society of Australia and New Zealand (TSANZ) specifically outline recommendations for commonly used medications by trimester based on known information about each therapeutic agent.[83]

Of critical importance, it is anticipated that up to 90% of the CF population will be treated with HEMT.[65,66] As noted earlier, CFTR modulators are likely to increase fertility in CF.[68] When the CFFPR was used to examine the impact of CFTR modulator therapies on pregnancy rates and outcomes from 2005 to 2014, it was clear that pregnancy rates increased in eligible patients following approval of the first CFTR modulator, ivacaftor.[84] Although animal data show no teratogenicity or fetal toxicity for CFTR modulators administered individually at normal human doses,[44,85–87] there are no prospective studies of the use of CFTR modulators in pregnant women.

There have been case reports of successful pregnancies in women on CFTR modulator therapy.[88–91] Furthermore, Nash and colleagues[92] recently reported the results of a multinational retrospective survey of CF care centers. In 61 women with CF, use of CFTR modulators during part or all of pregnancy resulted in 2 maternal complications that were deemed related to CFTR modulator therapy. No modulator-related complications were reported in infants exposed in utero and/or during lactation. Importantly, as previous reported in nonpregnant people with CF who suddenly discontinued modulators,[93,94] cessation of modulator therapy resulted in clinical decline in 9 women, prompting resumption of therapy during pregnancy. There is clear need for prospective data on maternal-fetal effects of CFTR modulators to make informed choices regarding use or discontinuation during pregnancy. Such a study, the MAYFLOWERS study (Maternal and Fetal Outcomes in the Era of Modulators), is planned to begin in the United States in the first quarter of 2021.

PARENTHOOD

As life expectancy and overall health increase for people with CF, a growing number are considering parenthood, including adoption and surrogacy. A recent survey of 188 young women with CF found that nearly 4 out of 5 young women said they wanted to have a child in the future.[4] In a retrospective, multicenter study of 605 women in Europe and the United Kingdom, 40% had attempted pregnancy.[68]

The decision of whether or not to become a parent is complex for people with CF, and associated complications of having CF have been identified as major factors in reproductive decision making.[59] A recent qualitative study found that parents and nonparents with CF expressed concerns around balancing roles as parent and patient, the impact of anticipated health decline and early mortality on their children, and communication with children about their CF.[95] In a qualitative study of Australian women with CF, participants reported that they have difficulty accessing current, accurate information about fertility, the safety and health impacts of pregnancy, and the safety of CF medications during pregnancy.[62]

In 2019, the UK patient registry reported that 58 women became mothers and 45 men became fathers, and CFFPR has documented a steady increase in pregnancy rates over time in women with CF (see **Fig. 2**).[14,96] Although sources such as the CF patient registries are key sources of epidemiologic information, they lack data regarding parenthood, including prevalence and longitudinal health impact. When reflecting on the experience of parenthood, parents with CF have identified they were "being a parent on compressed time," reflecting the challenge of parenting within both a limited life expectancy and a complex daily treatment regimen.[97] A recent systematic review found that, despite potential negative impacts on health, treatment adherence, the need for coping strategies for parenthood stresses, and the pressure of time related to mortality, people with CF report a positive outlook on parenthood.[98] Clinicians in the United States and Wales are working with community stakeholders to develop decision aids to facilitate the decision-making process regarding parenthood for people with CF.[99] In addition, qualitative studies are underway to better understand the impact of parenthood on those with CF.

BODY IMAGE

Survival and pulmonary function are directly associated with nutritional status in CF.[100] In addition to societal norms accentuating thin stature for women, the continual focus on eating and weight within CF care may increase the risk of people with CF developing maladaptive eating behaviors and unhealthy body image.[101–103] The perceptions and attitudes that people have toward their body shapes and features can affect their lived experiences.[101,104] Older reports have shown low prevalence of diagnosed eating disorders among people with CF,[102,105] although there have been individual case reports of anorexia in this population.[105,106] Good evidence exists relating to the relationship between perceived body image and quality of life in CF.[101,104] For example, appropriate body image can relate to self-esteem and influence people's compliance motivation. How this can influence health as it relates to CF has not been well studied.

Body image seems to be important to adolescents and adults with CF.[107,108] Although women with CF tend to have better body image on quality-of-life measures, they tend to have a lower BMI, and decreased quality of life in relation to chest symptoms and emotional function.[107,109,110] Adolescent women with CF have overall better body image scores than men, but it is of concern that they also are more likely to engage in maladaptive eating behaviors such as dieting in the form of restraining intake and disturbed eating attitudes, such as fear of weight gain and feeling fat.[102] This concern is likely to increase in the setting of HEMT given that the average weight gain in the most recent phase III trial was 3.4 kg (range 3.0–3.8 kg) over 6 months.[65]

CF providers should aim to routinely address body image with women with CF and improve their comfort and expertise on this topic.[111] Provider training may increase the frequency and comfort of addressing body image, and adolescents and young adults with CF have identified the use of a patient-centered, rather than a disease-centered, approach as important.[111] A survey identifying nutritional needs in a cohort of adults with CF emphasized that individualizing CF nutrition programs to provide a variety of resources from different platforms may be valuable to achieve better nutrition outcomes.[108] Further work on identifying the prevalence of body image concerns and disordered eating and the role of the CF team in the modern era of CF is needed.

INCONTINENCE

Urinary incontinence (UI) is a common extrapulmonary manifestation in women with CF.[112] Most of the existing studies incompletely describe the characteristics of UI and associations with CF disease severity. Inconsistent definitions of UI and poorly defined classification of patient burden have been used across previous research. Despite these limitations, the picture that emerges is significant. The prevalence of UI ranges from 16% to 76% among women with CF.[4,113,114] The most common triggers include coughing, laughing, sneezing, physical activity, airway clearance, and spirometry. UI has the potential to interfere with CF management (eg, reticence to perform chest physiotherapy, exercise, and/or spirometry), cause personal embarrassment and worry, and inhibit recreational, social, and intimate activities. In patients with CF and UI, it is important to rule out and appropriately treat urinary tract infections and CF-related diabetes as well as optimize the treatment of symptoms of constipation.

Although there are various management options for UI, the extent to which these are offered to and accepted by patients is unknown, and their benefits to people with CF are unclear. Evidence suggests that exercises for pelvic floor and core muscles may lessen patient burden.[115,116] Physical therapists (PTs) can be a valuable resource to evaluate and treat UI in CF clinics. Other nonsurgical options include intravaginal mechanical devices, disposable pads, and newer absorbent products.

Referral to a specialist PT or urogynecology for evaluation can also be considered.

Low rates of discussion of UI by CF health care providers have been reported, which limits women's access to treatment.[115] Adolescents and adults have reported various barriers to discussions of SRH, but the extent to which these issues also function as obstacles to discussion and treatment of UI is unclear.[5] Further research is needed to optimize discussion of this manifestation of CF, fully define prevalence in this population, and identify effective treatment modalities.

MENOPAUSE AND OSTEOPOROSIS

The age of menopausal transition classically starts late in the fifth decade of life[117,118] but has not been well characterized in the context of CF. Menopausal symptoms may include hot flashes, mood changes, sleep disturbance, depression, vaginal dryness, dyspareunia, sexual dysfunction, and irregular menstrual cycles. Menopause has been categorized into stages (Stages of Reproductive Aging Workshop [STRAW]) and usually begins within the 4 years before a woman's last menstrual period.[119]

In 2019, the CFFPR reported 8347 women aged 18 years or older, of whom 1246 were aged 47 years or older (14.9% in their perimenopausal/postmenopausal years), a percentage expected to increase as longevity in women with CF increases.[14] Only anecdotal information is available regarding the age at which women with CF experience menopausal symptoms. Little is documented regarding the treatment of menopause symptoms specific to women with CF, and information is commonly extrapolated from women without CF, such as the benefits and risks of hormone replacement therapy (HRT) to alleviate menopausal symptoms.[120] Hormonal replacement therapy can include estrogen versus estrogen and progesterone combination supplementation designed to alleviate menopausal symptoms such as hot flashes and vaginal dryness. Estrogens can be given orally, transdermally, or vaginally. When given orally, estrogens undergo hepatic metabolism and increase hepatic production of several proteins, including clotting factors. Women with CF may have altered hepatic metabolism, thus altering serum estrogen levels. Estrogen can also be used transdermally, sometimes with the addition of progestin. Topical estradiols are available in a variety of forms including gels, aerosols, and pumps for the treatment of vasomotor symptoms. Low-dose vaginal estrogen can be safely used to treat vaginal atrophy. In women without CF, the benefits of HRT for those aged 50 to 59 years may include a trend toward fewer fractures, less diabetes, and lower all-cause mortality, but there could also be a trend toward increased risk of cerebrovascular accidents, deep vein thrombosis, and pulmonary embolism. The balance of risks and benefits of HRT in women with CF needs to be further studied to determine the best approach to care for perimenopausal or postmenopausal women with CF.

People with CF, particularly women, are at increased risk for osteoporosis. This risk was hypothesized to be caused by malabsorption of vitamin D, and thus calcium, leading to low BMI and reduced exercise capacity.[121,122] Bone cells sense energy intake and stop forming if the energy intake is inadequate, often seen in the CF population. The hypothalamus also signals to stop bone formation if energy intake is inadequate. Osteoblasts have receptors for serotonin, secreted by the gut, which inhibits bone formation, giving another mechanism for poor bone health in people with CF. The risk of fracture in women with CF is determined by their T score and age. In women without CF with a T score of -2.5, at age 70 years, there is a 9% fracture rate over 10 years.[123] The CFFPR reports 40% of people with CF aged 50 years having bone disease (defined as osteopenia, osteoporosis, or bone fracture), increasing to 60% by age 70 years.[14] Extrapolating from the general population, there is a marked increase in the risk of fractures; for example, a T score of -3.0, compounded by age 60 years, has a 7.5% chance of fracture over 10 years. Preventive measures include adequate nutrition, vitamin D replacement, calcium, weight bearing, and consideration of bisphosphonates. Management of the multifaceted challenges of menopause and early bone loss in women with CF has not been well studied.

SUMMARY

Women with CF face a unique challenge in balancing their womanhood in the context of the disease burden of CF. As these women lead longer and healthier lives, they need more information to guide them on disease-specific SRH topics such as the effect of sex hormones on their health, the cause of the sex disparity in CF, management of fertility and pregnancy, and prevention of osteoporosis and UI. However, these topics have largely been understudied and overlooked. The landscape of CF is changing rapidly, and care and research must evolve to help address these critical topics. A group of physicians, researchers, and women with CF have joined to form the Women's Health Research Working Group, sponsored by the CF Foundation. The group's mission is to target questions specific to SRH with the goal of conducting well-designed studies to provide data-driven information to improve the lives of all women with CF.

CLINICS CARE POINTS

- Women with Cystic Fibrosis have increased pulmonary exacerbations, higher rates of colonization with *Pseudomonas aeruginosa* and worse long-term survival relative to men, which needs to be considered when caring for people with CF.

- Contraception is under-utilized in women with CF and should be discussed and considered more often, particularly given the potentially improved fertility in women with CF using CFTR modulator therapy and evidence that contraception may be associated with a decreased rate of pulmonary exacerbations.

- More women with CF are becoming pregnant and have good outcomes overall, however, they still need to be referred to high risk Obstetricians, such as Maternal Fetal Medicine specialists, for close monitoring with shared decision-making regarding risks and benefits of medication use while pregnant and breast feeding.

- As people with CF live longer and healthier lives due to therapies such as CFTR modulators, discussions regarding menopause, body image, urinary incontinence, and sexual and reproductive health are necessary.

DISCLOSURES

R. Jain receives consulting fees from Vertex Pharmaceuticals, Boehringer Ingelheim, and the CF Foundation unrelated to this work as well as grant support from the CF Foundation, Sound Pharmaceuticals, Genentech, Vertex Pharmaceuticals, Corbus, and Boehringer Ingelheim. T.M. Kazmerski receives consulting fees from the CF Foundation unrelated to this work as well as grant support from the CF Foundation and the Patient-Centered Outcomes Research Institute. K. Montemayor receives grant support from the CF Foundation and Johns Hopkins-Specialized Center for Research Excellence (SCORE) in Sex and Age Differences in Immunity to Influenza (SADII) and The Foundation for Gender-Specific Medicine. K. von Berg receives grant support and consulting fees from the CF Foundation, unrelated to this work. N. West receives consulting fees from Vertex Pharmaceuticals unrelated to this work, as well as grant support from the CF Foundation and Corbus. J.L. Taylor-Cousar receives grant support from Vertex Pharmaceutical, Proteostasis, Eloxx, and the CF Foundation as well as personal fees from Proteostasis, Santhera, 4DMT, Polarean, and Vertex for consulting, along with speaking fees from Vertex Pharmaceuticals unrelated to this work.

ACKNOWLEDGMENTS

The authors would like to thank the CF Foundation for support of the Women's Health Research Working Group.

REFERENCES

1. Harness-Brumley CL, Elliott AC, Rosenbluth DB, et al. Gender differences in outcomes of patients with cystic fibrosis. J Womens Health (Larchmt) 2014;23(12):1012–20.
2. Raghavan D, Jain R. Increasing awareness of sex differences in airway diseases. Respirology 2016; 21(3):449–59.
3. Sawyer SM, Phelan PD, Bowes G. Reproductive health in young women with cystic fibrosis: knowledge, behavior and attitudes. J Adolesc Health 1995;17(1):46–50.
4. Kazmerski TM, Sawicki GS, Miller E, et al. Sexual and reproductive health behaviors and experiences reported by young women with cystic fibrosis. J Cyst Fibros 2018;17(1):57–63.
5. Kazmerski TM, Sawicki GS, Miller E, et al. Sexual and reproductive health care utilization and preferences reported by young women with cystic fibrosis. J Cyst Fibros 2018;17(1):64–70.
6. Kazmerski TM, Borrero S, Tuchman LK, et al. Provider and patient attitudes regarding sexual health in young women with cystic fibrosis. Pediatrics 2016;137(6):e20154452.
7. Kazmerski TM, Borrero S, Sawicki GS, et al. Provider attitudes and practices toward sexual and reproductive health care for young women with cystic fibrosis. J Pediatr Adolesc Gynecol 2017; 30(5):546–52.
8. Kazmerski TM, Tuchman LK, Borrero S, et al. Cystic fibrosis program directors' attitudes toward sexual and reproductive health in young women with CF. Pediatr Pulmonol 2016;51(1):22–7.
9. Britto MT, Garrett JM, Dugliss MA, et al. Preventive services received by adolescents with cystic fibrosis and sickle cell disease. Arch Pediatr Adolesc Med 1999;153(1):27–32.
10. Frayman KB, Sawyer SM. Sexual and reproductive health in cystic fibrosis: a life-course perspective. Lancet Respir Med 2015;3(1):70–86.
11. Kazmerski TM, Prushinskaya OV, Hill K, et al. Sexual and reproductive health of young women with

cystic fibrosis: a concept mapping study. Acad Pediatr 2019;19(3):307–14.

12. FitzSimmons SC. The changing epidemiology of cystic fibrosis. J Pediatr 1993;122(1):1–9.

13. Rosenfeld M, Davis R, FitzSimmons S, et al. Gender gap in cystic fibrosis mortality. Am J Epidemiol 1997;145(9):794–803.

14. Cystic Fibrosis Foundation Patient Registry. 2019 Annual data report - Publication pending. Bethesda (MD): Cystic Fibrosis Foundation; 2020.

15. Montemayor K, Lambert AA, West NE. Pulmonary Exacerbations. In: Davis S, Rosenfeld M, Chmiel J, editors. New York: Springer International Publishing; 2020. p. 181-98.

16. de Boer K, Vandemheen KL, Tullis E, et al. Exacerbation frequency and clinical outcomes in adult patients with cystic fibrosis. Thorax 2011;66(8): 680–5.

17. Britto MT, Kotagal UR, Hornung RW, et al. Impact of recent pulmonary exacerbations on quality of life in patients with cystic fibrosis. Chest 2002;121(1): 64–72.

18. Sanders DB, Bittner RC, Rosenfeld M, et al. Failure to recover to baseline pulmonary function after cystic fibrosis pulmonary exacerbation. Am J Respir Crit Care Med 2010;182(5):627–32.

19. Carey MA, Card JW, Voltz JW, et al. It's all about sex: gender, lung development and lung disease. Trends Endocrinol Metab 2007;18(8):308–13.

20. Li Z, Kosorok MR, Farrell PM, et al. Longitudinal development of mucoid Pseudomonas aeruginosa infection and lung disease progression in children with cystic fibrosis. JAMA 2005;293(5):581–8.

21. Demko CA, Byard PJ, Davis PB. Gender differences in cystic fibrosis: Pseudomonas aeruginosa infection. J Clin Epidemiol 1995;48(8):1041–9.

22. Sutton S, Rosenbluth D, Raghavan D, et al. Effects of puberty on cystic fibrosis related pulmonary exacerbations in women versus men. Pediatr Pulmonol 2014;49(1):28–35.

23. Tam A, Wadsworth S, Dorscheid D, et al. Estradiol increases mucus synthesis in bronchial epithelial cells. PLoS One 2014;9(6):e100633.

24. Chotirmall SH, Smith SG, Gunaratnam C, et al. Effect of estrogen on pseudomonas mucoidy and exacerbations in cystic fibrosis. N Engl J Med 2012; 366(21):1978–86.

25. Evaluation of Dehydroepiandostrone Sulfate Levels in Cystic Fibrosis. Paper presented at: American Thoracic Society International Conference2019.

26. Han YY, Forno E, Celedon JC. Sex steroid hormones and asthma in a nationwide study of U.S. adults. Am J Respir Crit Care Med 2020;201(2): 158–66.

27. Marshall WATJ. Puberty. Boston (MA): Springer US; 1986.

28. Mahaney MC, McCoy KS. Developmental delays and pulmonary disease severity in cystic fibrosis. Hum Biol 1986;58(3):445–60.

29. Sproul A, Huang N. Growth patterns in children with cystic fibrosis. J Pediatr 1964;65:664–76.

30. Johannesson M, Gottlieb C, Hjelte L. Delayed puberty in girls with cystic fibrosis despite good clinical status. Pediatrics 1997;99(1):29–34.

31. Jin R, Hodges CA, Drumm ML, et al. The cystic fibrosis transmembrane conductance regulator (Cftr) modulates the timing of puberty in mice. J Med Genet 2006;43(6):e29.

32. Buntain HM, Greer RM, Wong JC, et al. Pubertal development and its influences on bone mineral density in Australian children and adolescents with cystic fibrosis. J Paediatr Child Health 2005; 41(7):317–22.

33. Kelly A, Schall JI, Stallings VA, et al. Deficits in bone mineral content in children and adolescents with cystic fibrosis are related to height deficits. J Clin Densitom 2008;11(4):581–9.

34. Iuliano-Burns S, Mirwald RL, Bailey DA. Timing and magnitude of peak height velocity and peak tissue velocities for early, average, and late maturing boys and girls. Am J Hum Biol 2001;13(1):1–8.

35. Abbassi V. Growth and normal puberty. Pediatrics 1998;102(2 Pt 3):507–11.

36. Bournez M, Bellis G, Huet F. Growth during puberty in cystic fibrosis: a retrospective evaluation of a French cohort. Arch Dis Child 2012;97(8):714–20.

37. Goldsweig B, Kaminski B, Sidhaye A, et al. Puberty in cystic fibrosis. J Cyst Fibros 2019;18(Suppl 2): S88–94.

38. Johannesson M, Carlson M, Brucefors AB, et al. Cystic fibrosis through a female perspective: psychosocial issues and information concerning puberty and motherhood. Patient Educ Couns 1998; 34(2):115–23.

39. Roe AH, Traxler S, Schreiber CA. Contraception in women with cystic fibrosis: a systematic review of the literature. Contraception 2016;93(1):3–10.

40. Whiteman MK, Oduyebo T, Zapata LB, et al. Contraceptive safety among women with cystic fibrosis: a systematic review. Contraception 2016; 94(6):621–9.

41. Curtis KM, Tepper NK, Jatlaoui TC, et al. U.S. medical eligibility criteria for contraceptive use. MMWR Recomm Rep 2016;65(3):1–103.

42. Festin M, Gaffield ML, Johnson S. WHO - medical eligibility criteria wheel for contraceptive use. 2008 update. Geneva (Switzerland): World Health Organization, April 1-4, 2008; 2009.

43. Deerojanawong J, Sawyer SM, Fink AM, et al. Totally implantable venous access devices in children with cystic fibrosis: incidence and type of complications. Thorax 1998;53(4):285–9.

44. Lumacaftor-ivacaftor prescribing information. In: Pharmaceuticals V. 2019. Available at: http://pi.vrtx.com/files/uspi_lumacaftor_ivacaftor.pdf. Accessed September 1, 2020.

45. Vertex Pharmaceuticals. Indications, important safety information, full prescribing information and patient information. Available at: https://www.vertextreatments.com/important-safety-information. Accessed September 1, 2020.

46. Kissner DG. Role of progestational agents in the treatment of undernourished patients with cystic fibrosis. Pediatr Pulmonol 2000;29(3):244.

47. Kernan NG, Alton EW, Cullinan P, et al. Oral contraceptives do not appear to affect cystic fibrosis disease severity. Eur Respir J 2013;41(1):67–73.

48. Gatiss S, Mansour D, Doe S, et al. Provision of contraception services and advice for women with cystic fibrosis. J Fam Plann Reprod Health Care 2009;35(3):157–60.

49. Plant BJ, Goss CH, Tonelli MR, et al. Contraceptive practices in women with cystic fibrosis. J Cyst Fibros 2008;7(5):412–4.

50. Roe AH, Traxler SA, Hadjiliadis D, et al. Contraceptive choices and preferences in a cohort of women with cystic fibrosis. Respir Med 2016;121:1–3.

51. Edenborough FP. Women with cystic fibrosis and their potential for reproduction. Thorax 2001;56(8):649–55.

52. Ahmad A, Ahmed A, Patrizio P. Cystic fibrosis and fertility. Curr Opin Obstet Gynecol 2013;25(3):167–72.

53. Ismail N, Giribabu N, Muniandy S, et al. Estrogen and progesterone differentially regulate the levels of cystic fibrosis transmembrane regulator (CFTR), adenylate cyclase (AC), and cyclic adenosine mono-phosphate (cAMP) in the rat cervix. Mol Reprod Dev 2015;82(6):463–74.

54. Hayslip CC, Hao E, Usala SJ. The cystic fibrosis transmembrane regulator gene is expressed in the human endocervix throughout the menstrual cycle. Fertil Steril 1997;67(4):636–40.

55. Shteinberg M, Lulu AB, Downey DG, et al. Failure to conceive in women with CF is associated with pancreatic insufficiency and advancing age. J Cyst Fibros 2019;18(4):525–9.

56. Edenborough FP, Borgo G, Knoop C, et al. Guidelines for the management of pregnancy in women with cystic fibrosis. J Cyst Fibros 2008;7(Suppl 1):S2–32.

57. Godfrey EM, Mody S, Schwartz MR, et al. Contraceptive use among women with cystic fibrosis: a pilot study linking reproductive health questions to the Cystic Fibrosis Foundation National Patient Registry. Contraception 2020;101(6):420–6.

58. Traxler SA, Chavez V, Hadjiliadis D, et al. Fertility considerations and attitudes about family planning among women with cystic fibrosis. Contraception 2019;100(3):228–33.

59. Kazmerski TM, Gmelin T, Slocum B, et al. Attitudes and decision making related to pregnancy among young women with cystic fibrosis. Matern Child Health J 2017;21(4):818–24.

60. Korzeniewska A, Grzelewski T, Jerzynska J, et al. Sexual and reproductive health knowledge in cystic fibrosis female patients and their parents. J Sex Med 2009;6(3):770–6.

61. Gage LA. What deficits in sexual and reproductive health knowledge exist among women with cystic fibrosis? A systematic review. Health Soc Work 2012;37(1):29–36.

62. Holton S, Fisher J, Button B, et al. Childbearing concerns, information needs and preferences of women with cystic fibrosis: an online discussion group. Sex Reprod Healthc 2019;19:31–5.

63. Fair A, Griffiths K, Osman LM. Attitudes to fertility issues among adults with cystic fibrosis in Scotland. The collaborative group of Scottish adult CF Centres. Thorax 2000;55(8):672–7.

64. Havermans T, Abbott J, Colpaert K, et al. Communication of information about reproductive and sexual health in cystic fibrosis. Patients, parents and caregivers' experience. J Cyst Fibros 2011;10(4):221–7.

65. Middleton PG, Mall MA, Drevinek P, et al. Elexacaftor-Tezacaftor-Ivacaftor for Cystic Fibrosis with a Single Phe508del Allele. N Engl J Med 2019;381(19):1809–19.

66. Heijerman HGM, McKone EF, Downey DG, et al. Efficacy and safety of the elexacaftor plus tezacaftor plus ivacaftor combination regimen in people with cystic fibrosis homozygous for the F508del mutation: a double-blind, randomised, phase 3 trial. Lancet 2019;394(10212):1940–8.

67. Hodges CA, Palmert MR, Drumm ML. Infertility in females with cystic fibrosis is multifactorial: evidence from mouse models. Endocrinology 2008;149(6):2790–7.

68. Jones GH, Walshaw MJ. Potential impact on fertility of new systemic therapies for cystic fibrosis. Paediatr Respir Rev 2015;16(Suppl 1):25–7.

69. Flume PA, Mogayzel PJ Jr, Robinson KA, et al. Cystic fibrosis pulmonary guidelines: pulmonary complications: hemoptysis and pneumothorax. Am J Respir Crit Care Med 2010;182(3):298–306.

70. Siegel BSS. Pregnancy and delivery in a patient with Cystic Fibrosis of the pancreas. Obstet Gynecol 1960;16(4):438–40.

71. Cohen LF, di Sant'Agnese PA, Friedlander J. Cystic fibrosis and pregnancy. A National Survey. Lancet 1980;2(8199):842–4.

72. Edenborough FP, Mackenzie WE, Stableforth DE. The outcome of 72 pregnancies in 55 women with cystic fibrosis in the United Kingdom 1977-1996. BJOG 2000;107(2):254–61.

73. Gillet D, de Braekeleer M, Bellis G, et al. Cystic fibrosis and pregnancy. Report from French data (1980-1999). BJOG 2002;109(8):912–8.

74. McMullen AH, Pasta DJ, Frederick PD, et al. Impact of pregnancy on women with cystic fibrosis. Chest 2006;129(3):706–11.

75. Reynaud Q, Rousset Jablonski C, Poupon-Bourdy S, et al. Pregnancy outcome in women with cystic fibrosis and poor pulmonary function. J Cyst Fibros 2020;19(1):80–3.

76. Thorpe-Beeston JG, Madge S, Gyi K, et al. The outcome of pregnancies in women with cystic fibrosis–single centre experience 1998-2011. BJOG 2013;120(3):354–61.

77. Giordani B, Quattrucci S, Amato A, et al. A case-control study on pregnancy in Italian Cystic Fibrosis women. Data from the Italian Registry. Respir Med 2018;145:200–5.

78. Goss CH, Rubenfeld GD, Otto K, et al. The effect of pregnancy on survival in women with cystic fibrosis. Chest 2003;124(4):1460–8.

79. Schechter MS, Quittner AL, Konstan MW, et al. Long-term effects of pregnancy and motherhood on disease outcomes of women with cystic fibrosis. Ann Am Thorac Soc 2013;10(3):213–9.

80. Patel EM, Swamy GK, Heine RP, et al. Medical and obstetric complications among pregnant women with cystic fibrosis. Am J Obstet Gynecol 2015;212(1):98 e91–99.

81. Jelin AC, Sharshiner R, Caughey AB. Maternal co-morbidities and neonatal outcomes associated with cystic fibrosis. J Matern Fetal Neonatal Med 2017;30(1):4–7.

82. Kroon M, Akkerman-Nijland AM, Rottier BL, et al. Drugs during pregnancy and breast feeding in women diagnosed with Cystic Fibrosis - an update. J Cyst Fibros 2018;17(1):17–25.

83. Middleton PG, Gade EJ, Aguilera C, et al. ERS/TSANZ Task Force Statement on the management of reproduction and pregnancy in women with airways diseases. Eur Respir J 2020;55(2):1901208.

84. Heltshe SL, Godfrey EM, Josephy T, et al. Pregnancy among cystic fibrosis women in the era of CFTR modulators. J Cyst Fibros 2017;16(6):687–94.

85. Ivacaftor prescribing information. In: Pharmaceuticals V. 2019. Available at: https://pi.vrtx.com/files/uspi_ivacaftor.pdf. Accessed September 18, 2020.

86. Tezacaftor-ivacaftor prescribing information. In: Pharmaceuticals V. 2019. Available at: https://pi.vrtx.com/files/uspi_tezacaftor_ivacaftor.pdf. Accessed September 18, 2020.

87. Elexacaftor-tezacaftor-ivacaftor prescribing information. In: Pharmaceuticals V. 2020. Available at: https://pi.vrtx.com/files/uspi_elexacaftor_tezacaftor_ivacaftor.pdf. Accessed September 18, 2020.

88. Kaminski R, Nazareth D. A successful uncomplicated CF pregnancy while remaining on Ivacaftor. J Cyst Fibros 2016;15(1):133–4.

89. Ladores S, Kazmerski TM, Rowe SM. A case report of pregnancy during use of targeted therapeutics for cystic fibrosis. J Obstet Gynecol Neonatal Nurs 2017;46(1):72–7.

90. Trimble A, McKinzie C, Terrell M, et al. Measured fetal and neonatal exposure to Lumacaftor and Ivacaftor during pregnancy and while breastfeeding. J Cyst Fibros 2018;17(6):779–82.

91. Mainz JG, Michl RK, Beiersdorf N, et al. Successful Pregnancy of a Patient with Cystic Fibrosis Genotype F508del/F508del and Progressed Pulmonary Destruction on lumacaftor/ivacaftor. Klin Padiatr 2019;231(5):271–3.

92. Nash EF, Middleton PG, Taylor-Cousar JL. Outcomes of pregnancy in women with cystic fibrosis (CF) taking CFTR modulators - an international survey. J Cyst Fibros 2020;19(4):521–6.

93. Trimble AT, Donaldson SH. Ivacaftor withdrawal syndrome in cystic fibrosis patients with the G551D mutation. J Cyst Fibros 2018;17(2):e13–6.

94. Carpino EAUA, Sawicki GS. Acute clinical outcomes following participation in short-term CFTR modulator trials in adults with cystic fibrosis: a retrospective chart review - a300. Pediatr Pulmonol 2018;53 S2:260–1.

95. Hailey CE, Tan JW, Dellon EP, et al. Pursuing parenthood with cystic fibrosis: reproductive health and parenting concerns in individuals with cystic fibrosis. Pediatr Pulmonol 2019;54(8):1225–33.

96. UK Cystic Fibrosis Registry 2019 Annual Data Report. 2020. Available at: https://www.cysticfibrosis.org.uk/.

97. Barker H, Moses J, O'Leary C. 'I've got to prioritise': being a parent with cystic fibrosis. Psychol Health Med 2017;22(6):744–52.

98. Jacob A, Journiac J, Fischer L, et al. How do cystic fibrosis patients experience parenthood? A systematic review. J Health Psychol 2020;26(1):60–81.

99. Kazmerski TM. Development of reproductive goals decision aid for women with cystic fibrosis. Paper presented at: International Conference on Communication in Healthcare2019; San Diego, CA, October 27-30, 2019.

100. Pedreira CC, Robert RG, Dalton V, et al. Association of body composition and lung function in children with cystic fibrosis. Pediatr Pulmonol 2005;39(3):276–80.

101. Tierney S. Body image and cystic fibrosis: a critical review. Body Image 2012;9(1):12–9.

102. Shearer JE, Bryon M. The nature and prevalence of eating disorders and eating disturbance in adolescents with cystic fibrosis. J R Soc Med 2004;97(Suppl 44):36–42.

103. Abbott J, Conway S, Etherington C, et al. Perceived body image and eating behavior in young adults with cystic fibrosis and their healthy peers. J Behav Med 2000;23(6):501–17.

104. Wenninger K, Weiss C, Wahn U, et al. Body image in cystic fibrosis–development of a brief diagnostic scale. J Behav Med 2003;26(1):81–94.

105. Gilchrist FJ, Lenney W. Distorted body image and anorexia complicating cystic fibrosis in an adolescent. J Cyst Fibros 2008;7(5):437–9.

106. Linkson L, Macedo P, Perrin FMR, et al. Anorexia nervosa in cystic fibrosis. Paediatr Respir Rev 2018;26:24–6.

107. Abbott J, Morton AM, Musson H, et al. Nutritional status, perceived body image and eating behaviours in adults with cystic fibrosis. Clin Nutr 2007; 26(1):91–9.

108. Kapnadak SG, Ramos KJ, Lopriore AM, et al. A survey identifying nutritional needs in a contemporary adult cystic fibrosis cohort. BMC Nutr 2019;5. https://doi.org/10.1186/s40795-018-0266-3.

109. Gee L, Abbott J, Conway SP, et al. Quality of life in cystic fibrosis: the impact of gender, general health perceptions and disease severity. J Cyst Fibros 2003;2(4):206–13.

110. Gee L, Abbott J, Hart A, et al. Associations between clinical variables and quality of life in adults with cystic fibrosis. J Cyst Fibros 2005;4(1):59–66.

111. Helms SW, Christon LM, Dellon EP, et al. Patient and provider perspectives on communication about body image with adolescents and young adults with cystic fibrosis. J Pediatr Psychol 2017;42(9):1040–50.

112. Frayman KB, Kazmerski TM, Sawyer SM. A systematic review of the prevalence and impact of urinary incontinence in cystic fibrosis. Respirology 2018;23(1):46–54.

113. Reichman G, De Boe V, Braeckman J, et al. Urinary incontinence in patients with cystic fibrosis. Scand J Urol 2016;50(2):128–31.

114. Blackwell K, Malone PS, Denny A, et al. The prevalence of stress urinary incontinence in patients with cystic fibrosis: an under-recognized problem. J Pediatr Urol 2005;1(1):5–9.

115. McVean RJ, Orr A, Webb AK, et al. Treatment of urinary incontinence in cystic fibrosis. J Cyst Fibros 2003;2(4):171–6.

116. von Berg K. Posture, pelvic floor and pistons: A look beyond "kegels" to treat urinary incontinence. S05.1. Paper presented at: The 30th Annual North American Cystic Fibrosis Conference2016; Orlando, FL, October 27-29, 2016.

117. McKinlay SM, Brambilla DJ, Posner JG. The normal menopause transition. Maturitas 1992;14(2): 103–15.

118. Randolph JF Jr, Crawford S, Dennerstein L, et al. The value of follicle-stimulating hormone concentration and clinical findings as markers of the late menopausal transition. J Clin Endocrinol Metab 2006;91(8):3034–40.

119. Harlow SD, Gass M, Hall JE, et al. Executive summary of the Stages of Reproductive Aging Workshop + 10: addressing the unfinished agenda of staging reproductive aging. J Clin Endocrinol Metab 2012;97(4):1159–68.

120. Stuenkel CA, Davis SR, Gompel A, et al. Treatment of symptoms of the menopause: an endocrine society clinical practice guideline. J Clin Endocrinol Metab 2015;100(11):3975–4011.

121. Aris RM, Merkel PA, Bachrach LK, et al. Guide to bone health and disease in cystic fibrosis. J Clin Endocrinol Metab 2005;90(3):1888–96.

122. Ott SM, Aitken ML. Osteoporosis in patients with cystic fibrosis. Clin Chest Med 1998;19(3): 555–67.

123. Kanis JA, Johnell O, Oden A, et al. Ten year probabilities of osteoporotic fractures according to BMD and diagnostic thresholds. Osteoporos Int 2001;12(12):989–95.

Interstitial Lung Diseases and the Impact of Gender

Theodoros Karampitsakos, MD, MSc, Ourania Papaioannou, MD, Matthaios Katsaras, MD, Fotios Sampsonas, MD, PhD, Argyris Tzouvelekis, MD, MSc, PhD*

KEYWORDS

- Interstitial lung diseases • Gender • Sex hormones • Pulmonary fibrosis

KEY POINTS

- Substantial epidemiologic evidence suggests that both sex and gender impacts prevalence, susceptibility and severity of interstitial lung diseases.
- Pneumoconioses and idiopathic pulmonary fibrosis are more common in men than women. A preponderance of sarcoidosis, lymphangioleiomyomatosis, and lymphocytic interstitial pneumonia in females has been reported.
- Experimental evidence has demonstrated sex-dependent differences in response to lung injury.
- Sex-stratified analyses should be implemented in future clinical trials.
- The idea of treating interstitial lung diseases with hormone analogs seems challenging and timely.

INTRODUCTION

Interstitial lung diseases (ILDs) encompass an amalgamated group of heterogeneous lung disorders, characterized by variable clinical and radiologic patterns.[1] A considerable proportion of patients with ILDs develop a progressive fibrosing phenotype, similar to idiopathic pulmonary fibrosis (IPF).[2–5] Despite an exponential increase in our knowledge for mechanistic insights associated with pulmonary fibrosis, the pathogenesis of ILDs remains largely unknown.[6,7]

Experimental evidence for the role of sex hormones in lung development coupled with epidemiologic associations of gender difference with ILDs prevalence fueled studies investigating the role of sex hormones and gender in the pathogenesis of pulmonary fibrosis.[8,9] In particular, sex hormones are critical regulators of human lung development before and during the neonatal period. Male neonatal lungs present with significant differences than female neonatal lungs in several aspects, such as surfactant production and alveolar surface area.[10] Gender has been associated with the prevalence, susceptibility, and severity of various chronic lung diseases including ILDs.[11] IPF is more prevalent with worse prognosis in males compared with females.[12] Lymphangioleiomyomatosis (LAM) affects almost exclusively young to middle-aged women[13,14] (**Fig. 1**). The aforementioned reports have led to mechanistic insights identifying a critical role of hormonal signaling in the pathogenesis of lung fibrosis.[8] This review article summarizes the experimental and clinical data on the impact of gender and sex hormones on ILDs.

SEX HORMONES AND LUNG DEVELOPMENT

Sex differences influence lung development and maturation.[11] Male fetuses exhibit increased alveolar surface area and alveoli compared with female fetuses at any given gestational age.[15,16] Large airway growth rates are higher than those of lung parenchyma in young females. On the other hand, growth rates of large airways in male lungs lag behind, thus leading to a phenomenon coined out as dysanaptic lung growth.[11,17]

Conflict of interest: None to declare.
Department of Respiratory Medicine, University Hospital of Patras, Greece.
* Corresponding author.
E-mail address: argyrios.tzouvelekis@fleming.gr

Clin Chest Med 42 (2021) 531–541
https://doi.org/10.1016/j.ccm.2021.04.011

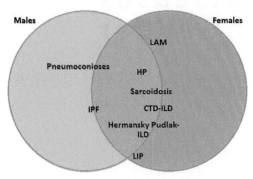

Fig. 1. Schematic representation of interstitial lung diseases occurring disproportionately between males and females. CTD, connective tissue disease; HP, hypersensitivity pneumonitis; LIP, lymphocytic interstitial pneumonitis.

Conducting airways of adult females are smaller compared with males of the same lung size.[11]

There is established experimental evidence showing that sex hormones are critical regulators of lung development.[10] Androgen receptors are increased in epithelial cells of budding sites and modulated bronchiole budding in the early human fetal lung.[18] Androgens inhibit surfactant production through direct or indirect effects of epidermal growth factor and transforming growth factor β1 (TGF-β1) on type II alveolar epithelial cells in a variety of animal models.[19] Surfactant production commences at earlier developmental stages in females than males.[20,21] Male neonates present with lower alveolar sodium transport than females in rats.[22] Estrogen levels influence lung development through effects of platelet-derived growth factor and granulocyte macrophage colony-stimulating factor signaling pathways on alveolar structure, lung elasticity and surfactant production.[23,24] The regulation of estrogen receptors (ERs) occurs through several microRNAs including microRNAs 221/222, 9, 193, 18, 625-5p, 22-3p, let-7 family modulating alveolar regeneration and extracellular matrix in mice.[8,25–28] Deletion of ERβ in female mice has been associated with increased alveolar size and decreased alveolar surface area.[29] Therapeutic effects of 17β-estradiol replacement against age-related lung disease in estrogen-deficient C57BL/6J mice has been demonstrated. In line with these findings, estrogens exhibit protective effects against cigarette smoke-induced lung injury in animal models.[30,31] Finally, the role of progesterone in lung development has been also studied. Reports have associated progesterone with decreased contractility and increased relaxation of bronchial smooth muscle, as well as with strong vasodilator effects in pulmonary arteries of both male and female rats.[32,33]

SEX HORMONES IN THE PATHOGENESIS OF PULMONARY FIBROSIS AND INTERSTITIAL LUNG DISEASES: EXPERIMENTAL DATA

Experimental evidence has demonstrated sex-dependent differences in response to lung injury[34–36] (**Table 1**). Profibrogenic pathways associated with metalloproteinases, AKT, and TGF-β have been shown to be mediated by sex hormones and mainly by ER activation.[10,37–40]

Studies have shown a female preponderance in mortality rates in modeled lung fibrosis, as indicated by increased levels of lung collagen deposition and profibrotic cytokine; however, follow-up data yielded contradictory results.[41] Another report demonstrated that aged male mice developed more severe fibrotic lung disease, as indicated by increased mortality, increased collagen deposition, and increased levels of profibrotic cytokines and neutrophils in bronchoalveolar lavage fluid compared with aged female mice or young mice of either sex.[42] In line with this finding, male sex hormones might exacerbate lung function impairment after bleomycin-induced lung fibrosis, because male mice presented with a more pronounced decrease in static lung compliance after bleomycin administration compared with females.[43] The effect of aging seem to favor female sex in terms of severity of modeled lung fibrosis.[41] Ovariectomy diminished pulmonary fibrosis in bleomycin-treated rats, whereas estradiol restored in vivo fibrotic responses.[41] Experimental data have shown that male hamsters immunized with trinitrochloro-1-benzene were less susceptible to lung fibrosis development compared with female littermates.[44] Sex-specific differences in osteopontin levels contributed to the differential sensitivity of male and female mice with regard to silica-induced lung fibrosis development.[45]

A recent seminal report showed upregulation of ERα expression in IPF lung tissue and fibroblasts both at the messenger RNA and protein levels.[8] Pharmacologic inhibition and mimicry of ERα and ERβ, respectively, attenuated bleomycin-induced pulmonary fibrosis. ERα antagonism exerted its antifibrotic effects through negative regulation of profibrotic pathways, such as Smad2 and AKT (protein kinase B). Furthermore, upregulation of let-7a and let-7d exerted antifibrotic effects through the downregulation of ERα and TGF-b and increased expression of Smad7 in IPF lung myofibroblasts.[8,46] Insulin-like growth factor-1, a profibrotic mediator and an ER signal transduction pathway stimulator, was upregulated in both IPF lungs and myofibroblasts, but mediated ER transcriptional activity only in the IPF lung fibroblasts.[8]

Table 1
Experimental data for the role of sex hormones in pulmonary fibrosis and interstitial lung diseases

Authors	Main Findings	Reference
Gharaee-Kermani et al	More severe fibrosis in female rats than males/Ovariectomy diminished pulmonary fibrosis in bleomycin-treated rats/Estradiol restored fibrotic response	41
Kimura et al	Female hamsters immunized with trinitrochloro-1-benzene more susceptible to lung fibrosis	44
Elliot et al	In vivo inhibition and mimicry of ERα and ERβ, respectively, attenuated bleomycin-induced pulmonary fibrosis/let-7a and let-7d downregulated ERα, TGF-b and increased Smad7	8
Glassberg et al	ER activation contributed to the progression of pulmonary lymphangioleiomyomatosis	51
Smith et al	TGFβ1 repressed ER expression	47
Tofovic et al	2-methoxyestradiol was protective against bleomycin-induced pulmonary fibrosis and PH	48
Flores-Delgado et al	Antifibrotic role of estrogens through Raf1 and ERK1/2 mitogen-activated protein	49
Morani et al	ERβ crucial for the maintenance of extracellular matrix composition in mice lungs	50
Redente et al	Aged male mice developed more severe fibrotic lung disease than females or young mice	42
Voltz et al	More pronounced post-bleomycin-decline in static lung compliance in male mice	43

In contrast with these findings, previous data showed a decreased expression of the ESR1 gene and ER protein in IPF lung tissues of patients undergoing lung transplantation.[47] In the same study, TGF-β1 repressed ER expression, suggesting a reciprocal interaction between profibrotic signal transduction pathways and sex hormones.[47] Nonestrogenic metabolite 2-methoxyestradiol showed protective effects in bleomycin-induced pulmonary fibrosis and associated pulmonary hypertension in male and female rats.[40] Nongenomic estrogen action exerted antifibrotic properties in adult, human, lung myofibroblasts through regulation of Raf1 and ERK1/2 mitogen-activated protein.[49] ERβ seemed to have a cardinal role for the maintenance of extracellular matrix composition in mice lungs.[50]

Similarly with pulmonary fibrosis, experimental data have implicated hormones in the pathogenesis of other ILDs, including LAM. ER activation contributed to the progression of pulmonary LAM through matrix metalloproteinase-induced cell invasiveness.[51,52] Estrogens accelerated angiomyolipoma cells' growth through AKT activation in a mouse xenograft model.[53] Similar proliferative effects of estrogens have been shown on Eker rat uterine leiomyoma-derived smooth muscle cells, as well as primary cultures of human LAM-associated angiomyolipoma cells.[54,55] In vitro studies on the tuberous sclerosis complex gene 2-null Eker rat embryonic fibroblasts demonstrated that prolactin increased cell proliferation through the activation of protein kinase pathways, including mitogen-activated kinase.[56] Unfortunately, hormone replacement therapies in experimental models of LAM yielded contradictory results.[52,55,57,58]

Taken together, abundant evidence has highlighted the critical role of sex hormones in experimental lung fibrosis. Their exact role seems complex and remains to be addressed. Contradictory results could be attributed to disease heterogeneity and extent, as well as the use of nonrepresentative of human disease animal models.

THE ROLE OF SEX IN THE EPIDEMIOLOGY OF INTERSTITIAL LUNG DISEASES: CLINICAL DATA
Idiopathic Pulmonary Fibrosis

It is well-known that IPF represents a disease paradigm with male predominance.[59] This knowledge has led to several misconceptions about and the underdiagnosis of this disease in female individuals.[60] In recent registries, real-life data, and clinical trials, males comprised between 50% and 82% of all patients diagnosed with

IPF.[61–69] Males presented with differences in terms of genetics that confer susceptibility to the disease.[70,71] The overall penetrance of pulmonary fibrosis in carriers of genes encoding telomerase was greater in males than females.[72]

Male patients with IPF have been linked to worse lung function and an increased burden of comorbidities, including cardiovascular disease at the time of diagnosis compared with female individuals.[73–75] Besides baseline functional status, gender impacts several patient-reported outcomes related to quality of life, degree of dyspnea, and cognitive and psychiatric disorders.[76]

With regard to treatment modalities, female sex and a lower baseline body mass index have been suggested as predictors of poor tolerance to antifibrotic drugs.[77] It remains to be addressed whether female sex is solely responsible for this or if the lower body surface area of female patients may provide an additional explanation. A recent study reported that older patients with IPF were more susceptible to antifibrotic dose reduction. This characteristic was unique to older male individuals; however, the number of females enrolled in the study (n = 17) was too limited to draw definite conclusions.[78] Importantly, males had significantly worse post-transplant survival.[79] Finally, several lines of evidence showed a "survival benefit" for females with IPF compared with males.[12,75,80–82]

On the basis of these findings, sex has been used as a reliable disease prognosticator either as a univariate variable or as a part of a multidimensional index and staging system for IPF, denominated as the Gender–Age–Physiology Index.[83]

Sarcoidosis

In contrast with IPF, sarcoidosis is a disease paradigm of female preponderance across all ethnic and racial groups in most reports.[84–88] Its incidence seemed to be even higher in African American women, with a reported yearly incidence of 71 per 100,000.[89] A bimodal age distribution of sarcoidosis incidence rates with the first peak of incidence between 20 and 39 years and the second between 50 and 60 years has been shown.[86,87] Interestingly, late-onset sarcoidosis was more common in females than males.[85,90–92]

Distinct clinical phenotypes based on sex have been reported[93] (**Table 2**). In particular, calcium metabolism abnormalities and pulmonary and cardiac involvement have been described more frequently in males, whereas females have been reported to be more prone to peripheral lymphadenopathy and the cutaneous, liver, and ocular manifestations of this disease.[94–97] Female-predominant characteristics of eye involvement included cystoid macular edema and scleritis.[94] Neurosarcoidosis has demonstrated an increased incidence in African American women.[98–100] The rare entity of bone sarcoidosis might be more common in women and especially in advanced disease.[101] Lupus pernio was encountered more frequently in women compared with men and was associated with chronic disease and extrapulmonary involvement.[102] The acute variant of sarcoidosis, called Löfgren's syndrome, presented differently in men and women.[103] Erythema nodosum was observed predominantly in females, whereas marked ankle periarticular arthritis or inflammation or arthritis without erythema nodosum was more common in males.[103]

Women with sarcoidosis have a lower health-related quality of life as well as greater degree of functional impairment compared with men.[104,105] Fertility and pregnancy have been important contributors to patients' quality of life in women of childbearing age. Current evidence suggests that

Table 2		
Clinical manifestations of sarcoidosis that are more common in males or females		
More Common Manifestations in Males	**More Common Manifestations in Females**	
Calcium metabolism abnormalities	Peripheral lymphadenopathy	
Pulmonary manifestations	Cutaneous manifestations	
Cardiac manifestations	Liver manifestations	
Ankle periarticular arthritis	Ocular manifestations	
	Neurologic manifestations	
	Musculoskeletal manifestations	
	Lupus pernio	
	Erythema nodosum	

sarcoidosis does not affect fertility and rarely affects the course of pregnancy.[81,106] However, treatment with steroid-sparing agents including methotrexate during pregnancy could be detrimental and may lead to teratogenicity.[94]

Finally, female sex has been associated with increased mortality compared with males.[107] Further features leading to poorer prognosis were diagnosis of sarcoidosis in African Americans and development of sarcoidosis-associated pulmonary hypertension.[107–109]

Connective Tissue Disease-Associated Interstitial Lung Disease

Female predominance in connective tissue disease-associated ILDs has been reported to be as high as 10:1 to 20:1,[110] with the highest ratios noted in systemic sclerosis, systemic lupus erythematosus, and Sjögren syndrome.[111,112] Rheumatoid arthritis is also more common in females, yet the female to male ratio is lower (2:1–3:1).[113–115]

Recent registries have shown female predominance not only in connective tissue disease ILDs, but also in lung-dominant connective tissue disease variants, including interstitial pneumonia with autoimmune features.[116–118] In contrast, female sex seems to confer a protective phenotype against fibrosis development in patients with connective tissue disease ILDs. In particular, male sex was a risk factor for pulmonary fibrosis development in rheumatoid arthritis, as well as for fibrotic lung disease and pulmonary hypertension in systemic sclerosis.[113–116,119,120] Studies investigating quality of life during the disease course showed increased rates of depression and worse quality of life in females with rheumatoid arthritis compared with males, but were inconclusive for sex-dependent differences in patients with systemic sclerosis.[119,121] Finally, male sex portended poorer prognosis in both rheumatoid arthritis and systemic sclerosis.[122–124]

Lymphangioleiomyomatosis

LAM has been established as an ILD occurring almost exclusively in females either sporadically or in association with tuberous sclerosis complex.[125] Pulmonary involvement in tuberous sclerosis has been strongly associated with premenopausal women.[125] The epidemiologic evidence that LAM was a typical paradigm of one of the strongest sex predispositions in human diseases fueled mechanistic investigations for the precise site of LAM cells' origin and for the effects of hormones on cell proliferation, cell metabolism, lymphangiogenesis and destruction of pulmonary parenchyma.[126] Expression of ER and progesterone receptor in pulmonary LAM specimens and renal angiomyolipoma cells was consistent with a hormone receptor-dependent model of disease progression.[127] Increased prolactin has been suggested as a negative prognosticator in LAM.[56] Recent data demonstrated that targeting ERs might be efficacious in the treatment of LAM either as combination with the mammalian target of rapamycin inhibitor sirolimus or as monotherapy.[58,128]

Other Interstitial Lung Diseases

Other ILDs occurring disproportionately between sexes include lymphocytic interstitial pneumonitis (LIP), ILD in Hermansky–Pudlak syndrome, and pneumoconioses.[52,129,130] LIP and ILD in Hermansky–Pudlak syndrome have been associated with a less pronounced female prevalence than LAM. The majority of patients with LIP are middle aged females, partially because LIP is strongly associated with Sjögren syndrome.[131] ILD in Hermansky–Pudlak syndrome is a rare entity with no effective treatment other than lung transplantation; it affects mainly females during childhood or between 30 and 40 years of age.[132–134] A slight female predominance has been recorded in hypersensitivity pneumonitis.[135–137] Men are more likely to develop pneumoconioses, possibly because they are more likely to have occupational exposures.[138,139] Most of the rest ILDs do not present with a clear sex predominance or the literature is still inconclusive.[52,140,141]

FUTURE PERSPECTIVES AND CONCLUDING REMARKS

There is substantial epidemiologic evidence that sex impacts the prevalence, susceptibility, and severity of ILDs. This evidence couples with recent experimental data suggesting a cardinal role of sex hormones in the pathogenesis of pulmonary fibrosis.

During the last years, we have experienced transformative events in the field of ILDs and guidelines have unified our clinical approach.[142–145] However, there is still a need to integrate sex and gender differences into personalized medicine approaches. Toward this direction, guidelines encompassing sex in the report of cellular and animal models are of paramount importance. Sex-stratified analyses should be implemented in future clinical trials. Recent findings highlight the need for further investigation of antifibrotics ideal dosage in females with low body mass index.[77] It remains to be addressed if hormone differences are associated with ILDs per se or represent an epiphenomenon. Sex-specified analyses of genome-wide association studies could improve our knowledge on the role of sex and gender on disease prognosis and treatment response. Sex-based approaches would be also fruitful for better understanding of the impact of hormone replacement therapy on ILDs including thyroid hormone, androgen analogues, and vitamin D.[130]

The idea of treating ILDs with hormone analogs seems challenging and timely.[146] Experimental reports for hormone analogues were promising and thus various hormone analogues have already entered the pipeline of clinical trials for lung diseases.[147] Lungs of patients with IPF are locally hypothyroid, whereas the aerosolized administration of active thyroid hormone and systemic delivery of sobetirome, a thyroid-hormone receptor agonist, alleviated experimental lung fibrosis through restoration of alveolar epithelial cell mitochondrial homeostasis.[148] The antidiabetic compound metformin exerted antifibrotic properties experimentally through positive regulation of adenosine monophosphate–activated protein kinase.[149] Potential therapeutic applicability of targeting progesterone deserves further investigation, given the expression of progesterone receptor within fibrotic areas of patients with usual interstitial pneumonia.[150] The androgen danazol reconstituted telomere length in patients with features of short-telomere syndrome, such as pulmonary fibrosis and bone marrow failure.[151,152] The steroid prohormones dehydroepiandrosterone and vitamin D were decreased in patients with IPF and exerted antifibrotic effects experimentally.[153,154]

Drug repositioning makes intuitive sense. Understanding local and systemic hormonal disparities and implementation of local hormone administration might provide clinical benefit with minimal adverse events.[9] Future well-designed, sex-based, and biologically enriched trials are sorely needed.

CLINICS CARE POINTS

- Pneumoconioses and Idiopathic Pulmonary Fibrosis are more common in men than women.
- A preponderance of Sarcoidosis, Lymphangioleiomyomatosis and Lymphocytic Interstitial Pneumonitis in females has been reported.
- Calcium metabolism abnormalities, pulmonary and cardiac involvement have been

described more frequently in males with sarcoidosis, while females with sarcoidosis have been reportedly more prone to peripheral lymphadenopathy, cutaneous, liver and ocular manifestations.

REFERENCES

1. Travis WD, Costabel U, Hansell DM, et al. An official American Thoracic Society/European Respiratory Society statement: update of the international multidisciplinary classification of the idiopathic interstitial pneumonias. Am J Respir Crit Care Med 2013;188(6):733–48.
2. Kolb M, Vasakova M. The natural history of progressive fibrosing interstitial lung diseases. Respir Res 2019;20(1):57.
3. Flaherty KR, Wells AU, Cottin V, et al. Nintedanib in progressive fibrosing interstitial lung diseases. N Engl J Med 2019;381(18):1718–27.
4. Cottin V, Wollin L, Fischer A, et al. Fibrosing interstitial lung diseases: knowns and unknowns. Eur Respir Rev 2019;28(151):180100.
5. Wells AU, Brown KK, Flaherty KR, et al. What's in a name? That which we call IPF, by any other name would act the same. Eur Respir J 2018;51(5):1800692.
6. Sgalla G, Iovene B, Calvello M, et al. Idiopathic pulmonary fibrosis: pathogenesis and management. Respir Res 2018;19(1):32.
7. Bagnato G, Harari S. Cellular interactions in the pathogenesis of interstitial lung diseases. Eur Respir Rev 2015;24(135):102–14.
8. Elliot S, Periera-Simon S, Xia X, et al. MicroRNA let-7 downregulates ligand-independent estrogen receptor-mediated male-predominant pulmonary fibrosis. Am J Respir Crit Care Med 2019;200(10):1246–57.
9. Tzouvelekis A, Bouros D. Estrogen signaling and MicroRNAs in lung fibrosis. Sex, hormones, and rock scars. Am J Respir Crit Care Med 2019;200(10):1199–200.
10. Carey MA, Card JW, Voltz JW, et al. The impact of sex and sex hormones on lung physiology and disease: lessons from animal studies. Am J Physiol Lung Cell Mol Physiol 2007;293(2):L272–8.
11. Carey MA, Card JW, Voltz JW, et al. It's all about sex: gender, lung development and lung disease. Trends Endocr Metab 2007;18(8):308–13.
12. Olson AL, Swigris JJ, Lezotte DC, et al. Mortality from pulmonary fibrosis increased in the United States from 1992 to 2003. Am J Respir Crit Care Med 2007;176(3):277–84.
13. Gleicher N, Barad DH. Gender as risk factor for autoimmune diseases. J Autoimmun 2007;28(1):1–6.

14. Gupta NFG, Kotloff RM, Strange C, et al. ATS Assembly on clinical Problems. Lymphangioleiomyomatosis diagnosis and management: high-resolution chest Computed Tomography, Transbronchial lung biopsy, and Pleural disease management. An official American thoracic society/Japanese respiratory society clinical practice guideline. Am J Respir Crit Care Med 2017;196(10):1337–48.

15. Binet ME, Bujold E, Lefebvre F, et al. Role of gender in morbidity and mortality of extremely premature neonates. Am J perinatology. 2012;29(3):159–66.

16. Thurlbeck WM. Postnatal human lung growth. Thorax 1982;37(8):564–71.

17. Llapur CJ, Martinez MR, Grassino PT, et al. Chronic hypoxia accentuates dysanaptic lung growth. Am J Respir Crit Care Med 2016;194(3):327–32.

18. Kimura Y, Suzuki T, Kaneko C, et al. Expression of androgen receptor and 5alpha-reductase types 1 and 2 in early gestation fetal lung: a possible correlation with branching morphogenesis. Clin Sci (Lond) 2003;105(6):709–13.

19. Dammann CE, Ramadurai SM, McCants DD, et al. Androgen regulation of signaling pathways in late fetal mouse lung development. Endocrinology 2000;141(8):2923–9.

20. Fleisher B, Kulovich MV, Hallman M, et al. Lung profile: sex differences in normal pregnancy. Obstet Gynecol 1985;66(3):327–30.

21. Townsel CD, Emmer SF, Campbell WA, et al. Gender differences in respiratory morbidity and mortality of preterm neonates. Front Pediatr 2017;5:6.

22. Kaltofen T, Haase M, Thome UH, et al. Male sex is associated with a reduced alveolar epithelial sodium transport. PLoS One 2015;10(8):e0136178.

23. Fuentes N, Silveyra P. Endocrine regulation of lung disease and inflammation. Exp Biol Med (Maywood) 2018;243(17–18):1313–22.

24. Massaro D, Massaro GD. Estrogen receptor regulation of pulmonary alveolar dimensions: alveolar sexual dimorphism in mice. Am J Physiol Lung Cell Mol Physiol 2006;290(5):L866–70.

25. Klinge CM. miRNAs regulated by estrogens, tamoxifen, and endocrine disruptors and their downstream gene targets. Mol Cell Endocrinol 2015;418(Pt 3):273–97.

26. Massaro D, Massaro GD. Estrogen regulates pulmonary alveolar formation, loss, and regeneration in mice. Am J Physiol Lung Cell Mol Physiol 2004;287(6):L1154–9.

27. Cochrane DR, Cittelly DM, Howe EN, et al. MicroRNAs link estrogen receptor alpha status and Dicer levels in breast cancer. Horm Cancer 2010;1(6):306–19.

28. Dong X, Xu M, Ren Z, et al. Regulation of CBL and ESR1 expression by microRNA-223p, 513a-5p and 625-5p may impact the pathogenesis of dust mite-induced pediatric asthma. Int J Mol Med 2016;38(2):446–56.

29. Patrone C, Cassel TN, Pettersson K, et al. Regulation of postnatal lung development and homeostasis by estrogen receptor beta. Mol Cell Biol 2003;23(23):8542–52.

30. Glassberg MK, Choi R, Manzoli V, et al. 17beta-estradiol replacement reverses age-related lung disease in estrogen-deficient C57BL/6J mice. Endocrinology 2014;155(2):441–8.

31. Glassberg MK, Catanuto P, Shahzeidi S, et al. Estrogen deficiency promotes cigarette smoke-induced changes in the extracellular matrix in the lungs of aging female mice. Transl Res 2016;178:107–17.

32. Perusquia M, Hernandez R, Montano LM, et al. Inhibitory effect of sex steroids on Guinea-pig airway smooth muscle contractions. Comp Biochem Physiol C, Pharmacol Toxicol Endocrinol 1997;118(1):5–10.

33. English KM, Jones RD, Jones TH, et al. Gender differences in the vasomotor effects of different steroid hormones in rat pulmonary and coronary arteries. Horm Metab Res 2001;33(11):645–52.

34. Sathish V, Martin YN, Prakash YS. Sex steroid signaling: implications for lung diseases. Pharmacol Ther 2015;150:94–108.

35. Garate-Carrillo A, Gonzalez J, Ceballos G, et al. Sex related differences in the pathogenesis of organ fibrosis. Transl Res 2020;222:41–55.

36. Card JW, Zeldin DC. Hormonal influences on lung function and response to environmental agents: lessons from animal models of respiratory disease. Proc Am Thorac Soc 2009;6(7):588–95.

37. Russo RC, Garcia CC, Barcelos LS, et al. Phosphoinositide 3-kinase gamma plays a critical role in bleomycin-induced pulmonary inflammation and fibrosis in mice. J Leukoc Biol 2011;89(2):269–82.

38. Park S, Ahn JY, Lim MJ, et al. Sustained expression of NADPH oxidase 4 by p38 MAPK-Akt signaling potentiates radiation-induced differentiation of lung fibroblasts. J Mol Med (Berlin, Germany) 2010;88(8):807–16.

39. Richter K, Kietzmann T. Reactive oxygen species and fibrosis: further evidence of a significant liaison. Cell Tissue Res 2016;365(3):591–605.

40. Craig VJ, Zhang L, Hagood JS, et al. Matrix metalloproteinases as therapeutic targets for idiopathic pulmonary fibrosis. Am J Respir Cell Mol Biol 2015;53(5):585–600.

41. Gharaee-Kermani M, Hatano K, Nozaki Y, et al. Gender-based differences in bleomycin-induced pulmonary fibrosis. Am J Pathol 2005;166(6):1593–606.

42. Redente EF, Jacobsen KM, Solomon JJ, et al. Age and sex dimorphisms contribute to the severity of

bleomycin-induced lung injury and fibrosis. Am J Physiol Lung Cell Mol Physiol 2011;301(4):L510–8.

43. Voltz JW, Card JW, Carey MA, et al. Male sex hormones exacerbate lung function impairment after bleomycin-induced pulmonary fibrosis. Am J Respir Cell Mol Biol 2008;39(1):45–52.

44. Kimura R, Hu H, Stein-Streilein J. Delayed-type hypersensitivity responses regulate collagen deposition in the lung. Immunology 1992;77(4):550–5.

45. Latoche JD, Ufelle AC, Fazzi F, et al. Secreted phosphoprotein 1 and sex-specific differences in silica-induced pulmonary fibrosis in mice. Environ Health Perspect 2016;124(8):1199–207.

46. Pandit KV, Corcoran D, Yousef H, et al. Inhibition and role of let-7d in idiopathic pulmonary fibrosis. Am J Respir Crit Care Med 2010;182(2):220–9.

47. Smith LC, Moreno S, Robertson L, et al. Transforming growth factor beta1 targets estrogen receptor signaling in bronchial epithelial cells. Respir Res 2018;19(1):160.

48. Tofovic SP, Zhang X, Jackson EK, et al. 2-methoxyestradiol attenuates bleomycin-induced pulmonary hypertension and fibrosis in estrogen-deficient rats. Vasc Pharmacol 2009;51(2–3): 190–7.

49. Flores-Delgado G, Bringas P, Buckley S, et al. Nongenomic estrogen action in human lung myofibroblasts. Biochem Biophys Res Commun 2001; 283(3):661–7.

50. Morani A, Barros RP, Imamov O, et al. Lung dysfunction causes systemic hypoxia in estrogen receptor beta knockout (ERbeta-/-) mice. Proc Natl Acad Sci U S A 2006;103(18):7165–9.

51. Glassberg MK, Elliot SJ, Fritz J, et al. Activation of the estrogen receptor contributes to the progression of pulmonary lymphangioleiomyomatosis via matrix metalloproteinase-induced cell invasiveness. J Clin Endocrinol Metab 2008;93(5):1625–33.

52. Shim B, Pacheco-Rodriguez G, Kato J, et al. Sex-specific lung diseases: effect of oestrogen on cultured cells and in animal models. Eur Respir Rev 2013;22(129):302–11.

53. Clements D, Asprey SL, McCulloch TA, et al. Analysis of the oestrogen response in an angiomyolipoma derived xenograft model. Endocr Related cancer 2009;16(1):59–72.

54. Howe SR, Gottardis MM, Everitt JI, et al. Estrogen stimulation and tamoxifen inhibition of leiomyoma cell growth in vitro and in vivo. Endocrinology 1995;136(11):4996–5003.

55. Yu J, Astrinidis A, Howard S, et al. Estradiol and tamoxifen stimulate LAM-associated angiomyolipoma cell growth and activate both genomic and nongenomic signaling pathways. Am J Physiol Lung Cell Mol Physiol 2004;286(4):L694–700.

56. Terasaki Y, Yahiro K, Pacheco-Rodriguez G, et al. Effects of prolactin on TSC2-null Eker rat cells and in pulmonary lymphangioleiomyomatosis. Am J Respir Crit Care Med 2010;182(4):531–9.

57. El-Hashemite N, Walker V, Kwiatkowski DJ. Estrogen enhances whereas tamoxifen retards development of Tsc mouse liver hemangioma: a tumor related to renal angiomyolipoma and pulmonary lymphangioleiomyomatosis. Cancer Res 2005; 65(6):2474–81.

58. Li C, Zhou X, Sun Y, et al. Faslodex inhibits estradiol-induced extracellular matrix dynamics and lung metastasis in a model of lymphangioleiomyomatosis. Am J Respir Cell Mol Biol 2013;49(1): 135–42.

59. Strek ME. Gender in idiopathic pulmonary fibrosis diagnosis: time to address unconscious bias. Thorax 2020;75(5):365–6.

60. Assayag D, Morisset J, Johannson KA, et al. Patient gender bias on the diagnosis of idiopathic pulmonary fibrosis. Thorax 2020;75(5):407–12.

61. Raghu G, Weycker D, Edelsberg J, et al. Incidence and prevalence of idiopathic pulmonary fibrosis. Am J Respir Crit Care Med 2006;174(7):810–6.

62. Raghu G, Chen SY, Hou Q, et al. Incidence and prevalence of idiopathic pulmonary fibrosis in US adults 18-64 years old. Eur Respir J 2016;48(1): 179–86.

63. Fernandez Perez ER, Daniels CE, Schroeder DR, et al. Incidence, prevalence, and clinical course of idiopathic pulmonary fibrosis: a population-based study. Chest. 2010;137(1):129–37.

64. Gribbin J, Hubbard RB, Le Jeune I, et al. Incidence and mortality of idiopathic pulmonary fibrosis and sarcoidosis in the UK. Thorax 2006;61(11):980–5.

65. Guenther A, Krauss E, Tello S, et al. The European IPF registry (eurIPFreg): baseline characteristics and survival of patients with idiopathic pulmonary fibrosis. Respir Res 2018;19(1):141.

66. Behr J, Kreuter M, Hoeper MM, et al. Management of patients with idiopathic pulmonary fibrosis in clinical practice: the INSIGHTS-IPF registry. Eur Respir J 2015;46(1):186–96.

67. Jo HE, Glaspole I, Grainge C, et al. Baseline characteristics of idiopathic pulmonary fibrosis: analysis from the Australian Idiopathic Pulmonary Fibrosis Registry. Eur Respir J 2017;49(2):1601592.

68. Richeldi L, du Bois RM, Raghu G, et al. Efficacy and safety of nintedanib in idiopathic pulmonary fibrosis. N Engl J Med 2014;370(22):2071–82.

69. King TE Jr, Bradford WZ, Castro-Bernardini S, et al. A phase 3 trial of pirfenidone in patients with idiopathic pulmonary fibrosis. N Engl J Med 2014; 370(22):2083–92.

70. Garcia CK. Idiopathic pulmonary fibrosis: update on genetic discoveries. Proc Am Thorac Soc 2011;8(2):158–62.

71. Borie R, Kannengiesser C, Nathan N, et al. Familial pulmonary fibrosis. Rev Mal Respir 2015;32(4): 413–34.

72. Diaz de Leon A, Cronkhite JT, Katzenstein AL, et al. Telomere lengths, pulmonary fibrosis and telomerase (TERT) mutations. PLoS One 2010;5(5):e10680.

73. Kalafatis D, Gao J, Pesonen I, et al. Gender differences at presentation of idiopathic pulmonary fibrosis in Sweden. BMC Pulm Med 2019;19(1):222.

74. Sese L, Nunes H, Cottin V, et al. Gender differences in idiopathic pulmonary fibrosis: are men and women equal or not? Eur Respir J 2020; 56(suppl 64):764.

75. Han MK, Murray S, Fell CD, et al. Sex differences in physiological progression of idiopathic pulmonary fibrosis. Eur Respir J 2008;31(6):1183–8.

76. Han MK, Swigris J, Liu L, et al. Gender influences health-related quality of life in IPF. Respir Med 2010;104(5):724–30.

77. Weir NA, Poreddy M, Scully A, et al. Gender and BMI Predict Antifibrotic Tolerance in IPF. B103. ILD: MANAGEMENT:A4259-A4259.

78. Harari S, Specchia C, Lipsi R, et al. Older idiopathic pulmonary fibrosis male patients are at a higher risk of nintedanib dose reduction. Respiration 2020;99(8):646–8.

79. Sheikh SI, Hayes D Jr, Kirkby SE, et al. Age-dependent gender disparities in post lung transplant survival among patients with idiopathic pulmonary fibrosis. Ann Thorac Surg 2017; 103(2):441–6.

80. Sauleda J, Nunez B, Sala E. Idiopathic pulmonary fibrosis: epidemiology, natural history, phenotypes. Med Sci (Basel) 2018;6(4):110.

81. Pandit P, Perez RL, Roman J. Sex-based differences in interstitial lung disease. Am J Med Sci 2020;360(5):467–73.

82. Zaman T, Moua T, Vittinghoff E, et al. Differences in clinical characteristics and outcomes between men and women with idiopathic pulmonary fibrosis: a multicenter retrospective cohort study. Chest 2020;158(1):245–51.

83. Ley B, Ryerson CJ, Vittinghoff E, et al. A multidimensional index and staging system for idiopathic pulmonary fibrosis. Ann Intern Med 2012;156(10):684–91.

84. Morimoto T, Azuma A, Abe S, et al. Epidemiology of sarcoidosis in Japan. Eur Respir J 2008;31(2):372–9.

85. Spagnolo P, Rossi G, Trisolini R, et al. Pulmonary sarcoidosis. Lancet Respir Med 2018;6(5): 389–402.

86. Govender P, Berman JS. The diagnosis of sarcoidosis. Clin Chest Med 2015;36(4):585–602.

87. Gerke AK, Judson MA, Cozier YC, et al. Disease burden and variability in sarcoidosis. Ann Am Thorac Soc 2017;14(Supplement_6):S421–8.

88. Valeyre D, Bernaudin JF, Jeny F, et al. Pulmonary sarcoidosis. Clin Chest Med 2015;36(4):631–41.

89. Cozier YC, Berman JS, Palmer JR, et al. Sarcoidosis in black women in the United States: data from the black Women's health study. Chest. 2011;139(1):144–50.

90. Rybicki BA, Major M, Popovich J Jr, et al. Racial differences in sarcoidosis incidence: a 5-year study in a health maintenance organization. Am J Epidemiol 1997;145(3):234–41.

91. Baughman RP, Field S, Costabel U, et al. Sarcoidosis in America. Analysis based on health Care use. Ann Am Thorac Soc 2016;13(8):1244–52.

92. Arkema EV, Grunewald J, Kullberg S, et al. Sarcoidosis incidence and prevalence: a nationwide register-based assessment in Sweden. Eur Respir J 2016;48(6):1690–9.

93. Iannuzzi MC, Rybicki BA, Teirstein AS. Sarcoidosis. N Engl J Med 2007;357(21):2153–65.

94. Birnbaum AD, Rifkin LM. Sarcoidosis: sex-dependent variations in presentation and management. J Ophthalmol 2014;2014:236905.

95. Yanardag H, Pamuk ON, Karayel T. Cutaneous involvement in sarcoidosis: analysis of the features in 170 patients. Respir Med 2003;97(8):978–82.

96. Ungprasert P, Crowson CS, Matteson EL. Influence of gender on epidemiology and clinical manifestations of sarcoidosis: a population-based retrospective cohort study 1976-2013. Lung 2017;195(1): 87–91.

97. Baughman RP, Teirstein AS, Judson MA, et al. Clinical characteristics of patients in a case control study of sarcoidosis. Am J Respir Crit Care Med 2001;164(10 Pt 1):1885–9.

98. Chapelon C, Ziza JM, Piette JC, et al. Neurosarcoidosis: signs, course and treatment in 35 confirmed cases. Medicine 1990;69(5):261–76.

99. Tavee JO, Stern BJ. Neurosarcoidosis. Clin Chest Med 2015;36(4):643–56.

100. Judson MA, Boan AD, Lackland DT. The clinical course of sarcoidosis: presentation, diagnosis, and treatment in a large white and black cohort in the United States. Sarcoidosis Vascu Diffuse Lung Dis 2012;29(2):119–27.

101. Aptel S, Lecocq-Teixeira S, Olivier P, et al. Multimodality evaluation of musculoskeletal sarcoidosis: imaging findings and literature review. Diagn Interv Imaging 2016;97(1):5–18.

102. Yanardag H, Pamuk ON, Pamuk GE. Lupus pernio in sarcoidosis: clinical features and treatment outcomes of 14 patients. J Clin Rheumatol 2003;9(2): 72–6.

103. Grunewald J, Eklund A. Sex-specific manifestations of Lofgren's syndrome. Am J Respir Crit Care Med 2007;175(1):40–4.

104. Bourbonnais JM, Samavati L. Clinical predictors of pulmonary hypertension in sarcoidosis. Eur Respir J 2008;32(2):296–302.

105. De Vries J, Van Heck GL, Drent M. Gender differences in sarcoidosis: symptoms, quality of life, and medical consumption. Women Health 1999; 30(2):99–114.

106. Budev MM, Arroliga AC, Emery S. Exacerbation of underlying pulmonary disease in pregnancy. Crit Care Med 2005;33(10 Suppl):S313–8.

107. Swigris JJ, Olson AL, Huie TJ, et al. Sarcoidosis-related mortality in the United States from 1988 to 2007. Am J Respir Crit Care Med 2011;183(11): 1524–30.

108. Karampitsakos T, Tzouvelekis A, Chrysikos S, et al. Pulmonary hypertension in patients with interstitial lung disease. Pulm Pharmacol Ther 2018;50: 38–46.

109. Parikh KS, Dahhan T, Nicholl L, et al. Clinical features and outcomes of patients with sarcoidosis-associated pulmonary hypertension. Sci Rep 2019;9(1):4061.

110. Ortona E, Pierdominici M, Maselli A, et al. Sex-based differences in autoimmune diseases. Ann Ist Super Sanita 2016;52(2):205–12.

111. Hayter SM, Cook MC. Updated assessment of the prevalence, spectrum and case definition of autoimmune disease. Autoimmun Rev 2012;11(10): 754–65.

112. Zandman-Goddard G, Peeva E, Shoenfeld Y. Gender and autoimmunity. Autoimmun Rev 2007; 6(6):366–72.

113. Koduri G, Norton S, Young A, et al. Interstitial lung disease has a poor prognosis in rheumatoid arthritis: results from an inception cohort. Rheumatology (Oxford) 2010;49(8):1483–9.

114. Gabbay E, Tarala R, Will R, et al. Interstitial lung disease in recent onset rheumatoid arthritis. Am J Respir Crit Care Med 1997;156(2 Pt 1):528–35.

115. Lake F, Proudman S. Rheumatoid arthritis and lung disease: from mechanisms to a practical approach. Semin Respir Crit Care Med 2014; 35(2):222–38.

116. Pan L, Liu Y, Sun R, et al. Comparison of characteristics of connective tissue disease-associated interstitial lung diseases, undifferentiated connective tissue disease-associated interstitial lung diseases, and idiopathic pulmonary fibrosis in Chinese Han Population: a Retrospective Study. Clin Dev Immunol 2013;2013:121578.

117. Sambataro G, Sambataro D, Torrisi SE, et al. Clinical, serological and radiological features of a prospective cohort of Interstitial Pneumonia with Autoimmune Features (IPAF) patients. Respir Med 2019;150:154–60.

118. Chartrand S, Swigris JJ, Stanchev L, et al. Clinical features and natural history of interstitial pneumonia with autoimmune features: a single center experience. Respir Med 2016;119:150–4.

119. Nguyen C, Berezne A, Baubet T, et al. Association of gender with clinical expression, quality of life, disability, and depression and anxiety in patients with systemic sclerosis. PLoS One 2011;6(3): e17551.

120. Ferri C, Valentini G, Cozzi F, et al. Systemic sclerosis: demographic, clinical, and serologic features and survival in 1,012 Italian patients. Medicine 2002;81(2):139–53.

121. Aurrecoechea E, Llorca Diaz J, Diez Lizuain ML, et al. Gender-associated comorbidities in rheumatoid arthritis and their impact on outcome: data from GENIRA. Rheumatol Int 2017;37(4):479–85.

122. Anderson ST. Mortality in rheumatoid arthritis: do age and gender make a difference? Semin Arthritis Rheum 1996;25(5):291–6.

123. Hesselstrand R, Scheja A, Akesson A. Mortality and causes of death in a Swedish series of systemic sclerosis patients. Ann Rheum Dis 1998; 57(11):682–6.

124. Al-Dhaher FF, Pope JE, Ouimet JM. Determinants of morbidity and mortality of systemic sclerosis in Canada. Semin Arthritis Rheum 2010;39(4):269–77.

125. Taveira-DaSilva AM, Pacheco-Rodriguez G, Moss J. The natural history of lymphangioleiomyomatosis: markers of severity, rate of progression and prognosis. Lymphatic Res Biol 2010;8(1):9–19.

126. Gu X, Yu JJ, Ilter D, et al. Integration of mTOR and estrogen-ERK2 signaling in lymphangioleiomyomatosis pathogenesis. Proc Natl Acad Sci U S A 2013; 110(37):14960–5.

127. Logginidou H, Ao X, Russo I, et al. Frequent estrogen and progesterone receptor immunoreactivity in renal angiomyolipomas from women with pulmonary lymphangioleiomyomatosis. Chest 2000; 117(1):25–30.

128. Bissler JJ, McCormack FX, Young LR, et al. Sirolimus for angiomyolipoma in tuberous sclerosis complex or lymphangioleiomyomatosis. N Engl J Med 2008;358(2):140–51.

129. Pinkerton KE, Harbaugh M, Han MK, et al. Women and lung disease. Sex differences and global health disparities. Am J Respir Crit Care Med 2015;192(1):11–6.

130. Han MK, Arteaga-Solis E, Blenis J, et al. Female sex and gender in lung/sleep health and disease. Increased understanding of basic biological, Pathophysiological, and behavioral mechanisms leading to better health for female patients with lung disease. Am J Respir Crit Care Med 2018;198(7): 850–8.

131. Swigris JJ, Berry GJ, Raffin TA, et al. Lymphoid interstitial pneumonia: a narrative review. Chest 2002;122(6):2150–64.

132. Hengst M, Naehrlich L, Mahavadi P, et al. Hermansky-Pudlak syndrome type 2 manifests with fibrosing lung disease early in childhood. Orphanet J Rare Dis 2018;13(1):42.

133. El-Chemaly S, O'Brien KJ, Nathan SD, et al. Clinical management and outcomes of patients with Hermansky-Pudlak syndrome pulmonary fibrosis evaluated for lung transplantation. PLoS One 2018;13(3):e0194193.

134. Vicary GW, Vergne Y, Santiago-Cornier A, et al. Pulmonary fibrosis in Hermansky-Pudlak syndrome. Ann Am Thorac Soc 2016;13(10):1839–46.

135. Lacasse Y, Selman M, Costabel U, et al. Clinical diagnosis of hypersensitivity pneumonitis. Am J Respir Crit Care Med 2003;168(8):952–8.

136. Fernandez Perez ER, Kong AM, Raimundo K, et al. Epidemiology of hypersensitivity pneumonitis among an insured population in the United States: a Claims-based cohort analysis. Ann Am Thorac Soc 2018;15(4):460–9.

137. Jacob J, Bartholmai BJ, Egashira R, et al. Chronic hypersensitivity pneumonitis: identification of key prognostic determinants using automated CT analysis. BMC Pulm Med 2017;17(1):81.

138. Zhao JQ, Li JG, Zhao CX. Prevalence of pneumoconiosis among young adults aged 24-44 years in a heavily industrialized province of China. J Occup Health 2019;61(1):73–81.

139. Amar RK, Jick SS, Rosenberg D, et al. Incidence of the pneumoconioses in the United Kingdom general population between 1997 and 2008. Respiration 2012;84(3):200–6.

140. Torre O, Elia D, Caminati A, et al. New insights in lymphangioleiomyomatosis and pulmonary Langerhans cell histiocytosis. Eur Respir Rev 2017; 26(145):170042.

141. Sieminska A, Kuziemski K. Respiratory bronchiolitis-interstitial lung disease. Orphanet J Rare Dis 2014;9:106.

142. Kawano-Dourado L, Glassberg MK, Molina-Molina M, et al. Gender equity in interstitial lung disease. Lancet Respir Med 2020;8(9):842–3.

143. Raghu GR-JM, Myers JL, Richeldi L, et al. Diagnosis of idiopathic pulmonary fibrosis. an official ATS/ERS/JRS/ALAT clinical practice guideline. Am J Respir Crit Care Med 2018;198(5):e44–68.

144. Crouser ED, Maier LA, Wilson KC, et al. Diagnosis and detection of sarcoidosis. an official american thoracic society clinical practice guideline. Am J Respir Crit Care Med 2020;201(8):e26–51.

145. Raghu G, Remy-Jardin M, Ryerson CJ, et al. Diagnosis of hypersensitivity pneumonitis in adults. an official ATS/JRS/ALAT clinical practice guideline. Am J Respir Crit Care Med 2020;202(3):e36–69.

146. Papaioannou O, Karampitsakos T, Barbayianni I, et al. Metabolic disorders in chronic lung diseases. Front Med 2017;4:246.

147. Available at: https://clinicaltrials.gov/ct2/show/NCT04115514?term=T3&cond=ARDS&draw=2&rank=1. Accessed March 23, 2021.

148. Yu G, Tzouvelekis A, Wang R, et al. Thyroid hormone inhibits lung fibrosis in mice by improving epithelial mitochondrial function. Nat Med 2018; 24(1):39–49.

149. Rangarajan S, Bone NB, Zmijewska AA, et al. Metformin reverses established lung fibrosis in a bleomycin model. Nat Med 2018;24(8):1121–7.

150. Mehrad M, Trejo Bittar HE, Yousem SA. Sex steroid receptor expression in idiopathic pulmonary fibrosis. Hum Pathol 2017;66:200–5.

151. Jouneau S, Kerjouan M, Ricordel C. Danazol treatment for telomere diseases. N Engl J Med 2016; 375(11):1095.

152. Townsley DM, Dumitriu B, Young NS. Danazol treatment for telomere diseases. N Engl J Med 2016; 375(11):1095–6.

153. Mendoza-Milla C, Valero Jimenez A, Rangel C, et al. Dehydroepiandrosterone has strong antifibrotic effects and is decreased in idiopathic pulmonary fibrosis. Eur Respir J 2013;42(5):1309–21.

154. Tzilas V, Bouros E, Barbayianni I, et al. Vitamin D prevents experimental lung fibrosis and predicts survival in patients with idiopathic pulmonary fibrosis. Pulm Pharmacol Ther 2019;55:17–24.

Gender Differences in Critical Illness and Critical Care Research

Tasnim I. Lat, DO*, Meghan K. McGraw, MD, Heath D. White, DO

KEYWORDS

- Gender • Female • Estrogen • Critical illness • Obstetrics • SARS-CoV-2 • Sepsis • ARDS

KEY POINTS

- Male patients gain admission to the intensive care unit and use resources in the intensive care unit more than female patients.
- Estrogen may have a protective effect in critical illness.
- Women receive less appropriate management of the acute respiratory distress syndrome than men.
- No consistent differences in sepsis outcomes by sex have been found, but women receive less timely initiation of antibiotics.
- Women are more likely to experience hypoactive delirium while in the intensive care unit and have worse functional outcomes after discharge.

INTRODUCTION

Research regarding the impact both social and genetic determinants of health play in admission to the intensive care unit (ICU) and outcomes from an ICU stay have gained traction in critical care literature in recent years. Determinants such as race and socioeconomic status are more commonly discussed; less explored is the impact of sex or gender on critical illness because women have historically been excluded from clinical trials or had limited participation, a problem that the US Food and Drug Administration has acknowledged previously and attempted to address.[1]

It is vital to understand the impact of gender on admission to the ICU as well as the influence of sex in various disease states in order for ICU clinicians to be able to apply the principles of precision medicine to their patients admitted to the ICU. In this article, we explore the research into and the impact of gender on admission into the ICU and the use of ICU resources, gender dimorphism in sepsis, the impact of gender on acute respiratory distress syndrome (ARDS), research regarding obstetrics critical care and outcomes, and the impact of gender on ICU mortality, delirium, and functional outcomes.

EPIDEMIOLOGY

Multiple epidemiologic studies have observed sex-related differences in admission to the ICU as well as the use of ICU resources. Many of these studies were performed in ICUs outside of the United States and have consistently demonstrated lower admission rates for women to ICUs despite similar severity of illness between men and women or even a greater severity of illness in women.[2–7] In a study performed by Blecha and colleagues[3] in Germany of more than 20,000 patients, male patients were more likely to undergo tracheostomy, dialysis, extracorporeal membrane oxygenation, and pulmonary artery catheter insertion despite similar severity of illness to female patients; additionally, the male patients had a longer duration of mechanical ventilation. Another study

Division of Pulmonary, Critical Care & Sleep Medicine, Baylor Scott & White Health, 2401 South 31st Street, Temple, TX 76508, USA
* Corresponding author.
E-mail address: Tasnim.Lat@BSWHealth.org

Clin Chest Med 42 (2021) 543–555
https://doi.org/10.1016/j.ccm.2021.04.012
0272-5231/21/© 2021 Elsevier Inc. All rights reserved.

performed in Austria by Valentin and colleagues[4] of more than 25,000 patients in 31 ICUs found that men were more likely to undergo invasive treatments with mechanical ventilation, vasopressor use, and intracranial pressure management compared with women, despite a higher severity of illness in women; this study also noted that 58.3% of patients admitted were male and 41.7% of admitted patients were female. This preponderance of males gaining admission to ICUs and using more ICU resources more than females may be due to several reasons. First, this difference may be a consequence of goals of care and end-of-life discussions; in a study by Sharma and colleagues,[8] male patients with advanced cancer who had of end-of-life discussions were more likely to receive aggressive, nonbeneficial care in the ICU than women with advanced malignancies who also participated in end-of-life discussions. This finding has been observed similarly in a population of postoperative patients admitted to the ICU, where women were less likely than men to remain at full code status at ICU discharge and death and were also more likely to be discharged or die after a change in code status to do not resuscitate as compared with men.[9] Interestingly, a study by Cooney and colleagues[10] found that divorced women and widowed women were more likely to have advanced directives and more likely to have designated a medical power of attorney compared with their married counterparts; this was conjectured to be due to familiarity with the end-of-life process for widowed women and due to dependence on nonkin ties for divorced women. The consumption of ICU resources predominantly by male patients is conjectured to be related to the role of sex hormones in the immune response in critical illness, which is discussed further elsewhere in this article.[11]

In the United States, studies have demonstrated that fewer women have been admitted to ICUs than men, despite higher severity of illness, although these studies are limited by their retrospective design.[12] Based on current epidemiologic studies of sex-related differences in admission to ICUs and the use of ICU resources, the questions of horizontal equity (equal use for equal need) and vertical equity (more treatment for those with greater need than those with lesser need) in relation to gender requires further research.

SEX HORMONES IN CRITICAL ILLNESS

Various in vitro and in vivo experimental models have shown gender differences in innate immune responses that may influence the trajectory of illnesses requiring admission to the ICU, such as shock, trauma, and sepsis. One such experimental study by van Eijk and colleagues demonstrated increased proinflammatory state with increased tumor necrosis factor-α and C-reactive protein levels in female patients after injection of lipopolysaccharide to simulate endotoxemia.[13] Estrogen has been suggested to be immunoprotective after trauma and severe blood loss, as well as in sepsis, whereas androgens have been demonstrated to suppress the immune system.[14–17] This finding is further bolstered by studies that outcomes in trauma, shock, and sepsis are better for women than men younger than the age of 50, when the protective effect of estrogen is presumably still present.[18] The findings in these studies are more complex than their conclusions; none of these gender-specific studies took oral contraceptives or hormone replacement therapy into account in investigating the outcomes in the critically ill patients. Furthermore, the cited studies did not account for variability in plasma sex hormone levels during menstrual cycles or menopause. The overall understanding of the impact of sex hormones on attenuating critical illness remains opaque at this time. The impact of sex-specific hormones in attenuating critical illness needs further research with specific attention to external factors impacting sex hormones.

GENDER DIFFERENCES IN ACUTE RESPIRATORY DISTRESS SYNDROME

ARDS is defined by the acute development of diffuse, bilateral pulmonary infiltrates after a direct or indirect lung injury with resultant hypoxia, a $Pao_2:Fio_2$ ratio of less than 300 on positive end-expiratory pressure of 5 cm H_2O, and often requiring mechanical ventilation, as defined by the Berlin criteria.[19] ARDS is further categorized into mild, moderate, and severe based on the $Pao_2:Fio_2$ ratio, with a $Pao_2:Fio_2$ of less than 300 defining mild, a $Pao_2:Fio_2$ of less than 200 defining moderate, and a $Pao_2:Fio_2$ of less than 100 defining severe disease.

Risk factors for the development of ARDS in the general population include direct lung injury—such as pneumonia, aspiration, drowning—and indirect lung injury through cytokine stimulation—such as trauma, sepsis, and pancreatitis. The development of ARDS is likely to be influenced by various mechanisms, including clinical, environmental, and genetic factors contributing to observed variations. Gender as a factor in the development of ARDS and ARDS outcomes is not well-studied. One study of critically injured patients who developed ARDS examined gender differences and found that women were more likely than men to develop ARDS after a major trauma, despite adjusting for age, mechanism of injury, injury severity, and blood product transfusion.[20] In contrast, the recent severe acute respiratory syndrome coronavirus 2 (SARS-CoV-2) pandemic has demonstrated a male bias mortality with higher incidence of ARDS and ARDS-related mortality in males, conjectured to be related to higher production of IL-6 in males as well as estrogen-related downregulation of angiotensin-converting enzyme 2 receptors, which the SARS-CoV-2 exploits to gain entry into host cells.[21] A higher incidence of death related to ARDS secondary to SARS and Middle East Respiratory Virus was also observed in males.[22,23] A study of trends of ARDS in the United States from 1990 to 2013 found that males had a higher average age-adjusted mortality than females.[24] Overall, gender as a risk factor for and sex bias in the development of ARDS has not been shown consistently in epidemiologic studies, but male sex does seem to confer higher risk of ARDS-related mortality.

The management of ARDS is entirely supportive until the underlying process driving ARDS has resolved or has been treated. Supportive care in the management of ARDS focuses on mitigating further lung injury that can be induced by mechanical ventilation. Major clinical trials in the treatment of ARDS have focused on decreasing further lung injury and have found that low tidal volume ventilation with goal plateau pressure of less than 30 mm Hg, as well as prone positioning, decrease mortality.[25,26] However, the major clinical trials of ARDS have historically included mostly male participants[25–27] or did not cite sex in the baseline characteristics[28] (**Table 1**).

Gender may impact the management of ARDS. The Large Observational Study to Understand the Global Impact of Severe Acute Respiratory Failure (LUNG-SAFE trial) was a multicenter, prospective, observational study of 459 ICUs from 50 countries across 5 continents looking at the epidemiology and patterns of management of patients who met the Berlin criteria for ARDS. Although there were no differences in the recognition of ARDS between the sexes, a secondary analysis of the LUNG-SAFE trial found that women were overall less likely to receive low tidal volume ventilation and were more likely to have higher driving pressures during mechanical ventilation for ARDS. Furthermore, in patients classified as having severe ARDS, women were found to have higher ICU and hospital mortality rates.[29] Further analyses of ARDS Network trials revealed that females were twice as likely to receive ventilation

Table 1
Participants by gender in major ARDS clinical trials

Trial	Participants by Gender

ARMA (Ventilation with Lower Tidal Volumes as Compared with Traditional Tidal Volumes for Acute Lung Injury and the Acute Respiratory Distress Syndrome)	861 total patients
	Intervention group (n = 432)
	  172 women
	  260 men
	Control group (n = 429)
	  175 women
	  254 men

PROSEVA (Prone Positioning in Severe Acute Respiratory Distress Syndrome)	466 total patients
	Intervention group (n = 229)
	  63 women
	  166 men
	Control group (n = 237)
	  85 women
	  152 men

ACURASYS (Neuromuscular Blockers in Early Acute Respiratory Distress Syndrome)	Not specified

ROSE (Early Neuromuscular Blockade in the Acute Respiratory Distress Syndrome)	1006 total patients
	Intervention group (n = 501)
	  210 women
	  291 men
	Control group (n = 505)
	  236 women
	  269 men

with tidal volumes in excess of 6 mL/kg of ideal body weight.[30,31] This gender inequity in the receipt of higher tidal volumes may simply be a function of shorter height and likelihood of overestimating height, ultimately affecting the application of low tidal volume ventilation.[32] There are no conclusive data to demonstrate whether there is sex-related susceptibility to ventilator-induced lung injury.[33] Nonetheless, it is clear that inexact measurements of height with an impact on delivering tidal volumes based on ideal body weight in the treatment of ARDS largely affects women and careful attention should be paid to the management of mechanical ventilation in this subgroup of patients.

One unique subset of female patients affected by ARDS and requiring further special attention is the obstetrics population. Very little literature has focused on the epidemiology and management of ARDS in obstetrics patients, who have also traditionally been excluded from ARDS clinical trials, although ARDS accounts for one of the most common etiologies of maternal death in the ICU.[34] Much of obstetrics-specific literature in ARDS resulted from the H1N1 influenza pandemic, in which pregnant women were found to have higher risk of development of complications from influenza A, with an increased rate of serious illness and hospitalization from influenza[35,36] and mortality rates estimated between 9% and 14%.[37] Complications related to pregnancy widen the differential for causes of ARDS, including amniotic fluid embolism, tocolytic-induced pulmonary edema, eclampsia, and puerperal sepsis. The physiologic changes of pregnancy, including decreased chest wall compliance, higher plateau pressures owing to diaphragmatic compression from the gravid uterus, and respiratory alkalosis pose a challenge in the management of ARDS, which often dictates plateau pressures of less than 30 mm Hg and lower tidal volumes with permissive hypercapnia to avoid ventilator-induced lung injury. Unfortunately, there are no clear-cut data on the role of permissive hypercapnia in the pregnant patient and its effect on uteroplacental and umbilical blood flow.

One of the most crucial aspects of ARDS management in the pregnant patient is the timing of delivery, during which the catecholamine surge and significant fluid shifts between the intravascular, intracellular, and interstitial compartments may influence trajectory of ARDS; very little literature examines or reviews the optimal timing of delivery in patients with ARDS.[38] Overall, the current literature provides expectant guidance on the management of the obstetrics patients suffering from ARDS, but clinical trials thus far have generally excluded pregnant patients. The treatment of ARDS in pregnancy is, therefore, extrapolated from the literature in the general population, with exceptions made for the physiologic changes of pregnancy and support for the fetus, including a higher SpO_2 goal of 94% and avoidance of permissive hypercapnia, because hypoxia and acidosis are poorly tolerated by the fetus.[39]

Overall, sex- and gender-specific literature in ARDS is limited at this time and remains an area requiring further research.

GENDER DIFFERENCES IN SEPSIS AND SEPTIC SHOCK

Sepsis and septic shock, conditions defined by life-threatening organ dysfunction as a result of a dysregulated host response to infection, are common clinical syndromes that require prompt identification and treatment. Multiple studies have attempted to ascertain whether gender differences exist in the presentation, treatment, and outcomes in patients with sepsis and septic shock.

There is some evidence that males are more likely to experience septic shock than females. Campanelli and colleagues[40] reviewed 36 articles of 498,146 patients and found that males were more likely than females to be admitted to the ICU for septic shock. A review of 1136 admissions by Azkárate and colleagues[41] also showed a male predominance, with 60% to 70% of the septic shock admissions per year being in males over the 6-year study period. A review of ICU admissions for severe sepsis in Italy similarly showed a male preponderance.[42]

Multiple studies have attempted to determine what sex-based factors may contribute to the risk and outcomes in critical illnesses, including infection and sepsis, with a focus on different hormonal responses, among other factors. Differences in sex hormone levels may be more important than gender alone. Male sex hormones (androgens) have been shown to have some immunosuppressive effects, in contrast with female sex hormones (estradiols), which have shown immunoprotective effects, as summarized by Angele and colleagues[43]; there remains speculation if therapies used to manipulate hormone status in septic patients could be beneficial, and efforts testing different treatments are ongoing.

Among the few interventions that have shown improved survival in sepsis and septic shock are completion of sepsis bundles[44] and a short time to the initiation of empiric antibiotics.[45] Two retrospective cohort studies have found that sepsis bundles were less likely to be completed in the emergency room if the patient was female.[46,47] In contrast, the DISPARITY study found no association between gender and bundle completion.[48] However, the DISPARITY study did find women were less likely to receive antibiotics within 3 hours.[49] Two other studies have also found that females had a longer time before antibiotic initiation for sepsis.[47,49] It is unclear why females have a delay to antibiotic initiation in sepsis and septic shock, and further research is needed to determine why there is inconsistency in sepsis and septic shock resuscitative efforts between the sexes.

There may be sex-based differences in mortality from sepsis. One large retrospective cohort study of more than 18,000 ICU patients in Canada, Brazil, and the United States found an increased mortality rate in females, even after adjusting for baseline characteristics.[50] Similarly, Nachtigall and colleagues[51] found an increase in mortality for female patients admitted to the ICU with sepsis, as did Sakr and colleagues in severe sepsis.[42] In contrast, other studies have found a male predominance in nonsurvivors of sepsis and septic shock.[52–54] Multiple other studies have found no difference in mortality between the sexes.[41,47,55–57] The difference in outcomes may be due to poor baseline characteristic matching; there was significant variability in sample size between the studies thus far. The development of multicenter, prospective registries would eliminate the biases wrought by retrospective studies.

Maternal sepsis is one of the major factors accounting for the admission of pregnant and postpartum patients to the ICU. Sepsis accounts for approximately 23% of all maternal deaths; a retrospective study by Hensley and colleagues[58] assessing for nationwide incidence and outcomes of maternal sepsis in 27 states in the United States within 42 days of delivery hospitalization discharge from 2013 to 2016 found that 2905 deliveries out of 5,957,678 deliveries were complicated by sepsis (0.04% of deliveries). Risk factors for sepsis in pregnancy include non-White ethnicity, obesity, impaired glucose tolerance and diabetes mellitus, protracted active labor, and prolonged rupture of membranes. Group A *Streptococcus* is one of the most common causes of infections in pregnant and postpartum patients. The immunologic changes of pregnancy to protect the fetus from the maternal inflammatory response includes downregulation of T-cell activity, additionally predisposing the pregnant patient to infections like *Listeria monocytogenes* and more severe manifestations of viral and fungal infections.[59] The physiologic changes of pregnancy may overlap with the physiologic changes seen in sepsis, leading

clinicians to a late identification of sepsis; this factor, in turn, may result in the late initiation of antibiotics, ultimately impacting morbidity and mortality.

Other differences between sepsis and septic shock outcomes that are sex specific have been observed. In a retrospective cohort study by Pietropaoli and colleagues,[50] females had a lower likelihood of independence at discharge and had more code status limitations during admission. Both Pietropaoli and colleagues[50] and Xu and colleagues[52] found that females were less likely to receive dialysis and invasive ventilation during admission for sepsis and septic shock. Xu and colleagues also found that males were more likely to receive vasopressors. Overall, the trend of these findings is for less aggressive care to be performed in female patients in sepsis and septic shock, although it is unclear if it is because females are less ill as compared with males and do not require aggressive care, if females are choosing to have less aggressive care, or if aggressive measures are not being offered to females. **Table 2** summarizes studies analyzing the gender in the treatment of sepsis.

OUTCOMES AND RESEARCH IN THE CRITICALLY ILL OBSTETRICS AND POSTPARTUM PATIENT

About 200 to 700 women per 100,000 deliveries require ICU admission in the United States.[60] Maternal mortality rates differ significantly in developing countries than in developed countries; the estimated maternal mortality rate ratio expressed as maternal deaths per 100,000 deliveries is 462 in developing countries versus 11 in developed countries. However, maternal mortality and severe morbidity is rising in the United States and is projected to increase[61,62] as advanced maternal age poses a risk factor for complications related to pregnancy requiring ICU admission, with the odds of maternal mortality increasing for obstetrics patients older than age 40.[63] Additional risk factors for poor outcome in the critically ill obstetrics patients include minority status (specifically, non-Hispanic Black patients) and those with lower socioeconomic status.[64] These outcomes are further complicated by care of the pregnant patient either by clinicians who are unfamiliar with the management of critically ill obstetrics and postpartum patients or by a lack of multidisciplinary care, including the intensivist.

Research regarding the care of the critically ill obstetrics patient has focused on identifying obstetrics patients at risk of requiring ICU-level care or multidisciplinary care, as well as the establishment of dedicated obstetrics critical care units

Table 2
Treatment differences in sepsis and septic shock in females

Author	Reference	Finding
Mikkelsen et al, 2010	46	Fewer sepsis bundles completed
Sunden-Cullberg et al, 2020	47	Fewer sepsis bundles completed, longer time to antibiotic initiation
Madsen et al, 2014	48	No difference in sepsis bundle completion, longer time to antibiotic initiation
Madsen et al, 2014	49	Longer time to antibiotic initiation
Pietropaoli et al, 2010	50	Less dialysis, less mechanical ventilation
Xu et al, 2019	52	Less dialysis, less mechanical ventilation, less initiation of vasopressors

owing to increasing maternal morbidity and mortality over the last 20 years.

Major maternal morbidity and mortality may be preventable in many cases; multiple reviews in various countries have suggested that up to 50% of maternal deaths are preventable and related to hemorrhage, hypertension, infection, and thromboembolic events.[65–67] Research of the critically ill obstetrics population in the last decade has focused on the use of early warning systems that can identify obstetrics patients at risk of progressing to critical illness as the physiologic changes of pregnancy may contribute to clinicians underestimating clinical deterioration. Three such scoring systems include the Modified Early Obstetric Warning System (MEOWS, used in the United Kingdom), the Maternal Early Warning Criteria (MERC), and the Maternal Early Warning Trigger (MEWT, used in the United States)[68] (**Table 3**). A validation study of the MEOWS of 676 obstetrics patients admitted to a single center in the United Kingdom found the implementation of the MEOWS in identifying patients at risk of deterioration to be 89% sensitive, 79% specific, have a positive predictive value of 39%, and negative predictive value of 98%.[69] The MEWT tool was implemented internally at multiple sites in the Dignity Health System in the United States and prospectively validated; the tool addressed the 4 most common conditions resulting in maternal morbidity: sepsis, cardiopulmonary dysfunction, preeclampsia–hypertension, and hemorrhage. Outcomes measured were the Centers for Disease Control and Prevention–defined severe maternal morbidity, composite maternal morbidity, and

ICU admission before the implementation of MEWT and after the implementation of MEWT. At the pilot sites, the use of the MEWT tool resulted in a significant decrease in severe morbidity as defined by the Centers for Disease Control and Prevention ($P<.01$) and in composite morbidity ($P<.01$); ICU admissions remained unchanged in the period after the implementation of the MEWT tool.[70] The use of obstetrics early warning systems have overall been shown to rapidly identify obstetrics patients at risk of clinical deterioration to mitigate morbidity; an evaluation of the effectiveness of these tools is ongoing, but preliminary reports suggest a positive impact on outcomes for obstetrics patients.[71]

In addition to the implementation of scoring tools to identify patients at risk of progressing to critical illness, a growing area of research in obstetrics critical care is the implementation of obstetrics-specific rapid response teams. The implementation of obstetrics rapid response teams was advocated by the US Department of Health and Human Services along with the American Hospital Association to improve delivery of emergency care on maternity wards. There is also an increasing national initiative by the American College of Obstetrics and Gynecologists, The Institute for Healthcare Improvement, The Joint Commission, and The Agency for Healthcare Research and Quality to implement rapid response teams[72] for obstetrics wards with translation to improved various patient outcomes, including decreasing ICU admissions and improved outcomes in postpartum hemorrhage.[73,74] A recent article

Table 3
Comparison of maternal early warning system

Early Warning System	Triggers for Evaluation

Modified Early Obstetric Warning System (MEOWS)	Either 1 red criterion or 2 yellow criteria must be yet to trigger evaluation
	Red
	  RR <10 or >30
	  SpO_2 <95
	  Temperature <35°C or >38°C
	  SBP <90 mm Hg OR >160 mm Hg
	  DBP >100 mm Hg
	  HR <40 or >120
	  Neurologic response either unresponsive or responsive to pain only
	Yellow
	  RR 21–30
	  Temperature 35–36°C
	  SBP 90–100 mm Hg OR 150–160 mm Hg
	  DBP 90–100 mm Hg
	  HR 40–50 or 100–120
	  Pain score 2–3
	  Neurologic response to voice only

Maternal Early Warning Criteria	Any of the following criteria should trigger evaluation RR <10 or >30 SpO_2 <95 on room air SBP <90 mm Hg or >160 mm Hg DBP >100 mm Hg HR <50 or >120 Oliguria <35 mL/kg for >2 h

Maternal Early Warning Trigger	Either 1 red criterion or 2 yellow criteria must be yet to trigger evaluation
	Red
	  RR >30
	  SpO_2 <90%
	  Temperature >38°C
	  SBP >60 mm Hg
	  DBP >110 mm Hg
	  Mean arterial pressure <55 mm Hg
	  HR >130
	  Nursing clinically uncomfortable with patient status
	Yellow
	  RR <12 or 25–30
	  Temperature <36 C
	  SBP <80 mm Hg OR 156–160 mm Hg
	  DBP <45 mm Hg or 106–110 mm Hg
	  HR <50 or 111–130
	  SpO_2 90%–93%
	  Altered mental status

Abbreviations: DBP, diastolic blood pressure; HR, heart rate; RR, respiratory rate; SBP, systolic blood pressure.

by the obstetrics-specific crisis team at the University of Pittsburgh Medical Center Magee Women's Hospital outlines the implementation, training, and maintenance of an obstetrics-specific rapid response team; although a detectable impact on the perinatal quality and safety data could not be ascertained owing to the short lead time between implementation and publication, the implementation of a crisis team familiar with obstetrics is expected to have a positive impact on care of the deteriorating or critically ill obstetrics patient.[75]

An area requiring further research is the impact of obstetrics ICU on maternal outcomes; very limited evidence is available for the establishment of obstetrics-specific critical care units[76,77]; nonetheless, the pregnant patient is expected to benefit from the establishment of multidisciplinary care with nursing resources dedicated to and familiar with obstetrics and postpartum complications requiring intensive care.

Finally, research regarding outcomes in the critically ill pregnant patient is not complete without commenting on the paucity of clinical trials allowing the inclusion of obstetrics patients. The Institute of Medicine published a report in 1994 recommending that pregnant patients be presumed eligible for inclusion in clinical studies unless there is (1) lack of medical benefit to the pregnant patient and (2) risk of significant harm to the fetus was known or could be plausibly inferred[78]; nonetheless, pregnant women continue to be excluded from pharmacologic trials and the treatment of this population is often inferred from outcomes in critically ill, nonpregnant patients. This has proven particularly problematic during the recent SARS-CoV-2 pandemic, during which obstetrics patients have proven vulnerable but have been excluded from clinical trials thus far. Advancements in the care of the critically ill obstetrics patient remain limited by the exclusion of pregnant patients from clinical trials.

GENDER DIFFERENCES IN INTENSIVE CARE UNIT OUTCOMES

Few studies have definitively concluded whether sex impacts survival in the ICU or functional outcomes after ICU admission. Retrospective studies are conflicting regarding differences in short-term mortality between men and women; although some investigators have concluded that short-term mortality does not differ between the sexes,[79–81] others have found that the odds of ICU mortality are higher in women and, in particular, women older than 50.[6] Only 1 prospective study has attempted to delineate long-term outcomes of critically ill patients on the basis of sex; the French and European Outcome Registry in Intensive Care Unit study (FROG-ICU study) was a prospective, multicenter, cohort designed to investigate the long-term mortality of critically ill patients, specifically, the 1-year mortality rate for women compared with men. The study included 2087 patients, 726 of whom were women with similar baseline characteristics and severity illness as compared with male participants. ICU mortality, 28-day mortality, and 1-year mortality did not differ significantly between men and women, even when adjusting for confounding factors such as comorbidities and severity of illness. Little has been published in regard to the short and long-term outcomes of critically ill patients on the basis of sex.[82]

Beyond survival, delirium and functional outcomes after critical illness may differ between the sexes, although research is limited in this area as well. Delirium is an acute condition characterized by disturbances in awareness, attention, and cognition that is particularly common in the ICU for many reasons, including the acuity and severity of patient illness, lack of family visitation, loud machines and noises, and frequent interventions. Delirium can have various manifestations, with some patients expressing agitation, impulsivity, and combativeness (hyperactive delirium), whereas others will express somnolence and decreased arousal (hypoactive delirium), and some will have both findings (mixed delirium). Delirium in the ICU has been shown to be associated with higher mortality rates at 6 months after discharge, longer hospital lengths of stay, increased incidence of cognitive impairment at hospital discharge, higher intensive care and overall hospital costs, and worse cognitive and functional impairment at 1 year after discharge.[83–85]

Given the prevalence and outcomes of delirium, many studies have been performed to evaluate the risk factors of those who develop delirium in the ICU. There is some variability in the literature as to whether there is a true gender predominance in the risk of ICU delirium, but multiple studies have shown no sex differences among patients who did develop delirium.[86,87] Furthermore, 1 study did not demonstrate any difference between men and women on the duration of ICU delirium.[88] However, a study in North American surgical and medical ICUs on delirium development in mechanically ventilated patients demonstrated more predominance of delirium in male patients.[89]

There may be sex differences in the subtype of delirium expressed. One review series of a pooled data set demonstrated that female patients were more likely to have a hypoactive delirium subtype as compared with the male patients studied, although this study was not conducted in ICU patients, but rather patients hospitalized in acute medicine settings.[90] The severity of the delirium in these hospitalized patients was noted to be similar between the sexes. Similarly, a retrospective review series found that male patients in the ICU had higher rates of documented agitation and hyperactive delirium as compared with females.[91] Additionally, the review series found that male patients in the ICU were more likely than females to be initiated on antipsychotics, presumably because hyperactive symptoms are more visible and invoke more safety concerns as compared with hypoactive symptoms. Similarly, another study on antipsychotic use in the ICU found that males admitted to the ICU were more likely than females to be newly initiated on antipsychotics, although this study did not focus specifically on delirious patients.[92] However, a different review series concluded there was no difference in ICU delirium subtype among the sexes.[93] Overall, the current literature does not demonstrate a consistent sex difference in the risk, duration, or severity of ICU delirium. Female patients who are mechanically ventilated may develop delirium less often as compared with their male counterparts. There may be differences in delirium subtypes expressed between the sexes, with female patients being more likely to express a hypoactive delirium.

Finally, sex- and gender-related disparities in functional outcomes after critical illness are not well-studied. A secondary analysis of the Bringing to Light the Risk Factors and Incidence of Neuropsychological Dysfunction in ICU survivors (BRAIN-ICU) attempted to examine disparities in functional outcome after a critical illness on the basis of sex; of the 821 participants enrolled in the study, 311 were female. The authors attempted to follow participants to 12 months of follow-up. At baseline, female participants had lower Sequential Organ Failure Assessment scores, but higher baseline depression and disability, as assessed by activities of daily living. At 3 months of follow-up, the female participants were found to have greater odds of activities of daily living disability, worse physical function-related quality of life, more depressive symptoms, more symptoms of post-traumatic stress disorder, and were less likely to be living at home at 3 months than male participants when adjusting for age, comorbidities, and baseline disability. At 12 months, most of these differences were no longer statistically significant, except for trauma symptoms and differences in global physical function, which the authors attributed to loss to follow-up and differences in trajectories of recovery by sex, although this aspect is not explored further. The authors concluded that females were more likely to experience disability, depression, trauma, and short-term institutionalization after critical illness than males.[94] Previous studies have confirmed susceptibility to physical and psychological impairments in female patients,[95,96] as well as lower socioeconomic status and a lack of an available caregiver, which impacts the ability to return home after a hospitalization.[97] These findings have yet to be confirmed by larger scale trials.

SUMMARY

Research on sex differences in critical illness is limited by reduced enrollment of both nonpregnant and pregnant females in clinical trials, retrospective studies, and gender dimorphism in 2 of the most common illnesses requiring intensive care—sepsis and ARDS. Men are admitted to the ICU more commonly than women and use more resources, with research suggesting better functional outcomes than women, although the short- and long-term survival rates are similar. Sex hormones seem to influence the trajectory of critical illness, but outcomes vary depending on the hormone cycle and disease state. Sepsis outcomes do not clearly differ by sex or gender, but women receive less timely treatment. Although males have higher ARDS-related mortality, women are subject to potentially inappropriate and harmful management with little research available on the treatment of the pregnant patients with ARDS. The critically ill obstetrics patients poses a management challenge owing to the physiologic changes of pregnancy and recent research has made efforts to develop obstetrics early warning systems, obstetrics-specific rapid response teams, and obstetrics critical care units to improve delivery of care and outcomes in the critically ill patient. The understanding of sex and gender differences in critical illness is currently limited, but expanded research will allow for increasing application of precision medicine in the ICU.

CLINICS CARE POINTS

- Male patients gain admission to the intensive care unit and utilize resources in the intensive care unit more than female patients.
- Estrogen may have a protective effect in critical illness.
- Women receive less appropriate management of the acute respiratory distress syndrome than men.
- No consistent differences in sepsis outcomes by gender have been found but women receive less timely initiation of antibiotics.
- Women are more likely to experience hypoactive delirium while in the intensive care unit and have worse functional outcomes following discharge.

DISCLOSURE

Dr T.I. Lat – no conflicts of interest to disclose. Dr M.K. McGraw – no conflicts of interest to disclose. Dr H.D. White – no conflicts of interest to disclose. This review was performed at Baylor Scott and White – Temple Memorial. No financial support was provided for this article.

REFERENCES

1. Goldstein RH, Walensky RP. Where were the women? Gender parity in clinical trials. N Engl J Med 2019;381(26):2491–3.
2. Raine R, Goldfrad C, Rowan K, et al. Influence of patient gender on admission to intensive care. J Epidemiol Community Health 2002;56(6):418–23.
3. Blecha S, Zeman F, Specht S, et al. Invasiveness of treatment is gender dependent in intensive care: results from a retrospective analysis of 26,711 Cases. Anesth Analg 2020. https://doi.org/10.1213/ANE.0000000000005082.
4. Valentin A, Jordan B, Lang T, et al. Gender-related differences in intensive care: a multiple-center cohort study of therapeutic interventions and outcome in critically ill patients. Crit Care Med 2003;31(7):1901–7.
5. Fowler RA, Sabur N, Li P, et al. Sex-and age-based differences in the delivery and outcomes of critical care. CMAJ 2007;177(12):1513–9.
6. Dodek P, Kozak JF, Norena M, et al. More men than women are admitted to 9 intensive care units in British Columbia. J Crit Care 2009;24(4):630.e1–6308.
7. Romo H, Amaral AC, Vincent JL. Effect of patient sex on intensive care unit survival. Arch Intern Med 2004;164(1):61–5.
8. Sharma RK, Prigerson HG, Penedo FJ, et al. Male-female patient differences in the association between end-of-life discussions and receipt of intensive care near death. Cancer 2015;121(16):2814–20.
9. Purcell LN, Tignanelli CJ, Maine R, et al. Predictors of change in code status from time of admission to death in critically ill surgical patients. Am Surg 2020;86(3):237–44.
10. Cooney TM, Shapiro A, Tate CE. End-of-life care planning: the importance of older adults' marital status and gender. J Palliat Med 2019;22(8):902–7.
11. Reinikainen M, Niskanen M, Uusaro A, et al. Impact of gender on treatment and outcome of ICU patients. Acta Anaesthesiol Scand 2005;49(7):984–90.
12. Mahmood K, Eldeirawi K, Wahidi MM. Association of gender with outcomes in critically ill patients. Crit Care 2012;16(3):R92.
13. van Eijk LT, Dorresteijn MJ, Smits P, et al. Gender differences in the innate immune response and vascular reactivity following the administration of endotoxin to human volunteers. Crit Care Med 2007;35(6):1464–9.
14. Angele MK, Schwacha MG, Ayala A, et al. Effect of gender and sex hormones on immune responses following shock. Shock 2000;14(2):81–90.
15. Klein SL. The effects of hormones on sex differences in infection: from genes to behavior. Neurosci Biobehav Rev 2000;24(6):627–38.
16. Federman DD. The biology of human sex differences. N Engl J Med 2006;354(14):1507–14.
17. Aulock SV, Deininger S, Draing C, et al. Gender difference in cytokine secretion on immune stimulation with LPS and LTA. J Interferon Cytokine Res 2006;26(12):887–92.
18. Wohltmann CD, Franklin GA, Boaz PW, et al. A multicenter evaluation of whether gender dimorphism affects survival after trauma. Am J Surg 2001;181(4):297–300.
19. ARDS Definition Task Force, Ranieri VM, Rubenfeld GD, Thompson B, et al. Acute respiratory distress syndrome: the Berlin Definition. JAMA 2012;307(23):2526–33.
20. Heffernan DS, Dossett LA, Lightfoot MA, et al. Gender and acute respiratory distress syndrome in critically injured adults: a prospective study. J Trauma 2011;71(4):878–85.
21. Scully EP, Haverfield J, Ursin RL, et al. Considering how biological sex impacts immune responses and COVID-19 outcomes. Nat Rev Immunol 2020;20(7):442–7.
22. Leong HN, Earnest A, Lim HH, et al. SARS in Singapore–predictors of disease severity. Ann Acad Med Singap 2006;35(5):326–31.
23. Alghamdi IG, Hussain II, Almalki SS, et al. The pattern of Middle East respiratory syndrome coronavirus in Saudi Arabia: a descriptive epidemiological analysis of data from the Saudi Ministry of Health. Int J Gen Med 2014;7:417–23.
24. Cochi SE, Kempker JA, Annangi S, et al. Mortality trends of acute respiratory distress syndrome in the United States from 1999 to 2013. Ann Am Thorac Soc 2016;13(10):1742–51.
25. Acute Respiratory Distress Syndrome Network, Brower RG, Matthay MA, Morris A, et al. Ventilation with lower tidal volumes as compared with traditional tidal volumes for acute lung injury and the acute respiratory distress syndrome. N Engl J Med 2000;342(18):1301–8.
26. Guérin C, Reignier J, Richard JC, et al. Prone positioning in severe acute respiratory distress syndrome. N Engl J Med 2013;368(23):2159–68.
27. National Heart, Lung, and Blood Institute PETAL Clinical Trials Network, Moss M, Huang DT, Brower RG, et al. Early neuromuscular blockade in the acute respiratory distress syndrome. N Engl J Med 2019;380(21):1997–2008.

28. Papazian L, Forel JM, Gacouin A, et al. Neuromuscular blockers in early acute respiratory distress syndrome. N Engl J Med 2010;363(12):1107–16.

29. McNicholas BA, Madotto F, Pham T, et al. Demographics, management and outcome of females and males with acute respiratory distress syndrome in the LUNG SAFE prospective cohort study. Eur Respir J 2019;54(4):1900609.

30. Walkey AJ, Wiener RS. Risk factors for underuse of lung-protective ventilation in acute lung injury. J Crit Care 2012;27(3):323.e1–3239.

31. Han S, Martin GS, Maloney JP, et al. Short women with severe sepsis-related acute lung injury receive lung protective ventilation less frequently: an observational cohort study. Crit Care 2011;15(6):R262.

32. L'her E, Martin-Babau J, Lellouche F. Accuracy of height estimation and tidal volume setting using anthropometric formulas in an ICU Caucasian population. Ann Intensive Care 2016;6(1):55.

33. López-Alonso I, Amado-Rodriguez L, López-Martínez C, et al. Sex susceptibility to ventilator-induced lung injury. Intensive Care Med Exp 2019;7(1):7.

34. Price LC, Slack A, Nelson-Piercy C. Aims of obstetric critical care management. Best Pract Res Clin Obstet Gynaecol 2008;22(5):775–99.

35. Jamieson DJ, Honein MA, Rasmussen SA, et al. H1N1 2009 influenza virus infection during pregnancy in the USA. Lancet 2009;374(9688):451–8.

36. Mak TK, Mangtani P, Leese J, et al. Influenza vaccination in pregnancy: current evidence and selected national policies. Lancet Infect Dis 2008;8(1):44–52.

37. Rush B, Martinka P, Kilb B, et al. Acute respiratory distress syndrome in pregnant women. Obstet Gynecol 2017;129(3):530–5.

38. Schnettler WT, Al Ahwel Y, Suhag A. Severe acute respiratory distress syndrome in coronavirus disease 2019-infected pregnancy: obstetric and intensive care considerations. Am J Obstet Gynecol MFM 2020;2(3):100120.

39. Cole DE, Taylor TL, McCullough DM, et al. Acute respiratory distress syndrome in pregnancy. Crit Care Med 2005;33(10 Suppl):S269–78.

40. Campanelli F, Landoni G, Cabrini L, et al. Gender differences in septic intensive care unit patients. Minerva Anestesiol 2018;84(4):504–8.

41. Azkárate I, Choperena G, Salas E, et al. Epidemiology and prognostic factors in severe sepsis/septic shock. Evolution over six years. Med Intensiva 2016;40(1):18–25.

42. Sakr Y, Elia C, Mascia L, et al. The influence of gender on the epidemiology of and outcome from severe sepsis. Crit Care 2013;17(2):R50.

43. Angele MK, Pratschke S, Hubbard WJ, et al. Gender differences in sepsis: cardiovascular and immunological aspects. Virulence 2014;5(1):12–9.

44. Nguyen HB, Corbett SW, Steele R, et al. Implementation of a bundle of quality indicators for the early management of severe sepsis and septic shock is associated with decreased mortality. Crit Care Med 2007;35(4):1105–12.

45. Ferrer R, Martin-Loeches I, Phillips G, et al. Empiric antibiotic treatment reduces mortality in severe sepsis and septic shock from the first hour: results from a guideline-based performance improvement program. Crit Care Med 2014;42(8):1749–55.

46. Mikkelsen ME, Gaieski DF, Goyal M, et al. Factors associated with nonadherence to early goal-directed therapy in the ED. Chest 2010;138(3):551–8.

47. Sunden-Cullberg J, Nilsson A, Inghammar M. Sex-based differences in ED management of critically ill patients with sepsis: a nationwide cohort study. Intensive Care Med 2020;46(4):727–36.

48. Madsen TE, Simmons J, Choo EK, et al. The DISPARITY Study: do gender differences exist in Surviving Sepsis Campaign resuscitation bundle completion, completion of individual bundle elements, or sepsis mortality? J Crit Care 2014;29(3):473. e7-11.

49. Madsen TE, Napoli AM. The DISPARITY-II study: delays to antibiotic administration in women with severe sepsis or septic shock. Acad Emerg Med 2014;21(12):1499–502.

50. Pietropaoli AP, Glance LG, Oakes D, et al. Gender differences in mortality in patients with severe sepsis or septic shock. Gend Med 2010;7(5):422–37.

51. Nachtigall I, Tafelski S, Rothbart A, et al. Gender-related outcome difference is related to course of sepsis on mixed ICUs: a prospective, observational clinical study. Crit Care 2011;15(3):R151.

52. Xu J, Tong L, Yao J, et al. Association of sex with clinical outcome in critically ill sepsis patients: a retrospective analysis of the large clinical database MIMIC-III. Shock 2019;52(2):146–51.

53. Adrie C, Azoulay E, Francais A, et al. Influence of gender on the outcome of severe sepsis: a reappraisal. Chest 2007;132(6):1786–93.

54. Pavon A, Binquet C, Kara F, et al. Profile of the risk of death after septic shock in the present era: an epidemiologic study. Crit Care Med 2013;41(11):2600–9.

55. Luethi N, Bailey M, Higgins A, et al. Gender differences in mortality and quality of life after septic shock: a post-hoc analysis of the ARISE study. J Crit Care 2020;55:177–83.

56. Wichmann MW, Inthorn D, Andress HJ, et al. Incidence and mortality of severe sepsis in surgical intensive care patients: the influence of patient gender on disease process and outcome. Intensive Care Med 2000;26(2):167–72.

57. van Vught LA, Scicluna BP, Wiewel MA, et al. Association of gender with outcome and host response in

critically ill sepsis patients. Crit Care Med 2017; 45(11):1854–62.

58. Hensley MK, Bauer ME, Admon LK, et al. Incidence of maternal sepsis and sepsis-related maternal deaths in the United States. JAMA 2019;322(9): 890–2.

59. Chebbo A, Tan S, Kassis C, et al. Maternal sepsis and septic shock. Crit Care Clin 2016;32(1):119–35.

60. Guntupalli KK, Hall N, Karnad DR, et al. Critical illness in pregnancy: part I: an approach to a pregnant patient in the ICU and common obstetric disorders. Chest 2015;148(4):1093–104.

61. Alkema L, Chou D, Hogan D, et al. Global, regional, and national levels and trends in maternal mortality between 1990 and 2015, with scenario-based projections to 2030: a systematic analysis by the UN Maternal Mortality Estimation Inter-Agency Group. Lancet 2016;387(10017):462–74.

62. Maternal mortality. 2019. Available at: https://www.who.int/news-room/fact-sheets/detail/maternal-mortality. Accessed July 07, 2020.

63. Enhancing reviews and surveillance to eliminate maternal mortality. Available at: https://www.cdc.gov/reproductivehealth/maternal-mortality/erase-mm/mmr-data-brief.html. Accessed July 07, 2020.

64. Cantwell R, Clutton-Brock T, Cooper G, et al. Saving mothers' lives: reviewing maternal deaths to make motherhood safer: 2006-2008. The eighth report of the confidential enquiries into maternal deaths in the United Kingdom [published correction appears in BJOG. 2015 Apr;122(5):e1] [published correction appears in BJOG. 2015 Apr;122(5):e1]. BJOG 2011; 118(Suppl 1):1–203.

65. Farquhar C, Sadler L, Masson V, et al. Beyond the numbers: classifying contributory factors and potentially avoidable maternal deaths in New Zealand, 2006-2009. Am J Obstet Gynecol 2011;205(4):331. e1–3318.

66. Saucedo M, Deneux-Tharaux C, Bouvier-Colle MH, French National Experts Committee on Maternal Mortality. Ten years of confidential inquiries into maternal deaths in France, 1998-2007. Obstet Gynecol 2013;122(4):752–60.

67. Creanga AA, Berg CJ, Syverson C, et al. Pregnancy-related mortality in the United States, 2006-2010. Obstet Gynecol 2015;125(1):5–12.

68. Friedman AM, Campbell ML, Kline CR, et al. Implementing obstetric early warning systems. AJP Rep 2018;8(2):e79–84.

69. Singh S, McGlennan A, England A, et al. A validation study of the CEMACH recommended modified early obstetric warning system (MEOWS) [published correction appears in Anaesthesia. 2012 Apr;67(4): 453]. Anaesthesia 2012;67(1):12–8.

70. Shields LE, Wiesner S, Klein C, et al. Use of maternal early warning trigger tool reduces maternal morbidity. Am J Obstet Gynecol 2016;214(4):527.e1–6.

71. Zuckerwise LC, Lipkind HS. Maternal early warning systems-Towards reducing preventable maternal mortality and severe maternal morbidity through improved clinical surveillance and responsiveness. Semin Perinatol 2017;41(3):161–5.

72. "Preparing for clinical emergencies in obstetrics and gynecology." ACOG. 2014. Available at: www.acog.org/clinical/clinical-guidance/committee-opinion/articles/2014/03/preparing-for-clinical-emergencies-in-obstetrics-and-gynecology. Accessed July 7, 2020.

73. Baek MS, Son J, Huh JW, et al. Medical emergency team may reduce obstetric intensive care unit admissions. J Obstet Gynaecol Res 2017;43(1): 106–13.

74. Skupski DW, Brady D, Lowenwirt IP, et al. Improvement in outcomes of major obstetric hemorrhage through systematic change. Obstet Gynecol 2017; 130(4):770–7.

75. Dalby PL, Gosman G. Crisis teams for obstetric patients. Crit Care Clin 2018;34(2):221–38.

76. Mabie WC, Sibai BM. Treatment in an obstetric intensive care unit. Am J Obstet Gynecol 1990;162(1):1–4.

77. Zwart JJ, Dupuis JR, Richters A, et al. Obstetric intensive care unit admission: a 2-year nationwide population-based cohort study. Intensive Care Med 2010;36(2):256–63.

78. Mastroianni AC, Faden R, Federman D. Women and health research: a report from the Institute of Medicine. Kennedy Inst Ethics J 1994;4(1):55–62.

79. Samuelsson C, Sjöberg F, Karlström G, et al. Gender differences in outcome and use of resources do exist in Swedish intensive care, but to no advantage for women of premenopausal age. Crit Care 2015; 19(1):129.

80. Schoeneberg C, Kauther MD, Hussmann B, et al. Gender-specific differences in severely injured patients between 2002 and 2011: data analysis with matched-pair analysis. Crit Care 2013;17(6):R277.

81. Park J, Jeon K, Chung CR, et al. A nationwide analysis of intensive care unit admissions, 2009-2014 - The Korean ICU National Data (KIND) study. J Crit Care 2018;44:24–30.

82. Hollinger A, Gayat E, Féliot E, et al. Gender and survival of critically ill patients: results from the FROG-ICU study. Ann Intensive Care 2019;9(1):43.

83. Ely E, Shintani A, Truman B, et al. Delirium as a predictor of mortality in mechanically ventilated patients in the intensive care unit. JAMA 2004;291(14): 1753–62.

84. Milbrandt EB, Deppen S, Harrison PL, et al. Costs associated with delirium in mechanically ventilated patients. Crit Care Med 2004;32(4):955–62.

85. Brummel NE, Jackson JC, Pandharipande PP, et al. Delirium in the ICU and subsequent long-term disability among survivors of mechanical ventilation. Crit Care Med 2014;42(2):369–77.

86. Jayaswal AK, Sampath H, Soohinda G, et al. Delirium in medical intensive care units: incidence, subtypes, risk factors, and outcome. Indian J Psychiatry 2019;61(4):352–8.

87. Zaal IJ, Devlin JW, Peelen LM, et al. A systematic review of risk factors for delirium in the ICU. Crit Care Med 2015;43(1):40–7.

88. Li Y, Yuan D, Li X, et al. [Risk factors for delirium in intensive care unit and its duration]. Zhonghua Wei Zhong Bing Ji Jiu Yi Xue 2020;32(1):62–6.

89. Mehta S, Cook D, Devlin JW, et al. Prevalence, risk factors, and outcomes of delirium in mechanically ventilated adults. Crit Care Med 2015;43(3):557–66.

90. Trzepacz PT, Franco JG, Meagher DJ, et al. Delirium phenotype by age and sex in a pooled data set of adult patients. J Neuropsychiatry Clin Neurosci 2018;30(4):294–301.

91. Karamchandani K, Schoaps RS, Printz J, et al. Gender differences in the use of atypical antipsychotic medications for ICU delirium. Crit Care 2018;22(1):220.

92. Marshall J, Herzig SJ, Howell MD, et al. Antipsychotic utilization in the intensive care unit and in transitions of care. J Crit Care 2016;33:119–24.

93. Krewulak KD, Stelfox HT, Ely EW, et al. Risk factors and outcomes among delirium subtypes in adult ICUs: a systematic review. J Crit Care 2020;56: 257–64.

94. Scheunemann LP, Leland NE, Perera S, et al. Sex disparities and functional outcomes after a critical illness. Am J Respir Crit Care Med 2020;201(7): 869–72.

95. Bienvenu OJ, Colantuoni E, Mendez-Tellez PA, et al. Depressive symptoms and impaired physical function after acute lung injury: a 2-year longitudinal study [published correction appears in Am J Respir Crit Care Med. 2012 Apr 15;185(8):900]. Am J Respir Crit Care Med 2012;185(5):517–24.

96. Newman AB, Brach JS. Gender gap in longevity and disability in older persons. Epidemiol Rev 2001; 23(2):343–50.

97. Van Pelt DC, Milbrandt EB, Qin L, et al. Informal caregiver burden among survivors of prolonged mechanical ventilation. Am J Respir Crit Care Med 2007;175(2):167–73.

Pharmacology Considerations in Women in Lung Disease and Critical Care

Claire C. Eng, PharmD, BCPS, BCCCP[a],*,
Mojdeh S. Heavner, PharmD, BCPS, BCCCP, FCCM[b]

KEYWORDS

- Sex • Gender • Pharmacology • Drug • Lung • Critical care

KEY POINTS

- A multitude of studies have shown that the physiologic distinctions between men and women can result in significant differences in the way certain drugs affect each sex.
- Males and females differ in specific drug pharmacokinetics and pharmacodynamics, including important drugs in lung disease and critical care.
- The impact of sex on pharmacokinetics and pharmacodynamics is frequently underestimated and should be considered in therapeutics.
- Pharmacokinetic disparities also exist at various points during a woman's life cycle, including pregnancy and menopause.

INTRODUCTION

Men and women have fundamental anatomic and physiologic differences. Until relatively recently, women had been underrepresented in drug trials. In part, this was to avoid enrollment of women of childbearing potential in clinical studies to avoid ethical risks to the fetus. The US Food and Drug Administration excluded this population from phase I and early phase II trials. This ban was ended in 1993.[1] A myriad of studies has shown that sex can result in significant differences in the way drugs affect males and females and vice versa. This article provides an overview of sex-related differences in drug pharmacokinetics and pharmacodynamics (PKPD) in respiratory disease and critical illness. A focus on PKPD differences throughout the female life cycle with attention to pregnancy and menopause is also provided.

DISCUSSION
Sex-Related Differences in Pharmacokinetics and Pharmacodynamics

PK is defined as the study of the time course of drug absorption, distribution, metabolism, and elimination. The following sections review data on overall PK differences between men and women. **Fig. 1** summarizes the highlights of this section.

Absorption

Women secrete less gastric acid and tend to have a prolonged gastrointestinal transit time compared with men.[2] Less gastric acid influences the rate of dissolution of drugs that have pH-dependent solubility in an acidic environment (decreases the absorption of weakly acidic drugs like aspirin and copper).[3] Differences in transit time may also lead to changes in absorption. Gastric emptying

[a] Clinical Pharmacy Specialist, Memorial Hermann Katy Hospital, Department of Pharmacy, 23900 Katy Freeway, Katy, TX 77494, USA; [b] Associate Professor and Vice Chair for Clinical Services, Department of Pharmacy Practice & Science, University of Maryland School of Pharmacy, 20 N. Pine Street, N427, Baltimore, MD 21201, USA
* Corresponding author.
E-mail address: Claire.Eng@memorialhermann.org

Clin Chest Med 42 (2021) 557–566
https://doi.org/10.1016/j.ccm.2021.04.013

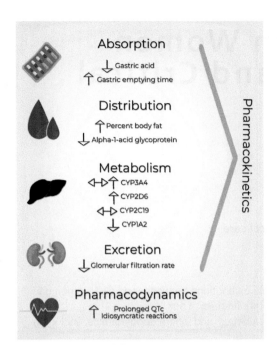

Fig. 1. Physiologic differences in women that can impact drug pharmacology. CYP, cytochrome P450.

time is longer in women than in men, resulting in prolonged gastric retention and delayed drug absorption from the small intestine. Additionally, progesterone and estrogens inhibit intestinal contractility and transit.[4] This factor can be especially impactful with modified-release dosage forms (ie, extended release, delayed release). Differences in drug absorption are not limited to the gastrointestinal system, but also involve transdermal or subcutaneous administration. Women have proportionally more adipose tissue than men. After correction for factors such as height, weight, and body surface area, sex differences have been observed for drugs including nicotine, aspirin, and heparin.[2] It is possible that a drug intended to be injected intramuscularly may be delivered to the adipose tissue instead. Owing to decreased blood flow, absorption from adipose is slower than that from muscle. This factor could be clinically significant if rapid onset is the intent of the ordered intramuscular route.

Distribution

The volume of distribution (V_d) relates the amount of a drug in the body to the concentration of the drug in the blood or plasma. Therefore, an altered V_d requires a modification in the dosing regimen to achieve therapeutic plasma concentrations.

$$\text{Maximum concentration } (C_{max}) =$$

$$(\text{Amount of drug in body})/(Vd)$$

Women tend to have a higher percentage of body fat than men, so women have a greater V_d for a lipophilic drug. Lipophilic drugs, including trazodone and diazepam, had a greater V_d in females than in males owing to the accumulation of these drugs in adipose tissue.[5,6] A higher V_d for a lipophilic drug can lead to a decreased plasma concentration and a prolonged plasma half-life. Conversely, hydrophilic drugs such as aminoglycosides and ethanol were found to have a lower V_d in women compared with men.[3]

In terms of drug protein binding, alpha-1-acid glycoprotein and the alpha-globulins are affected by estrogen, although albumin is not significantly affected.[2] alpha-1-acid glycoprotein is slightly lower in women, so if a drug binds primarily to this protein, it can create a difference since unbound (free) drug is what leads to a drug's effect. Estrogens also increase the levels of the serum-binding globulins (sex hormone–binding globulin, corticosteroid-binding globulin, and thyroxine-binding globulin).[7]

Metabolism

Hepatic metabolism is classified into phase I and phase II reactions (**Table 1**). Phase I includes the cytochrome P450 (CYP) enzymes, oxidation, reduction, and hydrolysis. Phase II consists of conjugation (eg, glucuronidation and sulfation), including uridine diphosphate glucuronosyltransferase (UGT) and N-acetyl-transferase enzymes. Genetic polymorphisms in expression of certain CYP enzymes cause significant effects on drug efficacy and toxicity but these are not expected to be sex dependent because they are not X-linked. There are however, sex-dependent differences in the activity of CYP and UGT enzymes.[8] The literature for certain CYP enzymes is conflicting, so this is an area for future study.

P-glycoprotein (Pgp), a drug transporter protein, decreases absorption and increases renal clearance of certain drugs. Because many drugs metabolized by CYP3A4 are also substrates of Pgp, the sex-related differences attributed to CYP3A4 have been hypothesized to actually be due to Pgp. The increased CYP3A metabolism seen in women compared with men might be the result of their lower Pgp activity relative to men rather than sex differences in CYP3A activity.[9]

Elimination

Drug elimination is generally via renal, hepatic, or pulmonary routes. The major method of drug excretion is renal. When adjusted for body surface area, renal blood flow, glomerular filtration, tubular secretion, and tubular reabsorption are all larger in men than nonpregnant women.[10] The glomerular

Table 1
Sex differences in hepatic metabolism

Molecular Mechanism	Sex-Specific Activity	Example Substrates of This Transporter/ Enzyme	Comments
Drug transporters			
P-glycoprotein	M > F	Dexamethasone, digoxin, tacrolimus, certain chemotherapy and antiretrovirals	
Phase I enzymes			
CYP1A2	M > F	Acetaminophen (minor), caffeine, clozapine, olanzapine, theophylline	
CYP2C9	M = F	Dapsone, glipizide, ibuprofen (minor), losartan, phenytoin, warfarin (S)	
CYP2C19	M = F	Citalopram, diazepam, lansoprazole, omeprazole, phenobarbital, phenytoin, propranolol	Controversial; some data suggest M > F, ethnicity and oral contraception use may be further factors
CYP2D6	M < F	Codeine, dextromethorphan, haloperidol, hydrocodone, metoprolol, paroxetine, sertraline	Data are conflicting, but more recent large studies describe a slightly but significantly higher activity in women
CYP2E1	M > F	Ethanol (minor), nicotine (minor)	
CYP3A	M = F, M < F	Alprazolam, atorvastatin, clarithromycin, cyclosporine, cyclophosphamide, dapsone, diazepam, diltiazem, fentanyl, losartan, methylprednisolone, midazolam, prednisone, simvastatin, verapamil	Responsible for metabolism of largest number of medications; conflicting study results may support sex differences in P-glycoprotein levels rather than CYP3A activity
Phase II enzymes			
UDP-glucuronosyl-transferases (UGT)	M > F	Acetaminophen, caffeine, ibuprofen, mycophenolate	

(continued on next page)

Table 1
(continued)

Molecular Mechanism	Sex-Specific Activity	Example Substrates of This Transporter/ Enzyme	Comments
Methyltransferases	M > F	Azathioprine, dopamine, epinephrine, norepinephrine	
N-acetyltransferases	M = F	Caffeine, catecholamine derivatives, dapsone, hydralazine, isoniazid	
Sulfotransferases	M > F	Caffeine	

Abbreviations: CYP, cytochrome P450; F, female; M, male; UDP, uridine 5-diphosphate.
Data from Soldin OP, Mattison DR. Sex Differences in Pharmacokinetics and Pharmacodynamics: *Clinical Pharmacokinetics.* 2009;48(3):143–157 and Meibohm B, Beierle I, Derendorf H. How Important Are Gender Differences in Pharmacokinetics?: *Clinical Pharmacokinetics.* 2002;41(5):329–342.

filtration rate (GFR) is 10% lower in females than males after adjustment for body size and age.[11] This factor has been demonstrated to impact renal clearance of certain antibiotics, which are largely cleared unchanged in the urine, including vancomycin, ceftazidime, and cefepime.[12] Digoxin is primarily renally eliminated and a study found that higher concentrations in women treated with digoxin for heart failure were associated with increased mortality.[13]

Pharmacodynamics

PD is defined as the relationship between drug concentration at the site of action and the resulting effect, including the time course and intensity of both therapeutic and adverse effects. Although there are a multitude of studies on the PK differences between males and females, there are few studies on PD differences. It is clear, however, that there is a higher incidence of adverse drug reactions in females.[8,14] Reasons hypothesized for this include differences in PD, differences in PK leading to overdose, a greater number of medications leading to more drug–drug interactions, and a higher reporting rate. Some of the most severe examples of the higher frequency of adverse effects in females include torsades de pointes and acute liver failure. In a review of articles on torsade de pointes associated with cardiovascular drugs, 70% occurred in women.[15] Seventy-four percent of drug-induced acute liver failure cases occur in women with a case fatality rate of 80%.[16]

Pharmacology in Critical Care

Central nervous system pharmacology
As discussed elsewhere in this article, women typically have a higher percent body fat compared with men. This point is particularly relevant as it pertains to drugs that act in the central nervous system, because many of these drugs are highly lipophilic. Drugs that partition to a greater extent in adipose tissue may, therefore, have a greater V_d in women.[8] This group includes benzodiazepines such as diazepam and midazolam, which should be used sparingly and with caution for intensive care unit (ICU) sedation. Anticipation that V_d may be increased for these drugs should prompt extra caution with repeated dosing, because the drugs can accumulate in adipose tissue and lead to prolonged effects, even after discontinuation. This point is perhaps most relevant with drugs that are administered as continuous infusions, such as midazolam, and needs to be considered with highly lipophilic sedatives and analgesics commonly used in the ICU, such as propofol and fentanyl. Alfentanil has been observed to result in a lower plasma level in women, which was attributed to differences in body adipose composition.[17] With increased V_d, the initial requirements may be higher as the drug distributes, with a depot effect and therefore a longer duration of action as the drug accumulates over time. In contrast, centrally acting drugs that are more hydrophilic would be expected to have a smaller V_d in women. This notion is confirmed in PD studies with rocuronium, a neuromuscular blocker that is notably hydrophilic. Women require 30% less rocuronium to achieve the same degree of neuromuscular blockade. Similar effects were seen for atracurium and vecuronium, but not with cisatracurium.[18] Perhaps this action was not observed with cisatracurium given its rapid metabolism to an inactive metabolite via plasma esterases. This finding highlights the importance of considering all PK and PD

factors that may differ by sex and thus impact differences observed in drug effects between women and men in clinical practice.

To highlight another complex example, propofol is highly lipophilic and one would expect that women would require higher amounts of drug up front, with more accumulation in adipose tissue over time. However, data with propofol are conflicting. Some studies have not indicated significant PK differences with propofol between men and women.[19] However, other studies have shown that women have a higher V_d compared with men, and there are also data that clearance is also higher.[20–22] The clinical impact of those differences would result in women having greater propofol requirements initially given the lipophilic nature, but with less risk than typically anticipated of having accumulation owing to increased clearance. This point was confirmed by several studies that showed that women required more propofol to have the same PD effects.[22–24] It has even been hypothesized with observations that women have a faster emergence from propofol-related anesthesia and that this effect is due to differences in progesterone levels.[25]

Given the complex interplay between these sex-based differences in drug pharmacology, it could be anticipated that women would experience different clinical outcomes related to sedation and analgesia in the ICU. Studies evaluating sex-based differences in both effect and toxicity related to sedation and analgesia have not been conducted but are warranted.

Cardiovascular pharmacology

A lower GFR in women has an important impact on cardiovascular pharmacology as well. Clearance of digoxin after oral administration has been shown to be 12% to 14% lower in women than men, likely because digoxin is predominantly eliminated renally. This finding was observed even after correction for body size and age, because both affect digoxin PK. Digoxin is also a substrate for Pgp, and men have higher Pgp than women. This sex-based difference can contribute to decreased absorption and, thus, decreased oral bioavailability, as well as decreased clearance of digoxin in women.[8] The clinical implications of these differences can be quite impactful. One study showed that women treated with digoxin for heart failure had a higher observed rate of death compared with placebo; this observation was not present for men. It was speculated in this study that the difference in clinical outcome was potentially related to PK and PD differences related to sex.[26] In a post hoc analysis of this study, a small but statistically significant difference

in the digoxin concentration was found to be associated significantly with the increased mortality observed. Dose-related effects with underlying differences in sex-based PK and PD effects were discussed as potential explanations for this unanticipated and alarming result.[13]

Unique differences in beta-blocker PK and PD changes have also been observed. Metoprolol and propranolol are primarily metabolized through CYP2D6. Although early studies indicated CYP2D6 activity was lower in women,[27,28] more recent studies have indicated this is actually higher.[2,9] Women also display a lower V_d of these 2 drugs, leading to increased C_{max} levels in women. Propranolol has been shown to reach a peak that is 80% higher in women than men, and some of this difference is hypothesized to be related to differences in sex hormones such as estrogen.[29] Differences with calcium channel blockers have also been observed. Verapamil is a CYP3A4 substrate, but is also a substrate of Pgp. Oral verapamil has been observed to have faster clearance in men.[30,31] In contrast, intravenous verapamil has faster clearance in women,[32] likely related to increased CYP3A4 activity.[9] The diminished clearance of verapamil in women is hypothesized to be related to a counterbalancing effect between decreased intestinal Pgp activity and increased CYP enzyme activity. The clinical implications of this difference are important when transitioning between oral and intravenous formulations frequently in ICU patients.

Furthermore, as briefly discussed elsewhere in this article, some PD differences may be driven by sex hormones. For example, estrogen increases angiotensin II (Ang II) levels and decreases negative feedback on angiotensin-converting enzyme and renin activity, with a decreased expression of Ang II type I receptor, as evidenced by greater blood pressure decreases in an experiment with female and male rats. This difference is hypothesized to be related to the expression and regulation of Ang II receptors by sex hormones such as estrogen.[33] The clinical implication of this is greater antihypertensive activity by drugs acting on the renin–aldosterone–angiotensin system. This process includes potential differences in the newer vasopressor, which is synthetically derived Ang II.

Differences in cardiovascular pharmacology between sexes can also be a factor in variable rates of adverse effects such as QTc prolongation. Women have a longer QTc at baseline, and female sex is an independent risk factor for development of torsades de point. In fact, two-thirds of all drug-induced cases of torsades have been reported in females.[34] Evidence exists for sex-based differences in QTc prolongation with amiodarone, ibutilide, quinidine, and sotalol.[35,36] The different rates of QTc prolongation and clinical adverse effects between men and women should be noted with noncardiovascular system medications, because the risk of QTc prolongation exists with many antiemetics, antipsychotics, and antibiotics that are used frequently in the ICU.

Miscellaneous pharmacology

Although the focus of this review was on systems related specifically to pulmonary and critical care, it should be noted that PKPD changes noted throughout apply similarly to other drug classes. As noted elsewhere in this article, the lower GFR in females is an important difference, given that many commonly used antibiotics are highly dependent on renal clearance (ie, vancomycin, piperacillin/tazobactam, and cefepime).[12] This difference in elimination is not commonly considered in clinical practice, which has the potential to lead to differing rates of drug-induced toxicities. An example, although there are not yet data to suggest this, could be a higher incidence of cefepime-induced neurotoxicity in women as compared with men.

Pharmacology in Respiratory Disease

Increasing evidence for sex-related differences in chronic obstructive pulmonary disease (COPD) risk, progression, and outcomes has recently been noted, suggesting a need to assess the impact of COPD interventions in male and female patients separately.[37] Differences have also been demonstrated in women compared with men in short-term responses to bronchodilators and inhaled corticosteroid therapy.[38,39]

Citing sex differences suggesting that both conjugative metabolism and renal tubular secretion of drugs may be lower in women than in men, Mohamed and colleagues[40] investigated albuterol PK differences across sex and race. The authors found that the apparent V_d of albuterol was significantly higher in men, but after correction for ideal body weight, was not different by sex.[40]

A dataset from the Lung Health Study was used to determine whether there are any sex differences in gene expression for muscarinic (M2 and M3) receptors in lungs of male and female patients. The authors found that female lungs have greater gene expression for the M3 receptor relative to M2 receptors than male lungs and that ipratropium induces a greater bronchodilator response in female than in male patients with particularly notable gains in nonobese females. They concluded that female patients are more likely to benefit from ipratropium than male patients with COPD.[41]

In a subgroup analysis of the UPLIFT trial, a 4-year randomized placebo-controlled trial of tiotropium in patients with COPD, a greater proportion of men than women exhibited a significant bronchodilator response overall, but there was no significant difference within each sex category between tiotropium and placebo. Men and women showed comparable benefits with respect to sustained improvements in forced expiratory volume in 1 second (FEV_1) and forced vital capacity, health-related quality of life, and COPD exacerbations.[42]

In a PK study of fluticasone and salmeterol in healthy subjects, sex was found to be a significant covariate on clearance with men having higher clearance than women. This finding might be attributed to greater enzymatic capacity of men to metabolize salmeterol and a difference in lung deposition between males and females.[43] A sensitivity analysis (n = 719) of the responses of male and female patients with COPD to 1 year of combination fluticasone/salmeterol versus placebo showed numerically larger FEV_1 responses in women than men, as well as slight sex differences in the reduction in COPD exacerbations and improvement in health-related quality of life, but none of these differences achieved statistical significance.[44] No significant sex differences were noted for the effect of salmeterol, fluticasone, or the salmeterol/fluticasone combination on FEV_1 decline in a post hoc analysis of the Toward a Revolution in COPD Health (TORCH) trial (n = 5343).[45]

In a post hoc subgroup analysis of pooled data from ACLIFORM and AUGMENT evaluating the efficacy of aclidinium/formoterol compared with placebo and monotherapies, improvements from baseline in FEV_1 were numerically greater in males compared with females with aclidinium/formoterol, but when assessing the percent predicted FEV_1, improvements were similar regardless of sex.[46]

Xu and colleagues[47] performed a randomized, double-blind, placebo-controlled, double dummy crossover multicenter trial (n = 32) to characterize PKPD of fluticasone and an active metabolite of ciclesonide. Ciclesonide is a prodrug, so has no activity itself; desisobutyryl-ciclesonide is its active metabolite and this study found that females had a significantly larger V_d than males. No covariate effects were found on fluticasone PK. Covariate analysis showed that females were found to have a higher maximum cortisol release rate, though it is unknown whether this effect was clinically significant.[47]

In a pooled analysis from the IGNITE Program, indacaterol/glycopyrronium showed better effects in women after 26 weeks of treatment, suggesting a potential sex difference in effects of bronchodilators on patient-related outcomes, which should be investigated further in prospective clinical trials.[48]

Theophylline has been shown to have a significantly shorter half-life in women compared with men (both smokers and nonsmokers).[49] Evidence of sex-related PK changes for corticosteroids is inconsistent. One study found that, after a single dose of methylprednisolone, clearance was increased in women compared with men, leading to a shorter half-life, although plasma binding and V_d were similar.[50] In another study, clearance of methylprednisolone was 3-fold higher in males compared with females.[51]

Sex differences to dexamethasone response were investigated in a post hoc analysis of a double-blind randomized, controlled trial of dexamethasone in bacterial meningitis. Although dexamethasone decreased the risk of unfavorable outcomes to a greater extent in women, on interaction testing, sex was not a significant modifier of the effect of dexamethasone.[52] Prednisolone PK and PD were investigated in relation to sex and race after a single dose of prednisone. Oral clearance and V_d were significantly higher in men compared with women.[53] This conflicted with a previous study, which found a higher clearance in females.[54]

Pregnancy-Induced Changes in Pharmacology

In addition to existing differences between women and men, pregnancy induces further physiologic changes that have the potential to impact drug pharmacology. This section highlights studies evaluating their absorption, distribution, metabolism, and excretion in pregnancy.

Given what we know about changes in decreased intestinal motility and increased gastric pH during pregnancy, we would expect an impact on bioavailability of enterally administered drugs. However, existing data do not indicate significant changes in absorption. Sotalol intravenous and oral administered during the third trimester and 6 weeks postpartum (n = 6) were not significantly different (overall was 85%–90%).[55] No difference in oral bioavailability was found for 3 beta-lactam antibiotics (ampicillin, cephradine, and cefazolin) when administered intravenously or enterally during the second or third trimester and 6 weeks postpartum in pregnant women with asymptomatic urinary tract infections (n = 18).[56,57]

Pregnancy increases the plasma volume and decreases protein levels. Albumin concentrations decrease during the second trimester and continue to decrease during pregnancy, reaching 70% to 80% of normal levels by delivery.[58] This process should cause an increased apparent V_d both through the increased total volume and decreased protein binding, with the most notable impact on C_{max} after initial doses of drugs are administered. This would necessitate higher than normal dosing initially of drugs that are highly protein bound. However, a unique effect could be anticipated for drugs such as phenytoin and valproic acid, which are both highly protein bound but are active via the unbound portion. Because lower protein binding is observed with these drugs, there would be a greater proportion of unbound and thus active drug. If drug monitoring involved only total drug levels, this could lead to an overdose in pregnancy. This finding is of clinical importance given that both phenytoin and valproic have a dose-related teratogenicity.[59]

Drug metabolism during pregnancy is quite altered and dynamic throughout. Some change is to be expected based on changes in protein binding already described, because a greater proportion of unbound drug will be available for hepatic metabolism than in a nonpregnant state. Pregnancy increases activity of CYP3A4, 2D6, 2C9, UGT1A4, and UGT2B7. Conversely, it decreases activity of CYP1A2 and 2C19.[60] The changes in activity of hepatic enzymes can have direct interactions and sometimes result in a counterbalancing effect. As an example, this occurs with theophylline metabolism, which is a major substrate for CYP1A2 and undergoes minor metabolism through CYP2E1 and CYP3A4. Despite the decrease in metabolism through its major pathway of CYP1A2, theophylline has increased unbound clearance during the third trimester compared with postpartum. Increased CYP3A4 activity may offset decreases in CYP1A2 activity.[61]

At least 1 study indicates that hepatic blood flow is increased significantly after 28 weeks gestation.[62] This change could result in increased clearance and decreased area under the curve, most notably for drugs that are administered intravenously and have high extraction ratio (eg, morphine, midazolam, and metoprolol), especially if changes in protein binding are also occurring.[60]

Although the GFR in women is typically lower than men, a 50% increase in the GFR is observed by the first trimester with continued increase throughout pregnancy, until the last 3 weeks when it begins to decrease. By the last week of pregnancy, the GFR typically returns to normal.[63] In this setting, drugs with low protein binding with high levels cleared unchanged would be expected to have increased clearance during pregnancy. An example of relevance to the ICU are beta-lactam antibiotics, which would be expected to have notably increased renal clearance in the setting of an increased GFR. Dosing could be optimized through strategies such as extended or continuous infusions, to ensure that drug levels are maintained above the minimum inhibitory concentration targets despite increased clearance. Underdosing could have significant clinical implications on a pregnant patient with an infection. Another relevant example for critically ill patients are low-molecular-weight heparins such as dalteparin and enoxaparin. These drugs are largely renally cleared unchanged and would therefore need to be dosed aggressively in pregnancy to avoid thrombosis.[60]

Overall, despite the well-described physiologic changes during pregnancy, data on pregnancy-related changes in drug PK remains sparse. The key to approaching the changes is understanding that there is a complex interplay between plasma volume increases, protein binding decreases, changes in enzymatic activity, and increases in the GFR. The conflicting interactions between these physiologic changes are further compounded by the dynamic nature of pregnancy. Wherever possible, therapeutic drug monitoring should be used, using the most appropriate methods (ie, free instead of total levels of antiepileptics) to ensure maximal therapeutic effect while minimizing toxicity.

Menopause-Induced Changes in Pharmacology

Compared with data on changes in pharmacology owing to pregnancy, literature on changes owing to menopause are lacking. Decreased hormone levels in menopause may cause PK changes, although data are conflicting. A study comparing rosuvastatin PK in premenopausal and postmenopausal women found that the C_{max} was lower, whereas the apparent V_d and oral clearances were higher in postmenopausal women. The lower C_{max} may be explained by gastrointestinal motility being slower in postmenopausal women. Additionally, the higher V_d may be due to lower plasma protein binding and increased clearance owing to uninhibited hepatobiliary efflux transporters in postmenopausal women.[64] Owing to any hormone replacement therapy that may be started after menopause, potential drug interactions with concomitant medications may result. Studies have shown significant changes with prednisolone and triazolam clearance after addition of hormone replacement therapy.[3] Studies have compared the PK of midazolam, erythromycin, and prednisolone clearance in premenopausal and postmenopausal women and found no significant differences in drug metabolism according to menopausal status.[7]

SUMMARY

Males and females differ in drug PKPD, including important drugs in lung disease and critical care. The impact of sex on PKPD is frequently underestimated and should be considered in therapeutics. However, inconsistencies in the findings of PKPD studies related to sex make it challenging to apply these principles in clinical practice. Overall, there is a dearth of research on sex-related differences in drug pharmacology, particularly in respiratory and critical care medicine. Further study is needed to accurately characterize sex-related differences and, even more important, understand how these differences may influence disparities in clinical outcomes between men and women.

CLINICS CARE POINTS

- The impact of sex on PKPD are frequently underestimated and should be considered in therapeutics.
- Current data indicate that significant differences exist between men and women in drug absorption, distribution, metabolism, excretion, and PD.
- PK and PD changes also develop at various points during a woman's life cycle, including during pregnancy and menopause.
- The ongoing challenge is limited and conflicting data on sex-related differences; emerging higher quality evidence should drive practice changes in medication use for lung disease and critical care.

DISCLOSURE

The authors have nothing to disclose.

REFERENCES

1. Merkatz RB, Temple R, Sobel S, et al. Women in clinical trials of new drugs – a change in food and drug administration policy. N Engl J Med 1993;329(4):292–6.
2. Soldin OP, Mattison DR. Sex differences in pharmacokinetics and pharmacodynamics. Clin Pharmacokinet 2009;48(3):143–57.
3. Xie CX, Piecoro LT, Wermeling DP. Gender-related considerations in clinical pharmacology and drug therapeutics. Crit Care Nurs Clin North Am 1997; 9(4):459–68.
4. Spoletini I, Vitale C, Malorni W, et al. Sex differences in drug effects: interaction with sex hormones in adult

life. In: Regitz-Zagrosek V, editor. Sex and gender differences in pharmacology, Vol 214. Berlin and Heidelberg, Germany: Springer; 2013. p. 91–105. https://doi.org/10.1007/978-3-642-30726-3_5.

5. Greenblatt DJ, Allen MD, Harmatz JS, et al. Diazepam disposition determinants. Clin Pharmacol Ther 1980;27(3):301–12.

6. Greenblatt DJ, Friedman H, Burstein ES, et al. Trazodone kinetics: effect of age, gender, and obesity. Clin Pharmacol Ther 1987;42(2):193–200.

7. Soldin OP, Chung SH, Mattison DR. Sex differences in drug disposition. J Biomed Biotechnol 2011; 2011:1–14.

8. Anderson GD. Chapter 1 gender differences in pharmacological response. In: International review of neurobiology, Vol 83. Amsterdam: Elsevier; 2008. p. 1–10.

9. Meibohm B, Beierle I, Derendorf H. How important are gender differences in pharmacokinetics? Clin Pharmacokinet 2002;41(5):329–42.

10. Silvaggio T, Mattison DR. Setting occupational health standards: toxicokinetic differences among and between men and women. J Occup Med 1994;36(8):849–54.

11. Gross JL, Friedman R, Azevedo MJ, et al. Effect of age and sex on glomerular filtration rate measured by 51Cr-EDTA. Braz J Med Biol Res 1992;25(2): 129–34.

12. Anderson GD. Sex and racial differences in pharmacological response: where is the evidence? Pharmacogenetics, pharmacokinetics, and pharmacodynamics. J Womens Health 2005;14(1):19–29.

13. Rathore SS. Association of serum digoxin concentration and outcomes in patients with heart failure. JAMA 2003;289(7):871.

14. Rademaker M. Do women have more adverse drug reactions? Am J Clin Dermatol 2001;2(6):349–51.

15. Makkar RR. Female gender as a risk factor for torsades de pointes associated with cardiovascular drugs. JAMA 1993;270(21):2590.

16. Miller MA. Gender-based differences in the toxicity of pharmaceuticals—the food and drug administration's perspective. Int J Toxicol 2001;20(3):149–52.

17. Pleym H, Spigset O, Kharasch ED, et al. Gender differences in drug effects: implications for anesthesiologists: gender differences in anesthesia. Acta Anaesthesiologica Scand 2003;47(3):241–59.

18. Adamus M, Gabrhelik T, Marek O. Influence of gender on the course of neuromuscular block following a single bolus dose of cisatracurium or rocuronium. Eur J Anaesthesiol 2008;25(7):589–95.

19. Schüttler J, Ihmsen H. Population pharmacokinetics of propofol: a multicenter study. Anesthesiology 2000;92(3):727–38.

20. Schnider TW, Minto CF, Gambus PL, et al. The influence of method of administration and covariates on the pharmacokinetics of propofol in adult volunteers. Anesthesiology 1998;88(5):1170–82.

21. Ward DS, Russell Norton J, Guivarc'h P-H, et al. Pharmacodynamics and pharmacokinetics of propofol in a medium-chain triglyceride emulsion. Anesthesiology 2002;97(6):1401–8.

22. Hoymork SC, Raeder J. Why do women wake up faster than men from propofol anaesthesia? Br J Anaesth 2005;95(5):627–33.

23. Vuyk J, Oostwouder CJ, Vletter AA, et al. Gender differences in the pharmacokinetics of propofol in elderly patients during and after continuous infusion. Br J Anaesth 2001;86(2):183–8.

24. Kreuer S, Biedler A, Larsen R, et al. Narcotrend monitoring allows faster emergence and a reduction of drug consumption in propofol–remifentanil anesthesia. Anesthesiology 2003;99(1):34–41.

25. Buchanan FF, Myles PS, Cicuttini F. Patient sex and its influence on general anaesthesia. Anaesth Intensive Care 2009;37(2):207–18.

26. Rathore SS, Wang Y, Krumholz HM. Sex-based differences in the effect of digoxin for the treatment of heart failure. N Engl J Med 2002;347(18): 1403–11.

27. Labbe L, Sirois C, Pilote S, et al. Effect of gender, sex hormones, time variables and physiological urinary pH on apparent CYP2D6 activity as assessed by metabolic ratios of marker substrates. Pharmacogenetics 2000;10(5):425–38.

28. Tanaka E. Clinically significant pharmacokinetic drug interactions between antiepileptic drugs. J Clin Pharm Ther 1999;24(2):87–92.

29. Walle T, Walle K, Mathur RS, et al. Propranolol metabolism in normal subjects: association with sex steroid hormones. Clin Pharmacol Ther 1994;56(2): 127–32.

30. Dadashzadeh S, Javadian B, Sadeghian S. The effect of gender on the pharmacokinetics of verapamil and norverapamil in human. Biopharm Drug Dispos 2006;27(7):329–34.

31. Krecic-Shepard ME, Barnas CR, Slimko J, et al. Gender-specific effects on verapamil pharmacokinetics and pharmacodynamics in humans. J Clin Pharmacol 2000;40(3):219–30.

32. Krecic-Shepard ME, Barnas CR, Slimko J, et al. In vivo comparison of putative probes of CYP3A4/5 activity: erythromycin, dextromethorphan, and verapamil. Clin Pharmacol Ther 1999;66(1):40–50.

33. Sartori-Valinotti JC, Iliescu R, Yanes LL, et al. Sex differences in the pressor response to angiotensin II when the endogenous renin-angiotensin system is blocked. Hypertension 2008;51(4):1170–6.

34. Hreiche R, Morissette P, Turgeon J. Drug-induced long QT syndrome in women: review of current evidence and remaining gaps. Gend Med 2008;5(2): 124–35.

35. Gowda RM, Khan IA, Punukollu G, et al. Female preponderance in ibutilide-induced torsade de pointes. Int J Cardiol 2004;95(2–3):219–22.

36. Drici MD, Clément N. Is gender a risk factor for adverse drug reactions? The example of drug-induced long QT syndrome. Drug Saf 2001;24(8):575–85.

37. Jenkins CR, Chapman KR, Donohue JF, et al. Improving the management of COPD in women. Chest 2017;151(3):686–96.

38. Kanner RE, Connett JE, Altose MD, et al. Gender difference in airway hyperresponsiveness in smokers with mild COPD. The lung health study. Am J Respir Crit Care Med 1994;150(4):956–61.

39. Soriano JB, Sin DD, Zhang X, et al. A pooled analysis of FEV 1 decline in COPD patients randomized to inhaled corticosteroids or placebo. Chest 2007;131(3):682–9.

40. Mohamed MHN, Lima JJ, Eberle LV, et al. Effects of gender and race on albuterol pharmacokinetics. Pharmacotherapy 1999;19(2):157–61.

41. Li X, Obeidat M, Zhou G, et al. Responsiveness to ipratropium bromide in male and female patients with mild to moderate chronic obstructive pulmonary disease. EBioMedicine 2017;19:139–45.

42. Tashkin D, Celli B, Kesten S, et al. Effect of tiotropium in men and women with COPD: results of the 4-year UPLIFT® trial. Respir Med 2010;104(10):1495–504.

43. Soulele K, Macheras P, Silvestro L, et al. Population pharmacokinetics of fluticasone propionate/salmeterol using two different dry powder inhalers. Eur J Pharm Sci 2015;80:33–42.

44. Vestbo J, Soriano JB, Anderson JA, et al. Gender does not influence the response to the combination of salmeterol and fluticasone propionate in COPD. Respir Med 2004;98(11):1045–50.

45. Celli BR, Thomas NE, Anderson JA, et al. Effect of pharmacotherapy on rate of decline of lung function in chronic obstructive pulmonary disease: results from the TORCH study. Am J Respir Crit Care Med 2008;178(4):332–8.

46. D'Urzo AD, Singh D, Donohue JF, et al. Efficacy of aclidinium/formoterol 400/12 µg, analyzed by airflow obstruction severity, age, sex, and exacerbation history: pooled analysis of ACLIFORM and AUGMENT. Int J Chron Obstruct Pulmon Dis 2019;14:479–91.

47. Xu J, Nave R, Lahu G, et al. Population pharmacokinetics and pharmacodynamics of inhaled ciclesonide and fluticasone propionate in patients with persistent asthma. J Clin Pharmacol 2010;50(10):1118–27.

48. Tsiligianni I, Mezzi K, Fucile S, et al. Response to indacaterol/glycopyrronium (IND/GLY) by sex in patients with COPD: a pooled analysis from the IGNITE Program. COPD 2017;14(4):375–81.

49. Nafziger AN, Bertino JS. Sex-related differences in theophylline pharmacokinetics. Eur J Clin Pharmacol 1989;37(1):97–100.

50. Lew KH, Ludwig EA, Milad MA, et al. Gender-based effects on methylprednisolone pharmacokinetics and pharmacodynamics. Clin Pharmacol Ther 1993;54(4):402–14.

51. Ayyar VS, DuBois DC, Nakamura T, et al. Modeling corticosteroid pharmacokinetics and pharmacodynamics, part II: sex differences in methylprednisolone pharmacokinetics and corticosterone suppression. J Pharmacol Exp Ther 2019;370(2):327–36.

52. Dias SP, Brouwer MC, van de Beek D. Sex-based differences in the response to dexamethasone in bacterial meningitis: analysis of the European dexamethasone in adulthood bacterial meningitis study. Br J Clin Pharmacol 2020;86(2):386–91.

53. Magee MH, Blum RA, Lates CD, et al. Prednisolone pharmacokinetics and pharmacodynamics in relation to sex and race. J Clin Pharmacol 2001;41(11):1180–94.

54. Meffin PJ, Brooks PM, Sallustio BC. Alterations in prednisolone disposition as a result of time of administration, gender and dose. Br J Clin Pharmacol 1984;17(4):395–404.

55. O'Hare MF, Leahey W, Murnaghan GA, et al. Pharmacokinetics of sotalol during pregnancy. Eur J Clin Pharmacol 1983;24(4):521–4.

56. Philipson A, Stiernstedt G, Ehrnebo M. Comparison of the pharmacokinetics of cephradine and cefazolin in pregnant and non-pregnant women. Clin Pharmacokinet 1987;12(2):136–44.

57. Philipson A. Pharmacokinetics of ampicillin during pregnancy. J Infect Dis 1977;136(3):370–6.

58. Dean M, Stock B, Patterson RJ, et al. Serum protein binding of drugs during and after pregnancy in humans. Clin Pharmacol Ther 1980;28(2):253–61.

59. Kaneko S, Kondo T. Antiepileptic agents and birth defects: incidence, mechanisms and prevention. CNS Drugs 1995;3(1):41–55.

60. Anderson GD. Pregnancy-induced changes in pharmacokinetics: a mechanistic-based approach. Clin Pharmacokinet 2005;44(10):989–1008.

61. Gardner MJ, Schatz M, Cousins L, et al. Longitudinal effects of pregnancy on the pharmacokinetics of theophylline. Eur J Clin Pharmacol 1987;32(3):289–95.

62. Nakai A, Sekiya I, Oya A, et al. Assessment of the hepatic arterial and portal venous blood flows during pregnancy with Doppler ultrasonography. Arch Gynecol Obstet 2002;266(1):25–9.

63. Davison JM, Dunlop W, Ezimokhai M. 24-Hour creatinine clearance during the third trimester of normal pregnancy. Br J Obstet Gynaecol 1980;87(2):106–9.

64. Nazir S, Iqbal Z, Nasir F. Impact of menopause on pharmacokinetics of rosuvastatin compared with premenopausal women. Eur J Drug Metab Pharmacokinet 2016;41(5):505–9.

Moving?

Make sure your subscription moves with you!

To notify us of your new address, find your **Clinics Account Number** (located on your mailing label above your name), and contact customer service at:

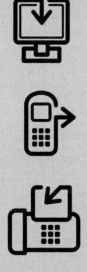

Email: journalscustomerservice-usa@elsevier.com

800-654-2452 (subscribers in the U.S. & Canada)
314-447-8871 (subscribers outside of the U.S. & Canada)

Fax number: 314-447-8029

Elsevier Health Sciences Division
Subscription Customer Service
3251 Riverport Lane
Maryland Heights, MO 63043

*To ensure uninterrupted delivery of your subscription, please notify us at least 4 weeks in advance of move.

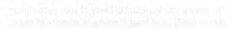

Printed and bound by CPI Group (UK) Ltd, Croydon, CR0 4YY

08/05/2025

01864694-0019